MW01001070

Nursing
TimeSavers

Cardiovascular Disorders

Nursing
TimeSavers

Cardiovascular Disorders

Springhouse Corporation
Springhouse, Pennsylvania

Staff

Executive Director, Editorial
Stanley Loeb

Senior Publisher
Matthew Cahill

Art Director
John Hubbard

Clinical Manager
Cindy Tryniszewski, RN, MSN

Senior Editor
Michael Shaw

Editors
Peter Dechnik, Traci A. Ginnona, Judd L.
Howard, Carol H. Munson, Art Ofner, Jean
Wallace, Pat Wittig

Copy Editors
Cynthia C. Breuninger (supervisor),
Priscilla H. DeWitt, Jennifer George
Mintzer, Dorothy E. Oren, Nancy Papsin,
Doris Weinstock

Designers
Stephanie Peters (associate art director),
Matie Patterson (senior designer), Donald
G. Knauss, Kaaren Mitchel, Amy Smith

Illustrators
Kevin Curry, Jacalyn Facciolo, Dan Fione,
Rhonda Forbes, Robert Jackson, Robert
Neumann, Judy Newhouse

Manufacturing
Deborah Meiris (director), Pat Dorshaw
(manager), Anna Brindisi, Kate Davis, T.A.
Landis

Production Coordination
Patricia McCloskey

Editorial Assistants
Maree DeRosa, Beverly Lane, Mary
Madden

Indexer
Barbara Hodgson

Library of Congress Cataloging-in-Publication Data
Cardiovascular disorders.
    p. cm. — (Nursing timesavers)
    Includes bibliographical references and
index.
    1. Cardiovascular system — Diseases —
Nursing.   I. Springhouse Corporation.
II. Series.
    [DNLM: 1. Cardiovascular Diseases —
nursing.   WY 152.5 C267461]
RC674.C363   1993
610.73'691 — dc20
DNLM/DLC   93-24341
ISBN 0-87434-611-8   CIP

Contents

Contributors and consultants

Contributors

Mary Chapman Gyetvan, RN, MSN
Nurse Consultant
Levittown, Pa.

Sandra M. Nettina, RN,C, MSN, CRNP
Adult Nurse Practitioner
Mercy Primary Care Group
Baltimore

Consultants

Sandra Bixler, RN, MSN, CCRN
Clinical Nurse Specialist
Berks Cardiologists, Ltd.
Reading, Pa.

David J. Blanchard, RPh, BS
Pharmacist Specialist
Mary Imogene Bassett Hospital
Cooperstown, N.Y.

Kathy Craig, RN, BA
Nurse Consultant
Collegeville, Pa.

Joan T. Granberry, RN, BS, CCRN
Clinical Nurse III
St. Francis Medical Center
Trenton, N.J.

Kristine A. Bludau Scordo, RN, PhD
Clinical Director
Clinical Nurse Specialist
The Cardiology Center of Cincinnati

Ann Smith, RN, MSN, CCRN
Clinical Nurse Specialist, Surgical ICU
Thomas Jefferson University Hospital
Philadelphia

Foreword

Providing effective cardiovascular care requires more skill now than ever before. Think, for instance, of the numerous tasks you have to carry out: besides investigating a patient's symptoms through a health history and a physical examination, you have to monitor electrocardiograms (ECGs) and hemodynamic status, give drugs, perform or assist with treatments, teach the patient, meet the emotional needs of the patient and members of his family, and document care. You also have to keep pace with recent advances in detecting and treating cardiovascular disorders — such as atherectomy or the use of implantable cardioverter defibrillators — and be ready to put this knowledge into practice. What's more, you must be able to quickly assess patients whose conditions may lead to cardiovascular complications or emergencies. And you must do all of this proficiently in a minimum amount of time.

Fortunately, you now have a trustworthy guide to help you meet this formidable challenge. *Cardiovascular Disorders,* the first book in the Nursing TimeSavers series, offers a wealth of clinical data and expertise. This remarkable book was developed by nursing professionals — clinicians with years of bedside know-how — who understand the time constraints you encounter every day.

Chapter 1 explains how to use the nursing process to provide expert cardiovascular care. It provides a thorough review of each step of the nursing process. You'll learn how to use the nursing process to identify patient problems, develop a plan of care, determine what kind of assistance the patient needs, and set outcomes for the patient and determine whether they've been achieved. You'll also find concise coverage of key nursing diagnoses encountered in cardiovascular care.

Chapter 2 provides guidelines for assessing your patient's chief complaint. If your patient says, "My chest hurts" or "My heart won't stop fluttering," turn to this chapter for a list of questions to ask and assessment techniques to perform. For each chief complaint, you'll find a discussion of potential causes to help you interpret the significance of your findings.

Chapter 3 provides step-by-step instructions for monitoring your patient's condition and response to interventions. You'll find guidelines for performing 12-lead ECG and cardiac monitoring and for monitoring intra-arterial pressure, pulmonary artery pressure, pulmonary artery wedge pressure, central venous pressure, and cardiac output. This chapter features tips for enhancing the efficiency of monitoring, interpreting waveforms, and troubleshooting problems with equipment.

Chapters 4 through 10 provide care guidelines for cardiovascular disorders. To save you time, each disorder is organized according to the nursing process with five easy-to-spot text headings:

• *Assessment.* This section tells you what health history findings, physical examination findings, and diagnostic test results to expect. Other pertinent assessment information is clearly labeled and easy to find.

• *Nursing diagnosis.* In this section, you'll find the most common nursing diagnoses and related etiologies for each disorder.

• *Planning.* This section provides a list of expected patient outcomes for each nursing diagnosis. This feature will ensure that your documentation includes accurate outcome statements.

• *Implementation.* In this section, you'll find complete, step-by-step nursing interventions.

• *Evaluation.* This section provides criteria to judge the effectiveness of nursing care and gauge your patient's progress toward meeting expected outcomes.

Throughout the book, you'll see special graphic devices called logos that direct you to important information and timesaving tips. The *FactFinder* logo provides key facts about a disorder, covering such topics as risk factors, demographics, and prognosis. The *Timesaving tip* logo alerts you to ways to save time as you proceed with your nursing care. The *Assessment TimeSaver* logo provides suggestions on how to organize and expedite the initial step of the nursing process. The *Treatments* logo summarizes the latest medical therapies for each disorder. The *Discharge TimeSaver* logo signals a checklist of teaching topics, referrals, and follow-up appointments to promote your patient's well-being after hospitalization.

Cardiovascular Disorders also includes two valuable appendices. The first outlines treatments for cardiovascular disorders, complete with concise descriptions, indications, and complications. The second contains a list of common cardiovascular drugs, with their dosages, indications, and adverse reactions.

By providing current clinical information in a focused, quick-reference format, *Cardiovascular Disorders* can help you immensely. Become familiar with this tool and use it anywhere — at home or at work. I'm sure you'll be pleased with the benefits: better care for your cardiovascular patients and, for you, the confidence to succeed in today's fast-paced world of health care.

Kristine A. Bludau Scordo, RN, PhD
Clinical Director
Clinical Nurse Specialist
The Cardiology Center of Cincinnati

Applying the nursing process to cardiovascular care

In North America, more than 70 million people have some form of cardiovascular disease. Because of this prevalence, nurses in almost any setting must be able to assess cardiac status, detect serious and potentially life-threatening changes, keep pace with new therapies, and monitor their patients' responses. What's more, because of the growing emphasis on disease prevention, nurses everywhere have increased responsibilities for patient teaching and follow-up.

By using the nursing process, you can provide cardiovascular care expertly and thoroughly while saving time. You'll use the nursing process to:
• identify patient problems you can treat
• identify patient problems you can help to prevent
• develop a plan that addresses the patient's actual and potential problems
• determine what kind of assistance the patient needs and who can best provide it
• select goals for the patient and determine whether they've been achieved
• document accurately your contribution to achieving patient outcomes.

The nursing process consists of a series of steps. Understanding each of these steps — assessment, nursing diagnosis, planning, implementation, and evaluation — will help you address the complex needs of cardiovascular patients in an orderly way. Keep in mind, however, that these steps are dynamic and flexible; they often overlap.

Assessment

The first step of the nursing process, assessment, is critical. That's because the quality of assessment data will determine the success of subsequent nursing process steps. Assessment usually includes taking a health history, performing a physical examination, and reviewing the results of diagnostic tests.

Timesaving tip: In cardiac care, a comprehensive assessment is ideal, but circumstances frequently require that you assess your patient quickly. In such circumstances, try to identify the most important clues to cardiac dysfunction. Let the patient's condition be your guide. For example, if the patient is admitted with unstable angina and exhibits diaphoresis while clutching his chest in pain, perform a brief, focused assessment and try to limit his movement as much as possible. If the patient has severe dyspnea, only ask questions that are absolutely necessary. Phrase them so the patient can nod or give one-word answers. You can obtain a more extensive history when the patient's condition improves or by interviewing a family member.

The onset of acute illness may cause anxiety. To calm the patient, ensure privacy and assume a gentle, confident manner. Identify yourself by name as well as by professional title. Speak in a conversational tone to put the patient at ease and to encourage him to share information.

Health history

The health history allows you to explore the patient's chief complaint and other symptoms, assess the impact of illness on him and his family, and begin to develop and implement a plan of care. It also allows you to gather information to guide diagnosis and treatment.

Chief complaint

Begin your health history interview by asking about the patient's chief complaint. If he can't identify a single chief complaint, ask "What made you seek medical care at this time?" Let the patient describe his problem in his own words. Avoid asking leading questions and be careful to use terms he understands.

Pay attention not only to what the patient says, but also to how he says it. Does he appear to be upset or in pain? Record the chief complaint in the patient's own words. Next, have him characterize the chief complaint. Ask about onset, frequency, and precipitating, alleviating, and influencing factors. Investigate any pain or discomfort by asking about its location, radiation, duration, and severity. Ask the patient if he has noticed any associated signs and symptoms or adverse effects of treatment.

Signs and symptoms of cardiovascular disease that may cause a patient to seek medical attention include chest pain, dyspnea, palpitations, syncope, paroxysmal nocturnal dyspnea, orthopnea, unexplained weakness and fatigue, ulcers or sores on the ankles or legs, irregular heartbeat, coughing, and weight changes with edema. For further information, see Chapter 2, Assessing chief complaints.

Past illnesses
Find out if the patient has any disorders that can affect the cardiovascular system or influence recovery. Consider asking the following questions:
• Have you ever had heart disease or been treated for it?
• Have you ever had hypertension, diabetes mellitus, hyperlipidemia, or other chronic or acute illness?
• Have you ever been hospitalized? Have you ever had surgery or an outpatient procedure?
• Have you ever experienced severe fatigue or syncope?
• Were you born with a heart problem? If so, when and how was it treated?
• Have you had a heart murmur?
• Have you ever had any serious injuries?
• Do you take any prescription or over-the-counter drugs?

• Are you allergic to any drugs, foods, or other products? If so, describe your reaction.

If your patient is female, ask whether she has begun menopause. If so, she faces an increased risk of coronary artery disease (CAD). Ask whether she takes oral contraceptives or receives hormone replacement therapy. Also, if she has had children, ask if she had any medical problems during pregnancy.

Family history
Because cardiovascular disease may recur in families, ask the patient about a family history of hypertension, diabetes mellitus, CAD, vascular disease, hyperlipidemia, or other cardiac illness. Also, ask if any relatives experienced sudden death from an unknown cause.

Life-style factors
Find out about the patient's daily activities, exercise habits, and diet. Consider asking the following questions:
• How much fried foods, meat, dairy products, and baked goods do you eat?
• Do you cook with salt? Do you add salt to your food? Do you eat high-sodium foods, such as french fries, smoked meats, and snack foods?
• Do you smoke or drink alcoholic or caffeine-containing beverages? If so, how much do you consume each day? When was the last time you smoked or drank alcoholic or caffeine-containing beverages?
• Do you use any drugs for recreational purposes?

Inquire about educational background, occupation, living arrangements, and family relationships. Explore any potentially stressful circumstances. Be aware that cardiovascular patients and their families are prone to stress, loneliness, depression, and other psychosocial problems. These problems may inhibit recovery.

Coping patterns

Assess the patient's ability to cope with cardiovascular illness. Consider asking the following questions:
• Has your illness required you to make drastic alterations in your lifestyle?
• How have you coped with crises in the past?
• Do you feel your current coping strategies are helping or hindering your progress?
• Are you having difficulty coming to terms with your illness?

Use your assessment of the patient's coping patterns to determine his teaching needs. Does he understand his diagnosis? Does he seem ready to accept change? How important is good health to him? Is he willing to work to regain it? If the patient isn't ready or willing to accept change, he's unlikely to respond to teaching.

Physical examination

Your next step is to perform a physical examination. Employing a systematic sequence of assessment techniques will help ensure that you don't miss important findings, even if you're rushed. However, if your patient is acutely ill and may require emergency intervention, you will need to remain flexible in your approach. (See *Organizing the physical examination.*)

Begin your assessment by observing the patient's general appearance. Then perform your examination, starting with the patient's head and ending with the lower extremities.

Choose a quiet room with privacy. If possible, close the door and windows, and turn off radios and noisy equipment. Adjust the thermostat, if necessary; cool temperatures may alter the patient's skin temperature and color, heart rate, and blood pressure.

General appearance

Look at the patient, noting his body type, overall health, and muscle composition. Is he well developed, well nourished, alert, and energetic? Also note his posture, gait, movements, and hygiene.

Measure and record the patient's height and weight. These measurements will help guide treatment, determine medication dosages, direct nutritional counseling, and detect fluid overload. Fluctuations in weight may prove significant, especially if they're extreme. For example, a patient developing heart failure may gain several pounds overnight.

Use this time to assess the patient's mental status. Are his responses appropriate? Does he speak clearly? As you proceed, watch his facial expressions for signs of discomfort, withdrawal, fear, or depression.

Vital signs

Take the patient's temperature, pulse and respiratory rates and rhythms, and blood pressure. Fever, for instance, can be a sign of cardiovascular inflammation or infection, such as infective endocarditis. Because compromised cardiac function increases the heart's work load, monitor the febrile patient for signs of poor tolerance, such as tachycardia and shortness of breath.

Palpate the patient's radial pulse for 1 minute. A normal resting pulse rate for an adult ranges from 60 to 100 beats/minute. The pulse rhythm should feel regular, with subtle slowing during expiration caused by changes in intrathoracic pressure and vagal response.

Respirations

A normal breathing pattern is regular, unlabored, and bilaterally equal. When assessing the patient's respiratory pattern, be alert for tachypnea, which may indicate low cardiac output, or dyspnea, which may indicate heart failure.

Assessment TimeSaver

Organizing the physical examination

Performing your cardiovascular assessment in a logical sequence, such as working from head to toe, will help you save time. You can also save time by combining steps whenever possible. For instance, you can inspect the patient's general appearance while taking the history and measuring vital signs. Or you can inspect the precordium as you begin auscultation.

The following list contains key cardiovascular assessment factors arranged in a head to toe sequence.

General appearance
- Body type and posture
- Weight
- Gait
- Hygiene
- Mental status
- Signs of distress (behavior or facial expressions)
- Speech

Vital signs
- Temperature
- Pulse rate and rhythm
- Respiratory rate and rhythm
- Blood pressure

Neck
- Jugular vein pulsations and distention
- Central venous pressure
- Carotid arteries: pulse rate, rhythm, equality, contour, and amplitude; thrills and bruits

Precordium
- Shape, size, and symmetry
- Retractions and accessory muscle use
- Point of maximal impulse
- Apical pulse rate and rhythm, thrills, gallops, and murmurs (type and grade)

Abdomen
- Abdominal pulsations or ascites
- Bruits of abdominal aorta or liver
- Abdominal tenderness
- Liver size and tenderness

Periphery
- Peripheral pulses: rate, rhythm, amplitude, and symmetry
- Dependent edema
- Bilateral temperature variation and sensation
- Tenderness
- Inflammation
- Arterial insufficiency (vascular filling time)
- Venous insufficiency
- Capillary refill time

Skin, nails, and mucous membranes
- Color
- Rashes
- Lesions
- Ulcers
- Texture
- Hair pattern
- Nail thickness and clubbing

Dyspnea may be hard to recognize if the patient is calm and resting. However, you may notice that he frequently pauses for breath when speaking. If the patient has severe heart failure, he may exhibit Cheyne-Stokes respiration.

Blood pressure
Always take the patient's blood pressure in both arms during the initial assessment. The results may vary slightly but should be within 10 mm Hg of each other. If time permits, first pal-

pate the pressure, wait 3 to 5 minutes, and then auscultate.

Normal blood pressure for a resting adult is 140/90 mm Hg or lower. Blood pressure above 140/90 mm Hg on several successive readings indicates hypertension. When interpreting your patient's results, keep in mind that simply undergoing a physical examination can cause enough emotional stress to provoke an increase in blood pressure. If the patient's blood pressure is high, allow him to relax for several minutes and then measure it again. (See *Detecting diagnostic clues when measuring blood pressure*.)

Pulse pressure
Calculate the patient's pulse pressure by subtracting diastolic pressure from systolic pressure. This value (normally 30 to 50 mm Hg) reflects arterial pressure during the resting phase of the cardiac cycle. Because pulse pressure increases when stroke volume increases, such factors as exercise, anxiety, and bradycardia can elevate pulse pressure. Pulse pressure also rises in response to decreased peripheral vascular resistance or aortic distention, which may accompany anemia, hyperthyroidism, fever, hypertension, aortic coarctation, or aging.

If the patient's pulse pressure is narrowed, suspect a mechanical obstruction. The obstruction may result from stenosis of the mitral or aortic valves, or peripheral vasoconstriction brought on by shock. Pulse pressure also diminishes in response to declining stroke volume, which may stem from heart failure, hypovolemia, or tachycardia. If the pulse pressure is widened, suspect aortic insufficiency.

Assessing the neck
Inspect the pulsations of the patient's internal and external jugular veins to determine adequacy of circulating volume, right ventricular function, and ve-

nous pressure. The external jugular vein is superficial and visible above the clavicle. The larger internal jugular vein lies deeper, along the carotid arteries, and transmits pulsations outward to the skin overlying these arteries. Normally, the jugular veins protrude when the patient lies down and flatten when he stands up.

Place the patient in semi-Fowler's position. If right ventricular function is normal, the jugular veins shouldn't be prominent. Next, have the patient turn his head slightly away from you. Use a small pillow to support the patient's head without flexing the neck sharply. Adjust the light to cast a small shadow along the neck. Bilateral jugular vein distention indicates elevated central venous pressure (CVP). Unilateral jugular vein distention may indicate local obstruction.

Assessing CVP
Elevated CVP may indicate impaired right ventricular function. CVP normally ranges from 6 to 8 cm H_2O. Factors that influence CVP include circulating blood volume, the tone of vessel walls, vein patency, respiratory function, pulmonary pressures, gravity, and right ventricular function. (See *Estimating central venous pressure*, page 8.)

Assessing central aortic pressure
Begin by auscultating each of the carotid arteries. Turn the patient's head slightly away from you. Place the bell of your stethoscope over the carotid artery and ask the patient to hold his breath. Normally, blood flow through the artery is silent, although you may hear a heart murmur that radiates to the carotid artery. If you detect bruits, the patient may have occlusive artery disease, arteriovenous fistula, or a condition that causes high cardiac output, such as anemia, hyperthyroidism, or pheochromocytoma. When bruits are present, gently palpate the artery with

Detecting diagnostic clues when measuring blood pressure

Measuring blood pressure in both arms during your initial assessment can provide important information about the patient's condition. For example, a difference of 10 mm Hg or more between arms may indicate thoracic outlet syndrome, dissecting aortic aneurysm, or another form of arterial obstruction.

If both measurements are within 10 mm Hg of each other but above 140/90 mm Hg, measure the patient's blood pressure in his thigh. To do so, have the patient lie on his abdomen, wrap a large cuff around the patient's leg an inch or more above the knee, and place your stethoscope over the popliteal artery (located on the posterior surface slightly above the knee). If this measurement is also high, it may simply confirm systemic hypertension. However, normal or low blood pressure in the legs coupled with high blood pressure in the arms suggests aortic coarctation. Normally, systolic pressure in the legs is up to 20 mm Hg higher than in the arms; diastolic pressure is about the same in the arms and legs.

As you measure blood pressure, you may hear an auscultory gap, a disappearance of Korotkoff sounds during inspiration. Check for pulsus paradoxus, a drop of more than 10 mm Hg in systolic pressure during inspiration. Pulsus paradoxus may indicate cardiac tamponade, chronic obstructive pulmonary disease, or constrictive pericarditis.

the pads of your fingers to detect the thrill that frequently accompanies the bruit. The presence of a thrill may indicate turbulence due to arterial obstruction.

You can easily palpate the carotid pulse, even if cardiac output is diminished. Place the patient in semi-Fowler's position and turn his head toward you. Place your fingers on the trachea and roll them laterally into the groove between the trachea and the sternocleidomastoid muscle. Palpate the carotid pulse for 15 to 30 seconds. Repeat this palpation on the opposite carotid artery. Assess for rate, rhythm, equality, contour, and amplitude. Observe the carotid area for exaggerated waves, which may indicate a hypervolemic or hyperkinetic left ventricle, possibly due to aortic insufficiency.

Assessing the precordium

To inspect the precordium, place the patient in low Fowler's or semi-Fowler's position. Stand to the right of the patient and adjust the light to cast a shadow across the patient's chest. First, identify key anatomic landmarks, including the suprasternal notch, the angle of Louis (sternal notch), the midsternal line, the midclavicular line, the anterior axillary line, and the posterior axillary line. Next, observe the patient's thorax for shape, size, symmetry, and obvious pulsations or retractions. Note the presence of left-chest prominence, which may signify congenital heart disease. Inspect the right and left lower sternum for excessive pulsations, bulging, lifting, heaving, or respiratory retraction.

Then locate and observe the point of maximal impulse (PMI) of the apical impulse. The apical impulse occurs almost simultaneously with the carotid

Estimating central venous pressure

Elevated central venous pressure (CVP) may signal impaired right ventricular function. By calculating the distance between the right atrium and the highest level of visible pulsation in the jugular vein, you can estimate CVP.

First, position the patient at a 45-degree angle and adjust the light to illuminate the pulse over the internal jugular vein. Note the highest level of visible pulsation. Then locate the angle of Louis (sternal notch). Palpate the clavicles at the suprasternal notch. Place two of your fingers on the suprasternal notch and slide them down the sternum until they reach a bony protuberance; this is the angle of Louis. The right atrium is approximately 2″ (5 cm) below this point. Measure the vertical distance between the highest level of visible pulsation and the angle of Louis (normally less than 1⅛″ [3 cm]). Then, add 2″ to estimate the distance between the highest level of pulsation and the right atrium. A distance of 4″ (10 cm) or more may indicate elevated CVP and elevated right ventricular pressure, which are characteristic of heart failure.

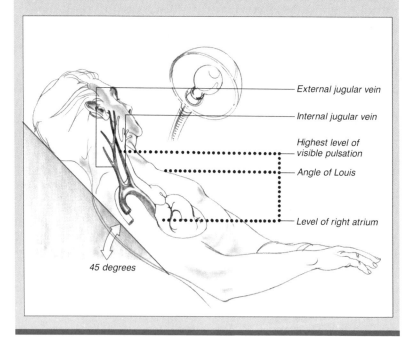

External jugular vein

Internal jugular vein

Highest level of visible pulsation

Angle of Louis

Level of right atrium

45 degrees

pulse and is evident in about half of all normal adults. To locate the PMI, place your right palm over the area of the apex—the fifth intercostal space at or near the midclavicular line. Palpate the apex to the left sternal border, the base of the heart, the epigastrium, the right sternal border, and the clavicular and left axillary areas. Identifying the PMI will help you evaluate heart size and hear heart sounds. Prominent pulsations may result from an enlarged left ventricle; also, an apical thrust greater than ¾″ (2 cm) suggests left ventricular enlargement.

After assessing the PMI, palpate the apex for thrills. A thrill results from loud, harsh murmurs having low-frequency sounds, such as mitral stenosis. Also palpate for thrills over the left sternal border and at the base of the heart, located at the second left and right intercostal space at the sternal borders.

Auscultation

Auscultating heart sounds proves particularly useful for identifying valvular abnormalities and gallops. Often, assessing the timing and rhythm of heart sounds can enable you to identify the valve affected and the specific problem. (See *What abnormal heart sounds mean*, page 10.)

Begin by identifying S_1, the *lub* of the *lub-dub* sound produced by the heart. S_1 occurs as the mitral and tricuspid valves close. Using the diaphragm of your stethoscope, auscultate the PMI while observing or palpating the carotid pulse. At the apex, S_1 is louder, longer in duration, and lower in pitch than S_2.

Next identify S_2, the *dub* of the *lub-dub* sound. S_2 occurs as the aortic and pulmonic valves close. Place the diaphragm of your stethoscope on the patient's chest over the second right intercostal space. S_2 will be the loudest sound you hear. Then, as you slowly move your stethoscope diagonally toward the PMI, S_2 should become softer. Listen for the normal splitting of S_2 during inspiration.

A third heart sound, S_3, may be audible early in diastole, as blood flows rapidly into the ventricles. To best hear S_3, position the patient on his left side and lightly place the bell of your stethoscope at the apex. An S_3 is normal in children, adolescents, and even young adults with thin chest walls. However, in most adults, an S_3 is ab-

normal. In ischemic heart disease, an S_3 suggests left ventricular failure.

You may also detect a fourth heart sound, S_4, late in diastole, signifying atrial contraction. S_4 can be heard most clearly using the same method you used to identify S_3.

Timesaving tip: If you hear an extra sound during atrial fibrillation, you can assume that it's not S_4. That's because S_4 results from atrial contraction. In atrial fibrillation, no effective atrial contraction takes place.

As you auscultate heart sounds, listen for murmurs, which result from turbulent blood flow. A murmur may indicate an increased rate of flow, an increased or decreased vessel diameter, decreased blood viscosity, or a vessel wall with a rough inner surface. Pathologic murmurs result from stenosis or insufficiency of any of the heart valves.

If you notice a murmur, record its location, intensity, and timing in the cardiac cycle. For example, the murmur may occur in the middle of systole (midsystolic), throughout systole (pansystolic), in early diastole, in the middle of diastole, or in late diastole. Refer to key anatomic landmarks when recording the location of the loudest sound, and indicate whether the murmur radiates toward other areas of the precordium. When recording your findings, describe the murmur's intensity as:
• grade I (very faint)
• grade II (soft and low)
• grade III (prominent but not palpable)
• grade IV (prominent and palpable; thrill present)
• grade V (very loud)
• grade VI (audible with the stethoscope off the chest).

Assessing the abdomen

Begin by inspecting the upper abdomen for evidence of cardiovascular disease. An enlarged, fluid-filled abdo-

What abnormal heart sounds mean

Abnormal heart sound	Timing	Possible causes
Accentuated S_1	Beginning of systole	• Hyperkinetic disorders, such as fever or mitral stenosis
Diminished S_1	Beginning of systole	• Mitral insufficiency • Severe mitral insufficiency with calcified, immobile valve • Heart block
Accentuated S_2	End of systole	• Pulmonary or systemic hypertension
Diminished or inaudible S_2	End of systole	• Aortic or pulmonary stenosis
Persistent S_2 split	End of systole	• Delayed closure of the pulmonic valve, usually from overfilling of the right ventricle causing prolonged systolic ejection time
Persistent S_2 split that widens during inspiration	End of systole	• Pulmonic valve stenosis • Atrial ventricular septal defect • Right bundle-branch block
Reversed or paradoxical S_2 split that appears in expiration and disappears in inspiration	End of systole	• Delayed ventricular stimulation • Left bundle-branch block • Prolonged left ventricular ejection time
S_3 (ventricular gallop)	Early diastole	• Normal in children and young adults • Overdistention of ventricle in rapid-filling segment of diastole • Mitral insufficiency • Ventricular failure
S_4 (atrial gallop or presystolic extra sound)	Late diastole	• Forceful atrial contraction from resistance to ventricular filling late in diastole • Left ventricular hypertrophy • Pulmonary stenosis • Hypertension • Coronary artery disease • Aortic stenosis
Pericardial friction rub (grating or leathery sound at left sternal border; usually muffled, high-pitched, and transient)	Throughout systole and diastole	• Pericardial inflammation

men typically indicates ascites due to heart failure. Visible or palpable pulsations in the epigastric area may be normal, particularly in unusually thin patients. However, abnormally large aortic pulsations may result from an aneurysm of the abdominal aorta or from aortic insufficiency. Similarly, exaggerated epigastric pulsations may result from right ventricular hypertrophy or an aortic abnormality. Determine the source of the pulsations by gently placing your palm on the epigastric area and sliding your fingers under the rib cage. You will feel aortic pulsations with your palm and right ventricular impulses with your fingertips.

Use the bell of the stethoscope to auscultate the epigastric area along the abdominal midline to the umbilicus. A bruit in this area indicates abdominal aortic aneurysm. Next, auscultate the right upper quadrant over the liver for a hepatic bruit, indicative of increased blood flow to the liver. A hepatic bruit may indicate heart failure. Then auscultate right and left of the umbilicus over the kidneys. A bruit in this area indicates obstructed blood flow to the kidneys.

Percussion of the liver may reveal hepatomegaly, which may occur during heart failure. Percuss the abdomen along the right midaxillary line to detect dullness in the borders of the liver. **Timesaving tip:** If you can't locate the inferior border of the liver using percussion, place the diaphragm of the stethoscope over the approximate location of the liver's lower border. Auscultate while lightly scratching along the midclavicular line from the right iliac crest upward. The scratching sound will be louder over the liver.

Palpating the abdomen may reveal areas of tenderness (possibly from an enlarged liver) and the contour of the palpable edge of the liver. A smooth edge suggests heart failure; a nodular edge may indicate cirrhosis.

Assessing the periphery

Start your assessment of the periphery by inspecting the color and condition of the patient's skin, especially the face, mouth, earlobes, and fingernails. Pallor or cyanosis may indicate poor cardiac output and poor tissue perfusion. If your patient has dark skin, examine the buccal membranes, lips, tongue, nail beds, and palms for an ashen gray color. Use this time to look for overt signs of cardiovascular risk factors. For example, yellow stains on the fingers often indicate that the patient smokes cigarettes; xanthomas may indicate that he has a high cholesterol level. Look for an earlobe crease, which is frequently seen in CAD.

Examine the patient's fingers and palms for petechial hemorrhages, Osler's nodes (tender, painful raised areas), or Janeway lesions (nontender nodules on the palms), all of which may suggest bacterial endocarditis. Inspect the patient's fingernails and toenails for changes in thickness, color, contour, consistency, and nail adherence. Signs of prolonged hypoxemia include clubbed fingers (chronic thickening and enlargement of the nails, bulbous enlargement of the fingertips). You may also find exaggerated curves in the nails and spongy softening of the root.

Skin texture and hair patterns

Observe your patient's skin for signs of poor circulation. For example, the skin may appear thin, waxy, fragile, or shiny. In addition, the patient may have little or no hair on his arms and legs, or he may remark that he's noticed a reduction in hair in these areas. Poor circulation may be caused by diabetes mellitus, an important risk factor for cardiovascular disorders. During your inspection, look for areas of unusual pigmentation, such as recent skin lesions, rashes, scarring, or ulceration, which may suggest arterial insufficiency.

Edema
Look for signs of edema in dependent parts of the body. For ambulatory patients, this involves inspecting the arms, hands, legs, feet, and ankles. However, if your patient is on bed rest, check for signs in the buttocks and sacral area. Palpate the suspected area against a bony prominence and record your findings. Describe characteristics of the patient's edema, such as extent and location, type (pitting or nonpitting), degree of pitting (when present), and symmetry (unilateral or symmetrical). The degree of pitting is determined by depth. When recording your findings, use the following scale:
  + 1 for mild pitting (less than ¼″ or 0.6 cm)
  + 2 for moderate pitting (¼″ to ½″ or 0.6 to 1.3 cm)
  + 3 for severe pitting (over ½″).

Skin temperature
The patient's skin should feel warm and dry. If the skin on his arms or legs is cool or clammy, suspect peripheral vasoconstriction. Such vasoconstriction typically occurs when cardiac output is low and is an early compensatory response in shock.

Arms and legs
As you assess the patient's arms and legs, check to see if the right and left limbs are of equal size. Then use light and deep palpation to test each limb for normal sensation. Note any areas of tenderness or areas that are warmer or cooler than normal.

Arterial blood flow
Determine the adequacy of arterial flow by testing vascular filling time in the patient's arms or legs. Have the patient lie down and raise his legs or arms 12″ (30 cm) above the level of his heart. Next, ask the patient to move the elevated limbs up and down for 60 seconds. Then have him sit up and

dangle his limbs over the edge of the examining table. Vascular refilling should take about 15 seconds. Suspect arterial insufficiency if either limb persistently shows marked pallor, delayed venous filling, a delay in the return of color causing a mottled appearance, or marked redness.

Venous blood flow
Assess the adequacy of venous flow by inspecting and palpating the patient's legs for superficial veins. Have the patient place his legs in a dependent position and check for signs of normal circulation, including venous distention, nodular bulges at venous valves (bifurcation of veins), and veins that collapse when the limb is elevated. Signs of venous insufficiency include dilated, tortuous veins with poorly functioning valves, peripheral cyanosis, peripheral pitting edema, skin thickening, unusual ankle pigmentation, and ulceration around the ankles.

Peripheral blood flow
Begin your assessment of peripheral blood flow by checking capillary refilling in the patient's fingernails or toenails. Apply pressure to a nail for 5 seconds. The area should blanch. Remove the pressure and observe how rapidly the normal color returns. If the patient has an adequate arterial supply, the color should return in less than 3 seconds. Delayed refilling suggests reduced peripheral circulation, which may result from low cardiac output and may lead to arterial insufficiency.
    Next, inspect and palpate for evidence of deep vein inflammation or clot formation. Ask the patient if he has pain, tenderness, or a sense of fullness in the calf. If so, ask if the feeling is aggravated by standing or walking. Check the patient's feet for edema and dependent cyanosis. Then gently press the calf muscle with your palm; pain may indicate thrombophlebitis. During

your assessment, test for Homans' sign: First, have the patient extend his leg. While supporting the entire leg, firmly and abruptly dorsiflex the patient's foot. Deep calf pain during this maneuver indicates thrombophlebitis.

Peripheral pulses

Assess peripheral pulses for rate, rhythm, amplitude, and symmetry. Palpate peripheral pulses lightly with the pads of the index, middle, and ring fingers of your dominant hand. Use three fingers where space permits; use two fingers to palpate small or angled areas (for example, over femoral pulses).

Always use a methodical approach when assessing peripheral pulses — start with the arms and move to the legs. Palpate the patient's brachial pulses medial to the biceps tendons. Then palpate the radial pulses on the palmar surface of the patient's relaxed, slightly flexed wrist, medial to the radial styloid processes.

Rate and rhythm. To determine rate, count all pulses for 30 seconds or longer (60 seconds when recording vital signs). A normal rate is 60 to 100 beats/minute. Determine rhythm by assessing the regularity of beats. If you detect an irregular radial pulse, take the apical-radial pulse.

Amplitude. Palpating the pulse amplitude provides information about the adequacy of the volume of circulating blood, vessel tone, strength of left ventricular contraction, and the elasticity of arterial walls. To assess pulse amplitude, palpate the vessel during ventricular systole. Normal arteries feel soft and pliable; sclerotic arteries feel beaded or corded and resist occlusion by external pressure. When recording your findings, describe pulse amplitude according to the following characteristics:

  + 3 for a bounding (increased) pulse
  + 2 for a normal pulse
  + 1 for a weak, thready (decreased) pulse
  0 if the pulse is absent.

Symmetry. When taking pulses, always palpate the pulse on both sides of the patient's body. Inequality between sides may indicate arterial occlusion.

Femoral pulses

Using the pads of your fingers, deeply palpate the area below the inguinal ligaments, midway between the anterior superior iliac spine and the symphysis pubis. Then auscultate each femoral area for bruits, which may indicate the presence of arteriosclerotic plaques.

Popliteal pulses

To assess popliteal pulses, which are located deep in the soft tissues behind the knees, place the patient in the supine or semi-Fowler position and have him flex his knees slightly. Using both hands, deeply palpate the pulses. Or place your thumbs on the front of the patient's knee, and palpate behind the knee with the first two fingers of both hands.

Pedal pulses

First, locate pedal pulses by placing your palm lightly on the dorsum. You should be able to feel the dorsalis pedis pulse points. Next, using the pads of your fingers, lightly palpate the dorsum of the feet. Be aware that heavy palpation can obscure the pulse. To prevent excessive traction on the arteries, dorsiflex the patient's foot (preferably 90 degrees) and palpate where the vessels pass over the dorsum. Then while the patient's foot is dorsiflexed, use the pads of your fingers to locate and assess the posterior tibial pulse on the posterior or inferior medial malleolus of the ankle.

Diagnostic tests

Diagnostic test findings complete the objective data base. Together with the health history and physical examination, they form a profile of your patient's condition. The list below reviews diagnostic tests commonly ordered for patients with known or suspected cardiac problems.

• Blood chemistry tests (sodium, magnesium, creatinine, potassium, chloride, calcium, carbon dioxide, glucose, blood urea nitrogen, cholesterol, high-density lipoprotein, low-density lipoprotein, and triglyceride levels) help to evaluate the cause and effects of cardiovascular disease and to identify chemical imbalances that may compromise cardiac function.

• Cardiac enzyme assays confirm acute myocardial infarction (MI) or severe cardiac trauma by measuring cellular proteins that are released into the blood because of cell membrane injury.

• Arterial blood gas (ABG) measurements evaluate gas exchange in the lungs and metabolic changes.

• Coagulation studies (bleeding time, platelets, prothrombin time, partial thromboplastin time, fibrinogen, plasminogen) aid diagnosis of bleeding disorders.

• Electrocardiography (ECG) can help detect MI, chamber enlargement, and arrhythmias.

• An ambulatory ECG or Holter monitor tracks cardiac activity over 12 to 24 hours. It may be used to determine cardiac status after MI, to assess the effectiveness of antiarrhythmic drugs, and to determine if arrhythmias are the cause of particular symptoms.

• Chest X-rays may reveal an enlarged heart and aortic dilation. They also help in the assessment of pulmonary circulation.

• Exercise testing, using a bicycle ergometer, treadmill, or short flight of stairs, can determine cardiac response to physical stress.

• Cardiac catheterization with selective coronary arteriography identifies the presence of CAD or valvular heart disease, the extent of heart failure, and the need for coronary artery bypass grafting (CABG) or percutaneous transluminal coronary angioplasty (PTCA).

• Digital subtraction angiography evaluates the coronary arteries, using X-ray images that are digitally subtracted by computer. Time-based color enhancement shows blood flow in nearby areas.

• Surface and transesophageal echocardiography uses pulsed high-frequency sound waves to evaluate chamber size, wall thickness, wall motion, and valve structure and function.

• Magnetic resonance imaging provides high resolution, three-dimensional images of valve leaflets and structures, pericardial abnormalities, ventricular hypertrophy, cardiac neoplasms, infarcted tissue, anatomic malformations, and structural deformities.

• Radionuclide imaging tests, such as positron emission tomography, technetium-99m Sestamibi (Cardiolite) scanning, thallium scanning, and multiple-gated acquisition scanning, use special cameras, computers, and intravenously injected radiopaque isotopes, or contrast media, to investigate coronary artery blood flow and ventricular contraction.

• Hemodynamic monitoring evaluates cardiac function and determines the effectiveness of therapy by measuring cardiac output, mixed venous oxygen saturation, intracardiac pressures, and blood pressure.

Nursing diagnosis

The next step of the nursing process, nursing diagnosis describes the patient's actual or potential response to a health problem. To formulate a nursing diagnosis, evaluate the essential information derived from your cardiac assessment. Consider such questions as:

• What are the patient's signs and symptoms?
• Which assessment findings are abnormal for this patient?
• How do particular behaviors affect the patient's cardiovascular health?
• Does the patient understand his illness and its treatment?
• How does his environment affect his health?
• How does he respond to his health problem? Does he want to change his state of health?

Chapters 4 through 10 contain common nursing diagnoses for many cardiovascular disorders. Keep in mind, however, that diagnostic statements must be tailored to your patient's individual needs. Each patient responds to illness and stress differently, and your nursing diagnoses should never become so standardized that individual differences and special needs aren't addressed.

Developing individual diagnoses for each patient can be difficult. You can make this task easier and save time by becoming familiar with the most frequently used nursing diagnoses.

Decreased cardiac output
This nursing diagnosis describes a cluster of cardiovascular and respiratory symptoms that occur when the amount of blood pumped by the heart fails to meet the needs of the body's tissues. Signs and symptoms of decreased cardiac output include blood pressure changes; arrhythmias; jugular vein distention; decreased peripheral pulse; cold, clammy skin; mucous membrane and skin color changes; oliguria; dyspnea, orthopnea, crackles; fatigue and restlessness; and change in mental status.

Decreased cardiac output may be associated with numerous cardiovascular disorders, such as Adams-Stokes syndrome, angina pectoris, aortic stenosis, arterial insufficiency, cardiac arrest, cardiac arrhythmias, cardiac tamponade, cardiogenic shock, heart failure, CAD, endocarditis, mitral stenosis or insufficiency, MI, pericarditis, tetralogy of Fallot, and others.

To foster greater accuracy, you should also write an etiology, or "related to" statement, for each nursing diagnosis. The etiology should identify conditions or circumstances that contribute to the development or continuation of the patient's health problem. For example, if you suspect that decreased cardiac output results from cardiac dysfunction caused by ischemia, you could formulate this diagnostic statement: *Decreased cardiac output related to reduced stroke volume caused by ischemia.*

Activity intolerance
This nursing diagnosis describes a patient's experience of extreme fatigue, dyspnea, or other symptoms when performing activities. The patient may also report general fatigue or weakness. His activity may be interrupted frequently because of breathlessness or pain. Activity intolerance affects all aspects of a patient's life and may lead to overwhelming fatigue, depression, powerlessness, and loss of purpose.

Activity intolerance can be associated with numerous cardiovascular disorders: cardiac tamponade, heart failure, CAD, endocarditis, MI, peripheral vascular disorder, tetralogy of Fallot, and others.

To assess for activity intolerance, evaluate the patient's response to activity. Check for dyspnea, excessive increase in respiratory rate, and an irregular breathing pattern. Be alert for tachycardia, bradycardia, arrhythmias, decreased pulse amplitude, and an excessive increase or decrease in blood pressure.

Altered cardiopulmonary tissue perfusion

This diagnosis refers to a cluster of symptoms that result when a decrease in capillary blood supply leads to a decrease in cellular nutrition. Altered cardiopulmonary tissue perfusion can result from aortic stenosis or insufficiency, CAD, cardiac tamponade, cardiogenic shock, heart failure, coronary artery spasm, mitral stenosis or insufficiency, and others.

When cardiopulmonary tissue perfusion is inadequate, the patient may experience such signs and symptoms as arrhythmias and abnormal ABG and cardiac enzyme levels. He may experience chest pain with or without activity. His skin may be cold and clammy. Your assessment may reveal crackles, cyanosis, decreased peripheral pulses, palpitations, fatigue, hypotension, tachycardia, mental status changes, pale mucous membranes, edema, rhonchi, shortness of breath, slow capillary refill time, and variations in hemodynamic readings.

Pain

A subjective state, pain refers to reported discomfort or an uncomfortable sensation. Unmanaged pain can be devastating and can have major psychological consequences. Pain is associated with numerous cardiovascular disorders: angina pectoris, aortic aneurysm, arterial insufficiency, arterial occlusion, cardiac tamponade, CAD, MI, pericarditis, rheumatic heart disease, thrombophlebitis, and others.

The patient's report of pain is the most important assessment information when formulating this diagnosis. Many patients perceive pain as a discomfort; therefore, ask the patient about discomfort when taking the health history. Physiologic indicators (such as changes in blood pressure and respiratory rate, dilated pupils, diaphoresis, and increased muscle tension) and behavioral clues (such as moaning, crying, restlessness, and grimacing) may provide further evidence for diagnosis.

Additional nursing diagnoses

When reviewing the list of nursing diagnoses, you'll find many additional diagnoses that may be appropriate to describe your patient's response to illness. (See *Identifying common nursing diagnoses in cardiovascular care*.)

During his illness, the cardiac patient will likely exhibit a broad range of emotional responses, including panic, depression, sleeplessness, anxiety, and anger. Emotional upset can be severe enough to interfere with compliance and recovery. Formulating nursing diagnoses may help you more accurately pinpoint the patient's psychosocial needs. Examples of possible diagnoses include *anxiety, ineffective denial, powerlessness,* and *hopelessness.* Although these diagnoses aren't specific to cardiac illness, their importance shouldn't be underestimated.

Patient teaching is a vital component of providing care for the cardiovascular patient. For example, you may need to teach your patient about diagnostic tests and therapeutic procedures. Your teaching may focus on encouraging life-style changes to alter the patient's cardiac risk factors — for example, teaching a hypertensive patient how to reduce the amount of salt in his diet. *Knowledge deficit* is the diagnosis used most frequently to document learning needs. Because this diagnosis is so broad, you should include a carefully worded etiology to ensure that the patient's specific needs are clearly communicated. For example, you might write in your plan of care *Knowledge deficit related to lack of understanding of hazards of high sodium intake.*

Identifying common nursing diagnoses in cardiovascular care

Certain nursing diagnoses can be used frequently to describe the response patterns of cardiovascular patients. This list identifies and defines these diagnoses.

Activity intolerance • Extreme fatigue or other physical symptoms resulting from simple activity.

Altered cardiopulmonary tissue perfusion • A decrease in cellular nutrition and respiration caused by reduced capillary perfusion.

Altered sexuality patterns • A state in which an individual expresses concern about engaging in sexual activity.

Anxiety • A feeling of threat or danger to oneself arising from an unidentifiable source.

Decreased cardiac output • Cardiovascular or respiratory symptoms resulting from insufficient blood being pumped by the heart.

Fatigue • An overwhelming sense of exhaustion and decreased capacity for physical and mental work, regardless of adequate sleep.

Fluid volume excess • An imbalance of water or sodium, causing increased total body fluid volume or fluid shift from one compartment to another.

Health-seeking behaviors • A state in which a patient in stable health seeks ways to alter personal health habits or his environment to move toward optimal health.

Impaired skin integrity • An interruption in skin integrity.

Ineffective denial • A conscious or unconscious attempt to disavow the knowledge or meaning of an event to reduce anxiety or fear, to the detriment of health.

Ineffective individual coping • An inability to use adaptive behaviors in response to difficult life situations, such as loss of health.

Knowledge deficit • An inadequate understanding of information or an inability to perform skills needed to practice health-related behaviors.

Noncompliance • Unwillingness to practice prescribed health-related behaviors.

Pain • Subjective sensation of discomfort derived from multiple sensory nerve interactions generated by physical, chemical, biological, or psychological stimuli.

Planning

The next step of the nursing process involves creating a plan of action that will direct your patient's care toward desired goals. This step includes writing a plan of care to serve as a record of your patient's nursing diagnoses, expected outcomes, nursing interventions, and evaluation data.

Early in the planning stage, you will need to determine priorities for nursing care. Most cardiovascular patients have multiple problems, which require multiple nursing diagnoses. Once you've formulated your patient's nursing diagnoses, you'll need to determine which problems require immediate attention and which can wait.

Always give highest priority to problems that pose immediate safety risks. Ask yourself: "Will my patient's life be endangered if this problem isn't addressed immediately?" Next, give priority to your patient's nonemergency needs. Lower-priority diagnoses involve needs that aren't related to the patient's specific illness or prognosis. (See *Setting priorities for nursing diagnoses.*)

Involving your patient in planning is crucial to ensuring successful nursing care. For example, a patient with CAD is more likely to comply with an activity regimen if you take time to ask what activities are meaningful to him.

Effective communication is essential when working with the patient and his family members. To enhance communication with the patient, create a quiet, private, and relaxed environment, and encourage the patient and his family members to ask questions about cardiovascular disorders and their treatment. Be sure to translate medical terms into simple, clear language.

Establishing patient outcomes

Next, you'll need to establish patient outcomes — measurable goals derived from the patient's nursing diagnoses. A patient outcome may specify an improvement in the patient's ability to function — for example, an increase in the distance a patient can walk each morning after cardiac surgery. Or it may specify an amelioration of a problem — for example, a reduction in pain for a patient who has angina pectoris. Each outcome statement should call for the greatest improvement possible for your patient.

A patient outcome statement should describe the specific behavior that will show the patient has reached his goal, include criteria for measuring the behavior, state conditions under which the behavior should occur, and include the target date or time by which the behavior should occur. It should be based on a nursing diagnosis. For example, if your patient's nursing diagnosis is *Activity intolerance related to an imbalance between oxygen supply and demand,* appropriate outcome statements might include:

• Patient will verbalize, in a discussion with nurse, an understanding of the need to increase his activity level gradually by 10/10/93.

• Patient will demonstrate his ability to walk down the hall without experiencing increases in dyspnea by 10/23/93.

• Patient will participate in developing a plan to increase his activity level. Plan will be completed by 10/25/93.

• Patient will demonstrate techniques for conserving energy while performing activities of daily living by 10/25/93.

Developing interventions

After establishing patient outcomes, you'll develop interventions designed to help the patient achieve these outcomes. Consider such factors as your patient's age, developmental and educational levels, environment, and cultural values. The more you know about the patient, the easier it will be to formulate appropriate interventions. For example, if your patient is scheduled for cardiac catheterization and has a reading disability, don't write an intervention for patient teaching that includes complex reading material.

When documenting interventions, state the necessary action clearly. Many interventions must be continued, and possibly evaluated and modified, by other nurses when you're not present. Also, if your patient and his family members are participating in his care, they'll need to understand the intervention. Write your intervention in precise detail. Include how and when to per-

Setting priorities for nursing diagnoses

For many patients, your assessment will reveal multiple problems that must be addressed. When planning care for these patients, you'll need to identify the multiple problems, establish appropriate nursing diagnoses, and rank them in order from highest to lowest priority. To help you set these priorities, consider the case of Miles Thomas, a 56-year-old municipal manager with a long history of hypertension.

Subjective data
Mr. Thomas was admitted for evaluation after experiencing chest pain at his desk. A myocardial infarction (MI) has been ruled out but an echocardiogram shows left ventricular hypertrophy and dilation from hypertension.

Mr. Thomas is tired and dyspneic on exertion. He tells you that he has had high blood pressure for 15 years and has taken diuretics "on and off." When he feels well, he often skips his medication. He tries to watch his salt intake but occasionally snacks on salted pretzels or popcorn. For the past several months, he has been feeling tired despite getting extra sleep and, within the past several weeks, he's been short of breath after climbing one flight of stairs. He's relieved that he didn't have an MI but confides that he's afraid he may not be so lucky next time.

Objective data
Your examination of Mr. Thomas reveals the following:
- height 5′ 10″ (1.8 m), weight 219 lb (99.3 kg)
- blood pressure 160/98 mm Hg; pulse rate 82 beats/minute, regular rhythm; respirations 26 breaths/minute, regular rhythm
- warm, dry skin; cyanosis absent
- ankle edema, trace bilateral
- peripheral pulses +2 and equal bilaterally; no jugular vein distention or carotid bruits
- point of maximal impulse displaced laterally 2 cm
- normal S_1 and S_2, no gallop, grade IV systolic murmur over mitral area
- fine bibasilar crackles

- soft, nontender abdomen
- nonpalpable liver; 10 cm by percussion.

Diagnostic test findings
- Serial cardiac enzyme, blood urea nitrogen, serum creatinine, and electrolyte levels within normal limits; serum cholesterol level is 234 mg/dl; low-density lipoprotein level is 150 mg/dl; and high-density lipoprotein level is 30 mg/dl.
- Electrocardiography indicates left ventricular hypertrophy with strain.
- Chest X-ray indicates cardiomegaly and increased vascular markings.
- Echocardiography indicates left ventricular hypertrophy and dilation and mitral valve insufficiency.

Identifying problems and establishing priorities
Results of the patient history, physical examination, and diagnostic tests suggest that Mr. Thomas has moderate hypertension, mild heart failure, and mitral insufficiency. You believe your primary nursing concern is the potential effect of these problems on Mr. Thomas's cardiac function. You decide your care must first be directed toward decreasing the heart's work load and preventing cardiac decompensation or an acute MI. To address these concerns in your plan of care, you select *decreased cardiac output related to reduced stroke volume* as your chief nursing diagnosis.

Your next concern is to address Mr. Thomas's fatigue and dyspnea on exertion. His activity intolerance may prolong his hospitalization, impair his abili-

(continued)

Setting priorities for nursing diagnoses *(continued)*

ty to resume regular activities, and harm his quality of life. So, you select *activity intolerance related to imbalance between tissue oxygen supply and demand* as your second-priority nursing diagnosis.

You're also concerned about Mr. Thomas's obesity, elevated cholesterol levels, and poor compliance with therapy. Mr. Thomas's willingness to confide that he fears an MI suggests that he may now be motivated to take action to improve his cardiac health.

Therefore, you decide he could benefit from learning more about hypertension and cardiac risk factors. You hope that this knowledge will enable him to modify his behavior. You select *knowledge deficit related to lack of awareness of the complications of hypertension* as your third-priority nursing diagnosis.

Having set priorities for Mr. Thomas's problems, you can now proceed to establish patient outcomes and implement care.

form the intervention as well as any special instructions.

Implementation

During the fourth step of the nursing process, you put your plan of care into action. Simply put, you'll intervene. During implementation, you usually have the most direct and prolonged contact with the patient. You must also coordinate and direct the activities of the health care team.

Treatment for cardiac problems is becoming increasingly sophisticated. More than 690,000 open-heart procedures are performed each year in the United States. Types of cardiac surgeries include CABG, permanent pacemaker insertion, valve replacement, vascular repair, atherectomy, and heart transplantation. Mechanical devices, such as a ventricular assist device, may be implanted in patients with heart failure. In addition, balloon catheter treatments are becoming increasingly common. For example, PTCA has become the treatment of choice for im-

proving coronary perfusion in many CAD patients. A new technology, laser angioplasty, shows great promise. Drugs used in the treatment of cardiac disorders include inotropic agents, adrenergics, antiarrhythmics, antianginals, antihypertensives, diuretics, antilipemics, and thrombolytics.

The increasing complexity of cardiovascular care has led to expanded nursing roles. Traditional nursing skills, such as close patient monitoring, prompt action at the bedside, and patient education, are taking on new dimensions. The following is a brief review of nursing interventions you may need to implement.

Therapeutic interventions

These interventions are geared toward alleviating the effects of illness or restoring optimal function. For example, if you administer quinidine to a patient with an arrhythmia, you're performing a therapeutic intervention for restoring health. Other common therapeutic interventions for cardiac patients include administering supplemental oxygen, elevating the patient's legs, performing range-of-motion exercises, promoting chest physiotherapy, and enforcing prolonged bed rest.

Emergency care
In a cardiac emergency, you may be called upon to perform such lifesaving measures as cardiopulmonary resuscitation or cardiac defibrillation.

Monitoring
Periodic or continuous evaluation of your patient's cardiac status and response to therapy is just as important as the initial assessment. Cardiac monitoring procedures include ECG, arterial pressure monitoring, pulmonary artery wedge pressure monitoring, and CVP monitoring. You may also need to periodically evaluate other indicators of your patient's health, such as pulse rate, blood pressure, capillary refill time, skin temperature and color, ABG levels, daily weight, intake and output, respirations, and mental status.

Patient teaching
Teaching can help the cardiac patient maintain his health and avoid future problems. Many of your lessons will focus on needed life-style adjustments — following activity and diet restrictions, maintaining a balance between activity and rest, establishing a routine for taking medication, and reducing stress. Timely information may help the patient to cope more successfully with hospitalization. For example, you may review the expected course of treatment with the patient and his family members, explain equipment used in the intensive care unit or recovery room, or reinforce the doctor's explanation of surgery or a medical procedure.

Preoperative care
Preoperative nursing measures may include enforcing food and fluid restrictions, shaving the patient's chest and scrubbing it with an antiseptic solution, obtaining necessary diagnostic test information, establishing an I.V. line, establishing baseline vital signs, establishing baseline ECG readings, providing teaching regarding preoperative and postoperative care, offering reassurance, and providing sedation.

Postoperative care
Interventions may include checking dressings for signs of bleeding or infection, changing dressings, assessing vital signs and level of consciousness (LOC), providing analgesics, providing ventilator support, communicating with family members, and maintaining chest tube drainage.

Emotional support
You may plan and implement interventions to enhance your patient's emotional well-being. For example, you may help the patient and his family members cope with anxiety by establishing a trusting and supportive relationship and setting aside time to listen to their concerns. For patients with severe emotional problems, you may need to provide a referral for psychological counseling.

Preparation for discharge
For many cardiovascular patients, leaving the hospital and adjusting to a medication regimen, life-style restrictions, or long-term care is difficult. By preparing the patient for discharge, you can help to make this transition safe and smooth and ensure continued quality of care.

Preparation for discharge may include instructing the patient to notify the doctor of any signs or symptoms of an adverse reaction or deteriorating health, providing a schedule for resuming normal activity, reminding the patient when to return for follow-up appointments, providing a referral to outside agencies such as the American

Heart Association, or making sure the patient understands the dose, schedule, and adverse effects of all prescribed drugs. You may also be responsible for communicating necessary information to a home health care agency.

Evaluation

During evaluation, the last step of the nursing process, you judge the effectiveness of nursing care and gauge your patient's progress toward meeting expected outcomes. Evaluating the patient gives you the chance to:
• determine if original assessment findings still apply
• uncover complications
• assess the patient's response to all aspects of care, including medications, changes in diet or activity, procedures, unusual incidents or problems, and patient teaching
• measure the effectiveness of your care.

An ongoing activity, evaluation usually overlaps with other phases of the nursing process. Your evaluation findings, in fact, may trigger a cycle of assessment, nursing diagnosis, planning, implementation, and further evaluation. You may also uncover new information that will help you implement the plan of care more effectively.

To ensure a successful evaluation, keep an open mind. Never hesitate to consider new patient data or to revise previous judgments. After all, no plan of care is perfect. In fact, you should anticipate revising the plan of care sometime during the course of treatment.

Reassessment
Reassessing the patient's status forms a crucial part of your evaluation. Techniques for gathering data include interviewing the patient, observing him, performing a physical examination, and reviewing the medical record.

Next, compare reassessment data with criteria established in the patient outcomes documented in your plan of care. For example, a patient with the nursing diagnosis *Pain related to imbalance between myocardial oxygen supply and demand* might have the following patient outcomes:
• Patient will verbalize relief from pain.
• Patient's blood pressure and heart rate will remain with normal limits (specify).
• Patient will demonstrate how to use a nitroglycerin disk during an anginal episode.

During reassessment, ask the patient about his current level of pain, measure his blood pressure and heart rate, and observe his ability to use a nitroglycerin disk. When evaluating your findings, consider whether the patient is moving toward or away from achieving outcomes. Also consider whether the patient's overall condition is improving or deteriorating.

You may find that the patient has achieved all documented outcomes by the projected dates. Or you may discover that some patient problems have been only partially resolved or haven't been resolved at all. If so, your next task is to assess factors interfering with goal achievement. Consider all possible reasons that a patient may not be able to achieve a desired outcome, such as those listed below.
• The purpose and goals of the plan of care aren't clear.
• The expected outcomes aren't realistic in light of the patient's condition.
• The plan of care is based on incomplete assessment data.
• Nursing diagnoses are inaccurate.
• The nursing staff experienced conflict with the patient or medical staff.
• Staff members didn't follow the plan of care.

• The patient failed to carry out activities outlined in the plan of care.

• The patient's condition changed.

Reviewing implementation

When trying to determine factors that are interfering with goal attainment, you'll want to take a closer look at whether the plan of care was implemented appropriately.

For example, suppose you're caring for a patient with the nursing diagnosis *Decreased cardiac output,* who now weighs 8 lb (3.6 kg) more than he did on admission. To find out why he has failed to achieve the expected outcome *Patient exhibits little or no edema or weight gain,* you'd review the nursing interventions listed on the plan of care. You'd ask yourself such questions as: Was a low-sodium diet prescribed and given? Was the patient taught to elevate his feet when out of bed? Did the patient carry out planned activities? Were medications administered on time? Finding out the answers to these questions would help you determine why the expected outcome hasn't been achieved.

Writing evaluation statements

Evaluation statements provide a method for documenting the patient's response to care. These statements indicate whether expected outcomes were achieved and list the evidence supporting your conclusions. The importance of clearly written evaluation statements can't be overemphasized: Documentation of patient outcomes is necessary to substantiate the rationales for nursing care and to justify the use of nursing resources. You'll record your evaluation statements in your progress notes or on the revised plan of care, according to your hospital's documentation policy.

Writing clear, concise evaluation statements is easy if you wrote precise patient outcome statements when planning care. Patient outcome statements provide a model for evaluation statements. When writing an evaluation statement, describe the patient's progress using active verbs, such as "demonstrate," "express," or "walk." Include criteria used to measure the patient's response to care, and describe the conditions under which the response occurred (or failed to occur). Write a separate evaluation for each patient response or behavior that you wish to describe. Don't forget to date the evaluation statement.

Examples of evaluation statements used in cardiovascular care include the following:

• Patient expresses an understanding of the importance of following his prescribed diet, drug regimen, and exercise program.

• His pulse rate and blood pressure remain within established limits (specify).

• Patient demonstrates stress reduction techniques.

• He describes signs and symptoms of decreased cardiac output, such as dizziness, fatigue, and dyspnea.

• He carries out activities of daily living without his heart rate exceeding or dropping below established limits (specify).

• He describes plans to alter his lifestyle to minimize cardiac risk factors.

• He participates in a cardiac exercise program.

• He reports achieving pain relief 5 to 20 minutes after receiving 10 mg morphine sulfate subcutaneously.

• His skin appears pink and less dusky after 20 minutes of oxygen administration at 2 liters/minute by nasal cannula.

• He demonstrates the ability to walk on a treadmill for 20 minutes without becoming fatigued.

• He demonstrates adequate cardiac output, as evidenced by a normal LOC, an absence of dizziness, and warm, dry skin.

• He shows adequate tissue perfusion, as evidenced by warm, dry skin and absence of cyanosis.
• His breath sounds are clear.
• He expresses fears associated with the diagnosis of abdominal aortic aneurysm.

Modifying the plan of care

During evaluation, you may discover that the plan of care needs to be modified. If patient outcomes have been achieved, make sure that this information is recorded. Revise other patient outcomes statements as necessary. Determine which nursing interventions need to be revised or discontinued. Assess whether changes are needed in the priorities assigned to nursing diagnoses. You may need to document that a nursing diagnosis has been resolved. Or you may find that a nursing diagnosis no longer accurately describes the patient's status. A new or revised diagnosis may be needed.

Like all steps of the nursing process, evaluation is ongoing. Continue to assess, diagnose, plan, implement, and evaluate for as long as you care for the patient.

CHAPTER 2

Assessing chief complaints

S everal important chief complaints — chest pain, dyspnea, tachypnea, palpitations, cyanosis, edema, fatigue, and syncope — tend to recur in cardiovascular patients. By fully investigating any of these complaints, you can form a diagnostic impression of your patient's problem and guide your subsequent care.

Chest pain

The most common complaint of cardiovascular patients, chest pain may signal an ischemic or inflammatory disorder. (See *Causes of chest pain*.) If your patient reports chest pain, take his health history and perform a physical examination according to the guidelines below.

History of the symptom
To further understand the patient's chest pain, consider asking the questions listed below:
• When did the pain begin?
• How would you describe the pain? Is it a dull, aching pressure or a sharp, stabbing pain?
• Is the pain on the surface or deep inside?
• Did it start suddenly or build gradually?
• Is it more severe now than when it started?
• Is it continuous or intermittent? If intermittent, how long does each episode last?
• Does the pain radiate to your neck, jaw, arms, or back?
• Do activities such as walking, exercising, changing position, or breathing affect the pain?
• Do certain foods affect the pain?
• Have you experienced this type of pain before?

• Are you taking any medication to relieve the pain?

Associated findings
Note whether the patient has experienced any of the following signs or symptoms:
• abdominal pain
• change in level of consciousness (LOC)
• persistent cough
• syncope
• weakness
• transient paralysis (especially in the legs)
• headache
• light-headedness
• problems with vision
• epistaxis
• belching
• anorexia
• nausea or vomiting
• dyspnea (particularly on exertion)
• palpitations
• myalgia
• undue fatigue.

Previous conditions and treatments
Consult with the patient, family members, or members of the health care team to determine if the patient has ever had any of the conditions or treatments listed below:
• acute myocardial infarction (MI)
• heart failure
• known coronary artery disease
• angina
• cardiogenic shock
• congestive cardiomyopathies
• pulmonary disease
• blunt or penetrating chest trauma
• lung cancer
• intestinal, renal, or connective tissue disease
• sickle cell anemia
• recent infection, especially in the upper respiratory tract
• thrombophlebitis
• hip or leg fracture

Causes of chest pain

Cardiovascular disorders that cause chest pain include angina, dissecting aortic aneurysm, myocardial infarction (MI), pericarditis, mitral insufficiency, mitral valve prolapse, aortic stenosis, cardiogenic shock, and aortic arch syndrome.

Angina
The patient with angina may report a painful tightness, heaviness, pressure, or expansion in the chest. It may be provoked by exertion, emotional stress, or eating a large meal. The patient may believe this pain is caused by indigestion. Anginal pain usually occurs in the retrosternal region and radiates to the neck, jaw, or arms (especially the inner aspect of the left arm). The pain usually lasts 2 to 10 minutes, building gradually to peak intensity, then slowly subsiding. Pain caused by Prinzmetal's angina typically occurs while the patient is resting and may awaken him at night.

Dissecting aortic aneurysm
This disorder causes extreme and sudden chest pain. The patient may report an excruciating tearing, ripping, or stabbing pain in the chest and neck that may radiate to the upper back, abdomen, or lower back and thigh as the aneurysm dissects. It may be dull or absent if neurologic function is compromised.

Myocardial infarction
MI may cause severe, crushing substernal ischemic chest pain that is not relieved by rest or nitroglycerin. It may radiate to the left arm, jaw, neck, abdomen, or shoulder blades.

Pericarditis
This disorder may cause sudden, persistent precordial or retrosternal chest pain that is aggravated by deep breathing, coughing, changing position (particularly by reclining), and sometimes by swallowing. The pain frequently is sharp or cutting and radiates to the shoulder, neck, and arms.

Mitral valve disorders
In mild and moderate cases of mitral insufficiency, the patient may be asymptomatic. In more severe cases, chest pain may occur. Mitral valve prolapse causes a sharp, stabbing precordial chest pain or precordial ache. The pain may last for seconds or hours and sometimes mimics the pain of ischemic heart disease.

Other cardiovascular disorders
Anginal pain may occur in aortic stenosis and cardiogenic shock. In aortic arch syndrome, chest pain may accompany recurrent loss of consciousness and other symptoms. Also, abruptly stopping a medication regimen of beta blockers may cause rebound angina in patients with coronary artery disease, especially if they have taken high doses for a prolonged period.

Noncardiovascular causes
Chest pain may be caused by anxiety, asthma, blastomycosis, bronchitis, cholecystitis, Chinese restaurant syndrome (related to the metabolism of monosodium glutamate), cholecystitis, coccidioidomycosis, costochondritis, distention of the splenic flexure, esophageal spasm, herpes zoster (shingles), hiatal hernia, interstitial lung disease, Legionnaire's disease, lung abscess, lung cancer, mediastinitis, muscle strain, nocardiosis, pancreatitis, peptic ulcer, pleurisy, pleuritis, pneumomediastinum, pneumonia, pneumothorax, psittacosis, pulmonary actinomycosis, pulmonary hypertension (primary), pulmonary embolism, rib fracture, sickle cell crisis, thoracic outlet syndrome, and tuberculosis.

- prolonged bed rest
- recent surgery or pregnancy
- recent subclavian vein cannulation or mechanical ventilation.

Drug use

Note past or current use of the drugs listed below:

- cocaine (may precipitate MI)
- nonsteroidal anti-inflammatory drugs, aspirin, or corticosteroids (may cause GI ulceration)
- octreotide (may lead to gallstones)
- oral contraceptives (may predispose the patient to thrombophlebitis and pulmonary embolism)
- procainamide or hydralazine (may lead to pericarditis).

Physical examination

Examine the patient according to the steps described below.

Inspection

- Check the patient's skin color. Note any paleness, cyanosis, pallor, mottling below the waist, peripheral edema, diaphoresis, or a capillary refill time greater than 2 seconds.
- Inspect the neck for jugular vein distention. Inspect the face and neck for puffiness.
- Observe the patient's breathing pattern, noting any dyspnea or audible wheezing. Inspect the chest for asymmetrical expansion or the use of accessory muscles.
- Observe the patient's neurologic status and LOC. Note anxiety, restlessness, or dizziness.
- If the patient coughs up sputum, examine its color, consistency, odor, and amount.
- If possible, inspect the retina for evidence of vascular changes.

Palpation

- Palpate over the lungs for vocal or tactile fremitus or subcutaneous crepi-

tation. If indicated, percuss over the affected lung to determine dullness.

- Palpate the neck for tracheal deviation and subcutaneous crepitation.
- Palpate peripheral pulses. Note the rate, rhythm, and intensity. Also note weak or absent radial, femoral, or pedal pulses and a decreased carotid artery pulse.
- Palpate the abdomen for masses or tenderness.
- Palpate the skin for warmth or coolness.

Percussion

- Percuss for hyperresonance and tympany.

Auscultation

- Auscultate the lungs for a pleural friction rub, crackles, wheezes, rhonchi, diminished or absent breath sounds, or whispered pectoriloquy.
- Auscultate the heart for murmurs, clicks, gallops, or a pericardial friction rub.
- Auscultate the abdomen and carotid arteries for bruits.
- Auscultate blood pressure in all four extremities. Note any discrepancy in values or quality. Note Korotkoff sounds.

Dyspnea

Dyspnea is the sensation of difficult or uncomfortable breathing. Its severity varies greatly and is often unrelated to the severity of the underlying disorder. Dyspnea may develop slowly or suddenly, and it may subside quickly or persist for years. (See *Causes of dyspnea*.)

If your patient complains of dyspnea, take his health history and perform a physical examination according to the guidelines below.

Causes of dyspnea

Cardiovascular disorders that cause dyspnea include aortic insufficiency, aortic stenosis, heart failure, mitral insufficiency, mitral stenosis, angina, cardiac arrhythmias, cardiogenic shock, dissecting abdominal aortic aneurysm, myocardial infarction (MI), and pericarditis.

Aortic insufficiency
In chronic severe aortic insufficiency, the patient may report dyspnea on exertion, paroxysmal nocturnal dyspnea with diaphoresis, or orthopnea.

Aortic stenosis
Dyspnea may occur in advanced stages of this disorder. As heart failure progresses, the patient may complain of orthopnea and paroxysmal nocturnal dyspnea. An insidious progression of fatigue and dyspnea may cause the patient to gradually reduce his activity level.

Heart failure
Dyspnea may occur suddenly but is more likely to develop gradually. Chronic paroxysmal nocturnal dyspnea due to heart failure also is common. The patient's health history may reveal prior dyspneic episodes of gradual or sudden onset.

Mitral valve disorders
Dyspnea on exertion may be caused by mitral insufficiency or the later stages of mitral stenosis. With mitral stenosis, the patient also may report paroxysmal nocturnal dyspnea or orthopnea with other signs and symptoms of this condition.

Other cardiovascular disorders
Dyspnea may accompany the pain or discomfort of angina. In many arrhythmias, acute or gradual dyspnea results from decreased cardiac output. If a patient is in cardiogenic shock, dyspnea may accompany tachypnea and other characteristic symptoms. Dyspnea may also occur in dissecting abdominal aortic aneurysm, MI, or pericarditis.

Noncardiovascular disorders
Dyspnea may be caused by adult respiratory distress syndrome, asthma, partial airway obstruction, epiglottitis, flail chest, inhalation injury, laryngotracheobronchitis, pneumonia, pneumothorax, amyotrophic lateral sclerosis (Lou Gehrig's disease), anemia, anxiety, cor pulmonale, emphysema, Guillain-Barré syndrome, interstitial lung cancer, pleural effusion, poliomyelitis (bulbar), pulmonary edema, pulmonary embolism, or tuberculosis.

Adverse drug effects
Dyspnea may occur as an adverse effect of many drugs, including bitolterol, dopamine, epinephrine, ergonovine, methylergonovine, muromonab-CD3, nitroprusside, naproxen, and recombinant interferon alfa-2a.
  Dyspnea also may occur during withdrawal from corticosteroid therapy or because of a disulfiram reaction. Also, if your patient has a history of asthma or laryngospasm, be aware that any drug capable of causing a hypersensitivity reaction can cause dyspnea.

History of the symptom

To further explore the patient's dyspnea, consider asking the questions listed below:
• Did your shortness of breath begin suddenly or gradually?
• Is it constant or intermittent?
• Have you had similar episodes in the past? How does this episode compare?
• How do you ease the discomfort caused by dyspnea?
• Are the attacks precipitated or aggravated by a specific activity?
• Does dyspnea occur when you're active or while you're resting?
• Does dyspnea worsen when you lie down?
• Has an episode ever caused you to awaken at night?

Associated findings

Note the presence of any of the following signs and symptoms:
• chest pain
• nausea or vomiting
• profuse sweating
• persistent cough
• weakness or light-headedness
• undue fatigue
• palpitations
• fever
• intolerance of cold temperatures.

Previous conditions and treatments

Consult with the patient, family members, or members of the health care team to determine if the patient has ever had any of the disorders, risk factors, or treatments listed below:
• heart disease
• chronic obstructive pulmonary disease
• upper respiratory tract infection
• asthma
• aspiration of a foreign body
• recent exposure to allergens, infectious organisms, fire, steam, superheated air, or chemical fumes
• deep vein thrombophlebitis

• varicose veins
• emotional stress
• trauma
• hip or leg fracture
• recent weight gain
• recent pregnancy
• recent cardiopulmonary resuscitation, subclavian cannulation, or mechanical ventilation.

Drug use

Ask the patient about past or current use of the drugs listed below; dyspnea may be an adverse effect of their use:
• bitolterol
• dopamine
• epinephrine
• ergonovine
• methylergonovine
• muromonab-CD3
• naproxen
• nitroprusside
• recombinant interferon alfa-2a or alfa-2b
• recombinant interleukin-2.

Dyspnea may also occur from using acetylcysteine, cholinergics, dinoprostone, esmolol, flecainide, labetalol, metocurine, tubocurarine, or vindesine.

The symptom may follow pulmonary fibrosis caused by:
• amiodarone
• busulfan
• melphalan
• mephenytoin.

What's more, dyspnea may represent a hypersensitivity reaction brought on by:
• cephalosporins
• penicillins
• quinidine
• salicylates.

Physical examination

Examine the patient according to the steps described below.

Inspection

• Observe the patient's respirations for dyspnea, tachypnea, pursed-lip exhalation, grunting, and the use of accessory muscles.

• Look for intercostal retraction during inspiration and intercostal bulging during expiration, flaring nostrils, or inspiratory stridor.
• Inspect for diaphoresis, distended neck veins, and oropharyngeal edema.
• Check for singed nasal hairs, orofacial burns, finger clubbing, peripheral edema, central or peripheral cyanosis, prolonged capillary refill time (more than 2 seconds), chest bruises, and ascites.
• Inspect for signs of chronic dyspnea, such as accessory muscle hypertrophy and barrel chest.
• Assess the patient's neurologic status for restlessness, anxiety, decreased mental acuity, or other abnormalities.
• If the patient has a productive cough, inspect the sputum for color, consistency, amount, and odor.

Palpation
• Palpate the patient's chest for asymmetrical chest expansion, decreased diaphragmatic excursion, subcutaneous crepitation, or decreased vocal or tactile fremitus.
• Gently palpate the neck for tracheal deviation.
• Palpate peripheral pulses and note the rate, rhythm, and intensity.
• Palpate the abdomen for hepatomegaly.
• Palpate the skin to assess for temperature and moisture.

Percussion
• Percuss the lungs for hyperresonance, dullness, and tympany.
• Percuss the liver for enlargement and tenderness.

Auscultation
• Auscultate the lungs for crackles, rhonchi, wheezing, decreased breath sounds or absent unilateral breath sounds, egobronchophony, broncho-

phony, whispered pectoriloquy, or a pleural friction rub.
• Auscultate the heart for tachycardia, abnormal heart sounds or rhythms (such as a ventricular or atrial gallop), or for a pericardial friction rub.
• Monitor the patient's blood pressure for changes in measurements, a paradoxical pulse, and differences in pulse pressures.

Tachypnea

A respiratory rate of 20 breaths/minute or more, tachypnea is a common symptom of cardiopulmonary disease. It may result from reduced partial pressure of oxygen in arterial blood (PaO_2) or arterial oxygen content, decreased perfusion, increased oxygen demand, increased partial pressure of carbon dioxide in arterial blood ($PaCO_2$), or acidosis. Common factors that increase the demand for oxygen include pain, exertion, anxiety, and fever. (See *Causes of tachypnea,* page 32.)

Generally, tachypnea indicates a need to increase minute volume (the amount of air breathed each minute). If tachypnea is accompanied by an increased tidal volume (the amount of air inspired and expired during one respiratory cycle), hyperpnea may result.

Tachypnea is easily detected by counting the rise and fall of the patient's chest as he breathes or by auscultating the movement of air in and out of his lungs.

If your patient complains of tachypnea, take his health history and perform a physical examination according to the guidelines below.

History of the symptom
To further explore the patient's tachypnea, consider asking the questions listed below:

Causes of tachypnea

Cardiovascular causes of tachypnea include arrhythmias, cardiac tamponade, cardiogenic shock, and heart failure.

Arrhythmias
Depending on the patient's heart rate, tachypnea may occur along with hypotension, dizziness, palpitations, weakness, and fatigue. The patient's level of consciousness may be decreased.

Cardiac tamponade
In this life-threatening disorder, tachypnea may accompany tachycardia, dyspnea, pulsus paradoxus, and other characteristic signs and symptoms.

Cardiogenic shock
In this medical emergency, tachypnea may accompany tachycardia and a decrease in systolic blood pressure (to less than 80 mm Hg or 30 mm Hg below baseline) along with other characteristic signs and symptoms.

Heart failure
Tachypnea occurs secondary to pulmonary congestion. It is accompanied by dyspnea, fatigue, tachycardia, and other signs and symptoms of heart failure.

Noncardiovascular causes
Tachypnea may be caused by alcohol withdrawal syndrome, adult respiratory distress syndrome, partial airway obstruction, anaphylactic shock, anemia, asthma, bronchiectasis, chronic bronchitis, pulmonary edema, pulmonary embolism, diabetic ketoacidosis, flail chest, increasing intracranial pressure, hyperosmolar nonketotic syndrome, hypovolemic shock, emphysema, febrile illness, interstitial fibrosis, lung abscess, malignant mesothelioma, metabolic acidosis, pneumonia, pneumothorax, primary pulmonary hypertension, septic shock, or lung, pleural, or mediastinal tumor. Also, an overdose of salicylates or theophylline can cause tachypnea.

• Are you having trouble breathing now?
• When did the episode of tachypnea begin? Was it preceded by a specific activity or incident?
• Have you had similar episodes before? How did you relieve the symptoms? Did you receive medical treatment?
• Do specific activities make it easier or more difficult to breathe? Is it more difficult to breathe when you lie down?

Associated findings
Note if the patient has experienced any of the following signs or symptoms:
• pain in the chest or other area
• persistent cough
• nausea and vomiting
• diarrhea
• a feeling of doom
• undue fatigue
• intolerance for cold temperatures
• anorexia
• excessive hunger or thirst
• excessive urination
• recent weight loss or gain.

Previous conditions and treatments
Check with the patient, family members, or members of the health care team to determine if the patient has ever had any of the disorders, treatments, or risk factors listed below:

- recent trauma (particularly involving the head, abdomen, or chest)
- leg or hip fracture
- cardiopulmonary resuscitation
- cardiovascular, pulmonary, or endocrine disorders
- diabetes mellitus or renal failure (both may cause metabolic acidosis)
- recent pregnancy
- recent systemic infection or exposure to an infectious organism
- exposure to hazardous fumes
- exposure to known or common allergens
- recent subclavian cannulation or mechanical ventilation.

Drug use

Note past or current use of the drugs listed below, which can cause tachypnea secondary to congestive heart failure:

- amiodarone
- angiotensin-converting enzyme inhibitors
- antihypertensives
- beta blockers
- calcium channel blockers
- carbamazepine
- corticosteroids
- doxorubicin
- flecainide
- recombinant interferon alfa-2a
- recombinant interleukin-2.

Tachypnea may also result from an overdose of salicylates or theophylline.

Physical examination

Examine the patient according to the steps described below.

Inspection

- Observe the patient's respirations, noting their rate and depth and whether the patient experiences difficulty.
- Note any change in the respiratory pattern. Also note stridor, grunting, flaring of the nostrils, nasal congestion, use of accessory muscles, asymmetrical or paradoxical chest wall movement, or intercostal bulging or retractions.
- Assess the patient's level of consciousness, noting changes such as restlessness, decreased mental acuity, lethargy, stupor, seizure, or coma.
- If the patient has a productive cough, note the color, amount, odor, and consistency of the sputum.
- Check for any abnormal breath odor.
- Assess for jugular vein distention.
- Check the skin for signs of trauma (such as bruising), pallor, cyanosis (a late sign of hypoxemia), edema, poor turgor, or presence of a rash.
- Assess the patient's fingers for clubbing.
- Test for a capillary refill time greater than 2 seconds.
- Monitor the patient for oliguria and anuria.

Palpation

- Palpate peripheral pulses. Note their rate, rhythm, and intensity.
- Gently check for any palpable rib or sternal fractures or any subcutaneous emphysema.
- Palpate over the lungs for decreased vocal or tactile fremitus and decreased diaphragmatic excursion.
- Palpate the abdomen for ascites and hepatomegaly.
- Palpate the neck for tracheal deviation. Gently palpate the eyeballs, noting any softness.
- Palpate the skin to assess for temperature and moisture.

Percussion

- Percuss over the lungs for any hyperresonance, tympany, or dullness.
- Percuss over the liver to detect enlargement or tenderness.

Auscultation

- Auscultate the chest for abnormal or adventitious breath sounds, such as crackles, rhonchi, wheezing, whis-

pered pectoriloquy, or a pleural friction rub.
• Auscultate the heart. Note any abnormal rate, rhythm, or sounds, particularly murmurs and gallops.
• Monitor for changes in blood pressure or pulse pressure. Detect orthostatic changes by measuring the patient's blood pressure while he reclines and then again after he sits up. Note the intensity of Korotkoff sounds.

Palpitations

The patient may describe palpitations as a pounding, jumping, turning, fluttering, or flopping in his chest, or as if his heart is missing or skipping beats. Usually, he feels palpitations in the precordium, throat, or neck. Palpitations may be regular or irregular, fast or slow, paroxysmal or sustained. (See *Causes of palpitations*.)

If your patient complains of palpitations, take his health history and perform a physical examination according to the guidelines below.

History of the symptom
To further explore an episode of palpitations, consider asking the questions listed below:
• What were you doing when you first noticed the palpitations? How long did the episode last?
• Have you experienced similar episodes in the past? Were the symptoms and precipitating factors similar?
• What did you do to alleviate the palpitations?

Associated findings
Ask the patient if he has experienced any of the following symptoms:
• chest pain
• dizziness
• weakness

• muscle cramps, tremor, or spasms in the feet or hands
• numbness or tingling in the fingertips, feet, or mouth
• anorexia
• belching
• undue fatigue
• dyspnea on exertion
• headache
• confusion.

Previous conditions and treatments
Consult with the patient, family members, or members of the health care team to determine if the patient has ever had any of the disorders, risk factors, or treatments listed below:
• hypertension or other cardiovascular disease
• pulmonary disease
• renal disease
• hypoparathyroidism or pseudohypoparathyroidism
• calcium or vitamin D deficiency
• malabsorption syndrome
• acute pancreatitis
• bone cancer
• thyroid disease
• hypoglycemia
• recent emotional stress
• recent multiple blood transfusions
• recent infusion of phosphate.

Drug use
Ask the patient about current or past use of the drugs or substances listed below:
• alcohol
• caffeine
• digitalis glycosides
• tobacco.
Also ask about use of the following drugs, which can cause arrhythmias:
• atropine
• beta blockers
• ganglionic blockers
• sympathomimetics.

Causes of palpitations

Cardiovascular disorders that cause palpitations include angina, aortic insufficiency, arrhythmias, mitral valve prolapse, mitral insufficiency, and mitral stenosis.

Angina
In this disorder, palpitations may accompany chest pain.

Aortic insufficiency
Palpitations may accompany an uncomfortable awareness of the heartbeat (especially when lying down), and a pounding sensation in the patient's head. You may notice that each heartbeat seems to jar the patient's body and that his head bobs during systole.

Arrhythmias
Paroxysmal or sustained palpitations may accompany dizziness, fatigue, weakness, or other signs and symptoms of arrhythmias.

Hypertension
The patient may report sustained palpitations alone or with headache, dizziness, tinnitus, and fatigue.

Mitral valve disorders
Palpitations may accompany pain associated with mitral valve prolapse. Palpitations may also occur in mitral insufficiency and the later stages of mitral stenosis.

Other causes
Palpitations may be caused by acute anxiety episodes, anemia, hypocalcemic tetany, hypoglycemia, thyrotoxicosis (thyroid storm), or pheochromocytoma. Transient palpitations may be caused by emotional or physical stress or the use of stimulants.

A newly implanted prosthetic valve can cause nonpathologic palpitations because the valve's clicking sound heightens the patient's awareness of his heartbeat. Palpitations may also be caused by medications capable of precipitating cardiac arrhythmia or that increase cardiac output, such as digitalis glycosides, sympathomimetics, ganglionic blockers, and atropine.

Physical examination
Examine the patient according to the steps described below.

Inspection
• Check the skin for pallor or diaphoresis. Note the presence of exophthalmos.
• Observe the patient's respirations, noting their rate and depth. Determine whether the patient is having difficulty breathing. Record any change in his normal respiratory pattern.
• Assess the patient's level of consciousness, noting any confusion, anxiety, nervousness, or irrational behavior.
• Inspect the nails for capillary nail bed pulsations.

Palpation
• Gently palpate the neck for thyroid enlargement.
• Palpate peripheral pulses, noting their rate, rhythm, and intensity.

Percussion
• Percuss over reflex points to determine hyperreflexia. Note whether the patient has Chvostek's or Trousseau's sign.

Auscultation

• Auscultate the patient's heart. Note any gallops or murmurs.
• Auscultate the lungs for abnormal breath sounds.
• Monitor the patient for changes in blood pressure and pulse pressure.

Cyanosis

Characterized by bluish or bluish black skin or mucous membranes, cyanosis results from an excess of unoxygenated hemoglobin in the blood. It's usually visible when the unsaturated hemoglobin level exceeds 5 g/dl. Severe cyanosis is readily apparent on inspection, whereas mild cyanosis may be more difficult to detect. In darkskinned patients, cyanosis is most apparent in the mucous membranes and nail beds. (See *Causes of cyanosis.*)

Central cyanosis reflects inadequate oxygenation of systemic arterial blood, which results in an excess of unsaturated hemoglobin in arterial blood. It may occur anywhere on the skin and on the mucous membranes of the mouth and lips. Central cyanosis may result from right-to-left cardiac shunting, pulmonary disorders, hematologic disorders, and reduced partial pressure of oxygen in arterial blood (PaO_2) at high altitudes.

Peripheral cyanosis reflects sluggish peripheral circulation due to vasoconstriction, reduced cardiac output, or vascular occlusion. Peripheral tissues remove excessive amounts of oxygen from the blood, causing reduced oxygen saturation in venous blood. Signs typically appear on exposed areas (such as fingers, nail beds, feet, nose, or ears) and may be widespread or local. Mucous membranes are not affected. Peripheral cyanosis may be aggravated by smoking, stress, or exposure to cold temperatures and may be alleviated by massage or warmth.

Cyanosis is an important sign of cardiovascular or cardiopulmonary disease, but it doesn't always provide an accurate gauge of oxygenation. Several factors contribute to the development of cyanosis: hemoglobin concentration, oxygen saturation, cardiac output, and PaO_2.

If your patient experiences cyanosis, take his health history and perform a physical examination according to the guidelines below.

History of the symptom

To further explore the patient's complaint of cyanosis, consider asking the questions listed below:

• When did you first notice skin discoloration?
• Does it subside and recur?
• Does it occur more often when you are tired or short of breath?
• What factors aggravate the condition? What factors alleviate it?

Associated findings

Ask if the patient's cyanosis has been accompanied by any of the following symptoms:

• chest, arm, or leg pain, especially when walking
• numbness or tingling
• weakness or temporary paralysis
• persistent cough
• trouble breathing at night
• weight gain
• fever.

Previous conditions and treatments

Consult with the patient, family members, or members of the health care team to determine if the patient has ever had any of the disorders, risk factors, or treatments listed below:

• myocardial infarction
• heart failure
• cardiogenic shock

- cardiomyopathy
- atherosclerosis
- rheumatic heart disease
- obstructive lung disease
- asthma
- allergies
- thrombophlebitis or varicose veins
- septicemia
- recent prosthetic heart valve surgery
- chest trauma
- hip or leg fracture
- recent injection of ergot or other intra-arterial injection
- recent subclavian vein cannulation
- mechanical ventilation
- recent pregnancy or emotional stress.

Drug use
Note past or current use of these drugs:
- aspirin
- indomethacin
- oral contraceptives.

Also ask about the use of the following drugs, which may bring on heart failure and produce cyanosis:
- amiodarone
- angiotensin-converting enzyme inhibitors
- antihypertensives
- beta blockers
- calcium channel blockers
- carbamazepine
- corticosteroids
- doxorubicin
- flecainide
- recombinant interferon alfa-2a
- recombinant interleukin-2.

Physical examination
Examine the patient according to the steps described below.

Inspection
- Inspect the skin and mucous membranes to determine the extent of cyanosis. Check for pallid skin, redness, and ulceration. Note whether any affected limb becomes blanched when elevated even slightly. Also inspect for

Causes of cyanosis

Cardiovascular disorders that cause cyanosis include acute peripheral arterial occlusion, heart failure, cardiogenic shock, thrombophlebitis, and Raynaud's disease.

Acute peripheral arterial occlusion
In this disorder, cyanosis may be seen in one arm or leg or both legs when the ischemic limb is in a dependent position. When elevated, the limb appears blanched. Cyanosis may be accompanied by a sharp pain or ache that becomes worse when the patient moves.

Heart failure
Cyanosis is a late sign of heart failure and may occur as central cyanosis, peripheral cyanosis, or both. Central cyanosis is associated with left ventricular failure, whereas peripheral cyanosis is associated with right ventricular failure.

Cardiogenic shock
Peripheral cyanosis may result from poor tissue perfusion.

Thrombophlebitis
Cyanosis may accompany redness and swelling in both deep vein and superficial vein thrombophlebitis.

Raynaud's disease
Cyanosis, usually in the hands, results from dilation of cutaneous arterioles and venules.

Other causes
Cyanosis may be caused by asthma, bronchiectasis, Buerger's disease, chronic obstructive pulmonary disease, pulmonary embolism, cystic fibrosis, epiglottitis, acute laryngotracheobronchitis, lung cancer, pulmonary embolism, methemoglobinemia, pneumothorax, or pneumonia.

finger clubbing, edema, and neck vein distention.
• Inspect the nail beds for a capillary refill time greater than 2 seconds.
• Assess the patient's respiratory rate and rhythm. Note any nasal flaring, stridor, audible wheezes, muffled voice, barking cough, retractions, or use of accessory muscles.
• Inspect for asymmetrical chest expansion or barrel chest.
• Assess the patient's level of consciousness and muscle strength.
• Inspect the abdomen for ascites and test for shifting dullness or fluid wave.

Palpation
• Palpate peripheral pulses, noting their rate, rhythm, and intensity.
• Palpate the liver for enlargement and tenderness.
• Palpate over the lungs to detect decreased vocal or tactile fremitus, decreased diaphragmatic excursion, or subcutaneous crepitation.
• Palpate the skin to assess for temperature and moisture.

Percussion
• Percuss for liver enlargement and tenderness.
• Percuss over the lungs for hyperresonance or tympany.

Auscultation
• Auscultate the heart rate and rhythm. Note any gallops or murmurs.
• Auscultate the abdominal aorta and femoral arteries for bruits.
• Listen for decreased or adventitious breath sounds. Note any wheezing, crackles, or whispered pectoriloquy.
• Auscultate blood pressure and note any abnormalities. Monitor for narrowing pulse pressure. Note the intensity of Korotkoff sounds.

Edema

An excessive accumulation of interstitial fluid, edema commonly occurs in severely ill patients and usually is chronic and progressive. Slight edema may be difficult to detect, especially in obese patients. Massive edema, in contrast, is immediately apparent. Generalized edema (anasarca) can be caused by congestive heart failure, pericarditis, or malnutrition and may result from factors that influence plasma osmotic pressure, such as hypoalbuminemia or excess sodium retention. (See *Causes of edema*.)

If your patient complains of edema, take his health history and perform a physical examination according to the guidelines below.

History of the symptom
To further explore the patient's complaint of edema, consider asking the questions listed below:
• When did you first notice the swelling? Is it painful?
• Does it seem better or worse at certain times of the day? Does it get worse when you stand up?
• What have you done to alleviate the swelling?

Associated findings
Ask the patient if edema occurs with any of the following signs and symptoms:
• chest pain
• shortness of breath, especially when reclining
• palpitations
• persistent cough
• undue fatigue
• intolerance of cold temperatures
• pain or weakness in the arms or legs
• recent weight gain
• decreased urine output.

Causes of edema

Cardiovascular disorders that cause edema include heart failure, mitral insufficiency, and chronic constrictive pericarditis.

Heart failure
Edema may occur concurrently with characteristic signs and symptoms of heart failure. Dependent edema may be one sign of left ventricular failure, whereas generalized edema may occur with other signs of right ventricular failure.

Mitral insufficiency
As mitral insufficiency progresses, peripheral edema may accompany other signs and symptoms of the disorder.

Chronic constrictive pericarditis
This disorder resembles right ventricular failure and usually begins with pitting edema in the arms and legs, which may progress to generalized edema. Edema may accompany other signs and symptoms, such as abdominal distention.

Noncardiovascular causes
Edema may be caused by cirrhosis, kwashiorkor, myxedema, nephrotic syndrome, protein-losing enteropathy, renal failure, or septic shock. It may be secondary to severe burns or renal, endocrine, or hepatic disease.

Angioneurotic edema, a periodic swelling of the skin, mucous membranes, viscera, and brain, appears to be associated with food allergies, urticaria, or stress or emotional factors. Generalized edema may be aggravated or caused by I.V. infusions and feedings (particularly I.V. saline administration or enteral feedings) or any drug that causes sodium retention. Cyclic edema associated with increased aldosterone secretion may occur in premenopausal women.

Previous conditions and treatments
Consult with the patient, family members, or members of the health care team to determine if the patient has ever had any of the disorders, risk factors, or treatments listed below:
• severe burns
• cardiovascular disorders
• renal disorders
• hepatic disorders
• endocrine disorders
• GI disorders
• recent severe infection
• recent I.V. infusion.

Drug use
Note past or current use of any of the drugs listed below, which may cause sodium retention and aggravate or lead to generalized edema:
• antihypertensives
• corticosteroids, androgenic steroids, or anabolic steroids
• estrogens
• phenylbutazone
• ibuprofen
• naproxen.

Also ask about the use of drugs that can precipitate heart failure, such as the following:
• amiodarone
• angiotensin-converting enzyme inhibitors
• antihypertensives
• beta blockers
• calcium channel blockers
• carbamazepine

- corticosteroids
- doxorubicin
- flecainide
- recombinant interferon alfa-2a
- recombinant interleukin-2.

Physical examination
Examine the patient according to the steps described below.

Inspection
- Observe the patient for dyspnea.
- Inspect the patient's arms and legs for symmetrical edema. Check the skin for ecchymoses, cyanosis, and diaphoresis.
- If the patient is on bed rest, assess the back, sacrum, hips, and pretibial area for dependent edema.
- Assess the nail beds. Note if the capillary refill time is greater than 2 seconds.
- Inspect the neck for jugular vein distention.

Palpation
- Palpate peripheral pulses, noting their rate, rhythm, and symmetry.
- Palpate the precordium, noting the presence of a systolic thrill or a diffuse apical impulse.
- Palpate the liver for hepatomegaly.
- Palpate the hands and feet for coolness.

Percussion
- Percuss the abdomen for ascites.
- Percuss the liver for enlargement and tenderness.

Auscultation
- Auscultate the lungs for abnormal and adventitious breath sounds, particularly crackles.
- Auscultate the heart for murmurs, gallops, or a pericardial friction rub.

Fatigue

When a patient experiences fatigue, it indicates that his cells lack the nutrients needed for energy and growth due to rapid depletion of nutrients, impaired replacement mechanisms, insufficient hormone production, or inadequate nutrient intake or metabolism. Fatigue represents an important normal response to physical overexertion, prolonged emotional stress, and sleep deprivation. However, it can be a nonspecific symptom of many physical and psychological disorders. Undue fatigue is a common complaint in cardiovascular disease. (See *Causes of fatigue.*)

If your patient complains of fatigue, take his health history and perform a physical examination according to the guidelines below.

History of the symptom
To explore the patient's complaint of fatigue, consider asking the following questions:
- When did you first feel unusually tired?
- Is your fatigue related to activity?
- Does rest help?

Associated findings
Ask the patient if fatigue is accompanied by any of the following signs and symptoms:
- shortness of breath or other breathing difficulty
- pain, especially chest pain, or discomfort
- loss of consciousness
- periodic weakness
- palpitations
- nausea or vomiting
- anxiety or restlessness
- dizziness
- feeling of impending doom
- persistent cough

Causes of fatigue

Cardiovascular disorders that cause fatigue include aortic stenosis, myocardial infarction (MI), heart failure, mitral valve prolapse, mitral insufficiency, and mitral stenosis.

Aortic stenosis
As aortic stenosis progresses, marked fatigue may accompany other symptoms such as dyspnea and syncope on exertion.

Myocardial infarction
Fatigue due to MI can be severe but is usually overshadowed by the characteristic pain of MI.

Heart failure
Increasing levels of fatigue may accompany insomnia, weakness, and other characteristic symptoms of heart failure.

Mitral valve disorders
Episodes of severe fatigue may accompany the characteristic pain or precordial ache of mitral valve prolapse. Associated complaints may include migraine headache, dizziness, weakness, and other symptoms. As mitral insufficiency or mitral stenosis progresses, a patient may report fatigue along with dyspnea on exertion, weakness, and other symptoms.

Noncardiovascular causes
Undue fatigue may be caused by acquired immunodeficiency syndrome, adrenocortical insufficiency, anemia, anxiety, cancer, chronic fatigue and immune dysfunction syndrome, chronic obstructive pulmonary disease, cirrhosis, depression, diabetes mellitus, hypercortisolism, hypopituitarism, infection, Lyme disease, malnutrition, myasthenia gravis, renal failure, restrictive lung disease, rheumatoid arthritis, systemic lupus erythematosus, and thyrotoxicosis.

Many drugs can cause fatigue, especially those identified during assessment. Also, most types of surgery cause temporary fatigue because of the combined effects of hunger, anesthesia, and sleep deprivation.

- intolerance for cold temperatures
- recent weight gain.

Previous conditions and treatments
Consult with the patient, family members, or members of the health care team to determine if the patient has ever had any of the disorders, risk factors, or treatments listed below:
- hypertension
- rheumatic fever
- congenital heart anomalies
- other cardiac illness
- emotional stress
- a recent change in daily routine.

Drug use
Ask the patient about past or current use of the drugs listed below:
- amiodarone
- antihypertensives
- carbamazepine
- corticosteroids
- digitalis glycosides
- doxorubicin
- flecainide
- recombinant interferon alfa-2a
- recombinant interleukin-2
- sedatives.

Physical examination
Examine the patient according to the steps described below.

Inspection
• Observe whether the patient is in distress or is having difficulty breathing.
• Inspect the skin for cyanosis or pallor.
• Inspect the nail beds. Note if the capillary refill time is longer than 2 seconds.
• Inspect for jugular vein distention.
• If the patient has a productive cough, inspect the sputum for color, consistency, odor, and amount.

Palpation
• Palpate peripheral pulses, noting their rate, rhythm, and symmetry.
• Palpate the precordium for a diffuse apical impulse or a systolic thrill.
• Palpate the abdomen for ascites and hepatomegaly.
• Palpate the skin to assess for temperature and moisture.

Percussion
• Percuss the liver for tenderness and enlargement.

Auscultation
• Auscultate the heart for murmurs, gallops, or a pericardial friction rub.
• Auscultate the lungs for abnormal or adventitious breath sounds, crackles, rhonchi, and wheezes.
• Auscultate peripheral pulses and note their symmetry.

Syncope

A brief lapse of consciousness, syncope is a common neurologic sign of impaired cerebral oxygenation. In most cases, the onset is abrupt and the episode lasts no longer than a few minutes. (See *Causes of syncope*.)

During syncope, the patient is hypotensive and has a strikingly pale appearance. Skeletal muscles are relaxed, the pulse may be slow and weak or very rapid and weak, and breathing is almost imperceptible. If the episode lasts 20 seconds or more, the patient may develop tonic-clonic movements. However, the confusion, headache, and drowsiness that follow a convulsive seizure, are absent in syncope.

The depth of unconsciousness varies during syncope. Some patients continue to hear voices and see blurred outlines of nearby objects; others are completely unconscious.

Syncope is much less common in children than in adults.

If your patient experiences syncope, take his health history and perform a physical examination according to the guidelines below.

History of the symptom
To explore the patient's episode of syncope, consider asking the following questions:
• Can you describe the episode? Did anyone witness it?
• How did you feel just before you fainted? For example, did you feel weak, light-headed, nauseous, or sweaty?
• What were you doing just before it happened? Did you get up suddenly from sitting or lying down?
• Did you notice any palpitations?
• How long were you unconscious?
• Did you experience any muscle spasms or incontinence?
• When you regained consciousness, did you feel alert or confused? Did you have a headache?
• Have you had similar episodes before? How often do they occur?

Associated findings
Ask the patient if he has recently experienced any of the following symptoms:

Causes of syncope

Cardiovascular disorders that cause syncope include aortic arch syndrome, aortic stenosis, arrhythmias, and dissecting aortic aneurysm.

Aortic arch syndrome
Characteristic symptoms of aortic arch syndrome include syncope when rising from a horizontal position, recurrent loss of consciousness, and other symptoms.

Aortic stenosis
As aortic stenosis progresses, syncope on exertion may accompany other symptoms of the disorder.

Arrhythmias
Any arrhythmia that decreases cardiac output and impairs cerebral circulation may cause syncope. The patient also may report dizziness or other related symptoms. Signs and symptoms that typically precede syncope include pallor, confusion, blurred vision, diaphoresis, dyspnea, and hypotension. In Adams-Stokes syndrome, the patient is asystolic during syncope due to incomplete heart block. Episodes may occur several times daily without warning, and the patient may experience spasms and myoclonic jerks during prolonged episodes.

Dissecting aortic aneurysm
Syncope may accompany the sudden onset of extreme chest pain caused by dissecting aortic aneurysm.

Other causes
Any condition that causes hypoxemia or orthostatic hypotension may lead to syncope. Tussive syncope may be caused by vigorous coughing. Vasovagal syncope may be caused by emotional stress, injury, shock, or pain. Syncope may also be caused by autonomic dysfunction, transient ischemic attack, or vagal glossopharyngeal neuralgia.

Adverse drug effects
Quinidine commonly causes syncope associated with ventricular fibrillation. Prazosin may cause severe orthostatic hypotension and syncope, usually after the first dose. Occasionally, griseofulvin, levodopa, and indomethacin produce syncope.

• pain in the chest, neck, shoulder, jaw, or abdomen
• sudden fatigue
• shortness of breath
• palpitations
• blurred vision.

• aortic arch syndrome
• aortic stenosis
• arrhythmias
• other cardiovascular illnesses
• hypoxemia
• transient ischemic attacks.

Previous conditions and treatments
Consult with the patient, family members, or members of the health care team to determine if the patient has ever had any of the disorders listed below:

Drug use
Ask the patient about past or current use of the following drugs:
• prazosin (which may cause severe orthostatic hypotension and syncope after the first dose)
• quinidine.

Also ask about use of the following drugs, which may occasionally cause syncope:
• griseofulvin
• indomethacin
• levodopa.

Physical examination
Examine the patient according to the steps described below.

Inspection
• Observe the patient's level of consciousness.
• Note whether the patient is in severe distress, possibly due to dyspnea or pain. Check for weakness or paralysis in his arms or legs.
• Inspect the patient's skin for pallor, cyanosis, diaphoresis, or discoloration (below the waist).
• Inspect the nail beds for a prolonged capillary refill time (more than 2 seconds).
• Perform an ophthalmoscopic examination and note any retinal atrophy or loss of retinal pigmentation.
• Inspect for jugular vein distention or tracheal deviation.

Palpation
• Palpate the carotid pulse and all peripheral pulses. Note their quality, rate, rhythm, and symmetry.
• Gently palpate the abdomen for tenderness or masses.
• Palpate the neck for tracheal deviation.
• Palpate the skin to assess for temperature and moisture.

Percussion
• Gently percuss the abdomen for masses.

Auscultation
• Auscultate the heart for an abnormal rate or rhythm. Note murmurs, bruits, gallops, or a pericardial friction rub.

• Auscultate blood pressure in all four extremities and note any differences. Note hypotension.

CHAPTER 3

Monitoring cardiovascular status

Ongoing evaluation of your patient's condition is an essential component of cardiovascular care. Depending on your patient's disorder, you'll probably be called on to assist in one or more forms of electrocardiography (ECG), which monitors the heart's electrical activity. Other procedures — those that monitor intra-arterial pressure, pulmonary artery pressure (PAP), pulmonary artery wedge pressure (PAWP), central venous pressure (CVP), and cardiac output — enable you to assess the heart's pumping ability.

Electrocardiography

In ECG, a series of electrodes placed at specific points on the patient's limbs and chest detect the heart's electrical activity and transmit this data to the ECG unit. The equipment records the electrical activity over a specified duration and then displays this information as a characteristic waveform, either on the ECG monitor or as a tracing on a strip of paper. The ECG is used to analyze the heart's rate and rhythm, determine response to drug therapy, and identify any complications of diagnostic procedures or surgery. (See *Variations of electrocardiography*.)

Standard 12-lead ECG
The standard 12-lead ECG provides 12 distinct views of the heart. Routinely performed to establish a baseline of the heart's electrical activity, an ECG is also commonly used to monitor all patients ages 45 or older who are undergoing surgery. Subsequent tracings can be compared to the baseline to monitor changes in heart rate and rhythm brought on by activity or treatment, or to detect heart disease.

In emergencies, the 12-lead ECG helps assess symptoms such as the onset of chest pain that radiates to the jaw, left shoulder, or left arm; increased severity of chest pain; sudden onset of an irregular heart rhythm, bradycardia, or tachycardia; significant changes in blood pressure; or signs of cardiac crisis or decompensation, including light-headedness, diaphoresis, confusion, anxiety, or a change in level of consciousness.

Daily or periodic 12-lead ECGs may be ordered for a recent myocardial infarction (MI), chronic arrhythmias, cardiac decompensation from cardiomyopathy, congestive heart failure, valvular disorders, electrolyte imbalances, or drug toxicity.

Implementation
• Place the ECG leads on the inner aspects of both wrists, the medial aspects of the lower legs, and in the six specific spots on the chest. (See *Placing leads in a 12-lead ECG,* page 48.)
• Explain the procedure to your patient to allay his fears and promote cooperation. Inform him that no special preparation is required and that the procedure takes no longer than 15 minutes.
• Check the patient's health history for cardiac medications. Note current drug therapy on the test request form.
• Place the patient in the supine position. If he can't tolerate this position, use the semi-Fowler position.
• Expose the patient's chest, ankles, and wrists to attach the electrodes. If using disposable electrodes, remove the paper backing before positioning. For reusable electrodes, apply electrode gel and position the electrodes. If necessary, shave a small area of skin or clean it with an alcohol sponge before applying the electrodes to ensure proper skin contact.

Timesaving tip: If your patient's skin is oily, scaly, or diaphoretic, rub the site with an alcohol sponge followed by a dry 4″ × 4″ gauze pad

Variations of electrocardiography

Several important monitoring and diagnostic techniques employ electrocardiography (ECG) equipment. Each monitors the heart for an established period and may be used in a hospital or ambulatory care setting.

Exercise ECG

Exercise ECG (stress ECG, treadmill test, graded exercise test) is a variation of the standard 12-lead ECG. This procedure is used to monitor heart rate, blood pressure, and ECG waveforms during a period of physical stress. During the test, the patient pedals a stationary bicycle, walks on a treadmill, or climbs a set of stairs until he achieves a predetermined heart rate. The test is stopped immediately if the patient experiences chest pain or exhibits signs of exercise intolerance, such as fatigue, shortness of breath, increase in or new onset of arrhythmias, significant ST-segment depression or elevation, or hypotensive response.

Exercise ECG is used to help assess the effects of physical stress on patients experiencing chest pain, atypical angina, arrhythmias, or shortness of breath. It's used to investigate how cardiovascular disease, such as coronary artery disease or peripheral vascular disease, affects the heart. In patients recovering from myocardial infarction (MI), exercise ECG may be used to evaluate rehabilitation, patient's ability to return to work, and tolerance for isometric activity. Exercise ECG may also be used to evaluate patients after coronary artery bypass grafting or percutaneous transluminal coronary angioplasty or to assess the effects of various drugs, such as antiarrhythmics, antihypertensives, and antianginals.

Ambulatory ECG

Ambulatory ECG monitoring (such as Holter monitoring) records the patient's heart rate and rhythm continuously for an established period (for example, 24 to 72 hours). During this period, the patient keeps an activity diary. The diary and ECG record are used to evaluate how daily physical and psychological stress affect the patient's heart, as well as to provide information about the heart's response to a specific activity that causes discomfort.

Signal-averaged ECG

Signal-averaged ECG is a surface ECG that detects and amplifies low-amplitude (1 to 20 microvolts [µV]) late potentials. Late potentials represent electrical activity that occurs after normal depolarization of the ventricles. The presence of late potentials indicates areas of slow ventricular conduction. This electrical instability occurs in ischemic areas and is the major cause of ventricular tachycardia. During signal-averaged ECG, a portable computerized ECG unit averages literally hundreds of ECG complexes to produce a QRS complex that's free of artifacts resulting from respiratory and body movements. With all artifacts removed, the cardiologist can see late potentials.

Signal-averaged ECG is most often used for patients with unexplained syncope, idiopathic ventricular tachycardia, or cardiomyopathy and after MI. Identifying late potentials can help distinguish patients who have a high risk of ventricular tachycardia and sudden death.

Placing leads in a 12-lead ECG

A standard 12-lead ECG records the heart's electrical potential from 12 different views:
• Standard bipolar leads (I, II, II) detect variations in electrical potential at two points (the negative pole and the positive pole) and record the difference.
• The unipolar augmented limb leads (aV$_R$, aV$_L$, and aV$_F$) measure electrical potential between one augmented limb lead and the electrical midpoint of the remaining two leads.
• Six unipolar chest leads (V$_1$ through V$_6$) view electrical potential from the horizontal plane, helping to locate abnormality in the heart's lateral and posterior walls.

Limb leads
Attach the leads as follows:
• Place the RA or white lead on the inner aspect of the patient's right wrist.
• Place the LA or black lead on the inner aspect of the patient's left wrist.
• Place the RL or green lead on the medial aspect of the patient's right lower leg.
• Place the LL or red lead on the medial aspect of the patient's left lower leg.

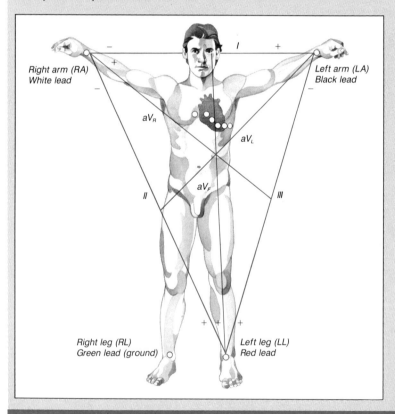

Right arm (RA)
White lead

Left arm (LA)
Black lead

aV$_R$

aV$_L$

II

aV$_F$

III

Right leg (RL)
Green lead (ground)

Left leg (LL)
Red lead

Chest leads

- Place the V_1 lead at the fourth intercostal space on the right sternal border.
- Place the V_2 lead at the fourth intercostal space on left sternal border.
- Place the V_3 lead halfway between V_2 and V_4.
- Place the V_4 lead at the fifth intercostal space on the midclavicular line.
- Place the V_5 lead at the fifth intercostal space on the anterior axillary line (halfway between V_4 and V_6).
- Place the V_6 lead at the fifth intercostal space on the midaxillary line, level with V_4.

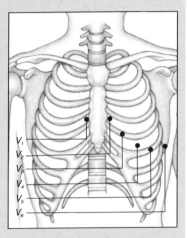

Multichannel and single-channel ECGs

A multichannel ECG uses 6 unipolar chest leads. All electrodes are attached at the same time, and the 12 views are recorded simultaneously.

A single-channel ECG uses only one chest lead. After each view is recorded, the dial on the machine is turned to the standby position, the chest lead is repositioned for the next view, and a printout is obtained.

before applying the electrode to help reduce electrical interference.

- Attach the leadwires to the electrodes.
- Turn on the machine, and check the paper supply.
- Make sure the paper speed selector is set to the standard 25 mm/second and that the machine is set to full voltage. The machine will record a normal standardization mark on the recording paper.
- Tell the patient to relax, lie still, and breathe normally. Explain that any movement (twitching, shivering, talking) can distort the ECG tracing. Remember that electrodes that are improperly attached or placed also can produce a poor tracing.
- Activate the machine and obtain the tracing.
- Remove the electrodes from the patient's skin.

Timesaving tip: If frequent ECGs will be necessary, use a marking pen to indicate lead positions on your patient's chest to ensure consistent placement.

Cardiac monitoring

In cardiac monitoring, or continuous ECG monitoring, the patient is connected to an ECG for an extended period to permit analysis of the heart's electrical activity. Cardiac monitoring usually uses three electrodes placed on the chest in one of three patterns. Four or five leads may be used to increase the area of electrical activity being monitored. (See *Placing leads in cardiac monitoring,* page 50.)

In *hardwire* monitoring, leads connect the patient directly to a bedside ECG monitor. Information is also displayed on a central monitor at the nurses' station. In *telemetry* monitoring, the patient wears a transmitter that relays signals through an antenna in the ceiling to a monitor at the nurses' station.

Placing leads in cardiac monitoring

Placement of leads and electrodes varies depending on the cardiac monitoring system you're using.

Three-electrode system
The most common system used in cardiac monitoring is the three-electrode system. The most commonly used limb lead is lead II. The most commonly used chest leads are MCL$_1$ and MCL$_6$ (modified versions of V$_1$ and V$_6$). In general, a three-electrode monitoring system has one positive lead and one negative lead. A third lead serves as the ground.

Lead II
To establish lead II, place the negative electrode at the first intercostal space on the right sternal border, the positive electrode at the fourth intercostal space on the left midclavicular line, and the ground electrode at the fourth intercostal space on the right sternal border.

Lead II measures the electrical flow from the right arm to the left leg, producing good QRS complexes, which reflect ventricular activity, and positive P waves, which show atrial activity.

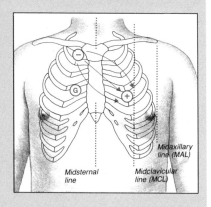

Midsternal line

Midclavicular line (MCL)

Midaxillary line (MAL)

Lead MCL$_1$
To establish lead MCL$_1$, position the negative electrode on the left side of the patient's chest just below the clavicle. Position the positive electrode at the right sternal border at the fourth intercostal space. Position the ground electrode on the right side of the chest just below the clavicle.

Lead MCL$_1$ records the sequence of ventricular depolarization better, so it's used to differentiate between right or left bundle-branch block and ectopy. Note that the positive electrode should be positioned directly over the right ventricle.

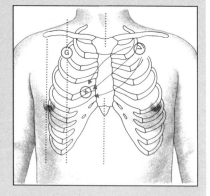

Placing leads in cardiac monitoring *(continued)*

Lead MCL₆

To establish lead MCL₆, position the negative electrode just below the left clavicle at the midclavicular line. Position the positive electrode at the left fifth intercostal space on the midaxillary line (over the apex of the left ventricle). Position the ground electrode just below the right clavicle on the midclavicular line.

Lead MCL₆ allows you to easily see tall QRS complexes so that you can identify right bundle-branch block and ST-segment and T-wave changes.

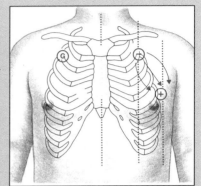

Four- and five-electrode system

In a four-electrode system, a right leg (RL) electrode is added to provide a permanent ground for all leads used in the three-electrode system. Place this electrode at the 4th or 5th intercostal space on the right midclavicular line.

A five-electrode system uses an additional exploratory chest electrode. By placing the exploratory chest electrode on different areas of the patient's precordium, you can obtain a reading from any of the modified chest leads, as well as the standard limb leads.

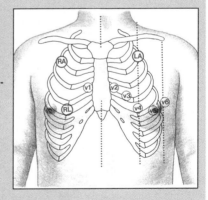

Like a 12-lead ECG, a continuous ECG can display information about the heart's rhythm and rate on a monitor or generate a permanent record on a printed strip. Additionally, the monitor has alarms that sound automatically if the patient develops an arrhythmia or if his heart rate exceeds a predetermined limit. The system can be programmed to record arrhythmias as they occur, or to obtain a tracing manually by pressing a button on the monitor.

Cardiac monitoring allows ongoing evaluation of patients with conduction disturbances or possible life-threatening arrhythmias. What's more, it allows evaluation of the effects of treatment.

Because telemetry monitoring allows the patient some freedom of movement, it's especially helpful for evaluating symptoms commonly associated with activity, such as intermittent arrhythmias, dizziness, syncope, chest pain, and palpitations. Telemetry monitoring may be used to investigate adverse drug reactions, exercise tolerance after MI, and rhythm disturbances during anginal attacks, or to evaluate the efficacy of treatments such as pacemaker implantation or antiarrhythmic or antianginal drugs.

Implementation
• Explain the procedure to your patient, including placement of the electrodes.

Timesaving tip: Avoid opening packages containing pregelled electrodes until just before using them to prevent the gel from drying.

• Firmly apply the pregelled electrodes to your patient's skin at the predetermined points. If necessary, shave a small area of skin or clean it with an alcohol sponge before applying the electrodes to ensure proper skin contact.

Timesaving tip: To save time during an emergency, avoid placing the electrodes on areas of your patient's chest that may be needed for placement of defibrillator pads or for chest compression.

Timesaving tip: If your patient is diaphoretic, use tincture of benzoin on his skin to help secure the electrodes.

• If you're connecting the patient to a hardwire monitor, turn on the bedside monitor.

• If you're using telemetry monitoring, insert a battery in the transmitter, making sure the polarity markings on the transmitter match those on the battery. Check the battery's charge by pressing the battery test button on the transmitter. Make sure that the leadwire cable is securely attached to the transmitter. Place the transmitter in the carrying pouch and securely tie the pouch strings around the patient's neck and waist.

• When the electrodes are in place, observe the waveforms on the monitor. Assess the quality of the waveforms and, if necessary, use the gain control to change waveform size. Adjust the waveform position on the recording paper. Set the upper and lower limits of the heart-rate alarm.

• Record the date and time, the positions of the leads, and a sample rhythm strip. Always label the rhythm strip with your patient's name, room number, date, and time. Analyze the strip for rate, rhythm, and any abnormal features.

• Document a rhythm strip each time your patient's condition changes and at least once every 8 hours, or according to your hospital's policy.

• Assess the patient's skin integrity and reposition or apply new electrodes every 24 hours, or as necessary.

A high-rate alarm may signify excessive movement by the patient or a gain that's set too high (causing the monitor to count both P waves and QRS complexes). A low-rate alarm may signify electrodes that need to be replaced or repositioned, or a gain that's set too low. A fuzzy baseline may indicate 60-cycle electrical interference from improper grounding of the patient's bed.

Interpreting ECG results
To correctly interpret an ECG strip, you must be able to recognize the components of a normal waveform. (See *Identifying ECG waveform components.*) Then estimate the patient's heart rate and analyze the strip.

Estimating heart rate
Heart rate can be measured in several ways depending on whether your patient's rhythm is regular or irregular. Normal heart rate is 60 to 100 beats/minute. Five different methods for de-

Identifying ECG waveform components

Each ECG waveform has three major sections: a P wave, a QRS complex, and a T wave. These sections are further divided into the PR interval, J point, ST segment, U wave, and QT interval.

P wave and PR interval
The P wave represents atrial depolarization. The PR interval (measured from the beginning of the P wave to the beginning of the QRS complex) indicates the time needed for an impulse to travel from the atria through the atrioventricular node and bundle of His.

QRS complex
The QRS complex represents ventricular depolarization or the time needed for an impulse to travel through the bundle branches to the Purkinje fibers.

The Q wave is the first negative deflection in the QRS complex, and the R wave is the first positive deflection. The S wave is the second negative deflection (or the first negative deflection after the R wave). The QRS complex is measured from the beginning of the Q wave to the end of the S wave.

J point and ST segment
The J point marks the end of the QRS complex and the beginning of the ST segment. The J point signifies the end of depolarization and the beginning of repolarization. The ST segment represents part of ventricular repolarization.

T wave and U wave
The T wave represents ventricular repolarization and usually follows the same deflection pattern as the P wave. The U wave follows the T wave (representing repolarization of the Purkinje system); however, it isn't always seen.

QT interval
The QT interval represents ventricular depolarization and repolarization. It extends from the beginning of the QRS complex to the end of the T wave.

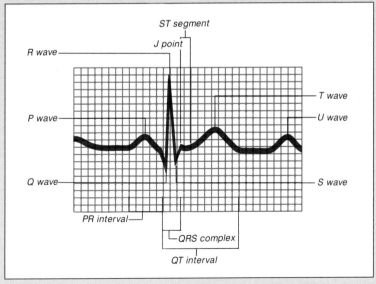

Estimating heart rate quickly

To estimate the ventricular rate, find an R wave that peaks on a dark grid line of the graph paper. Then find the line on which the next R wave peaks. Count the number of boxes between R wave peaks; then use the table to find the rate. To calculate the atrial rate, use the same method with P waves, instead of R waves.

Number of small blocks	Rate
5 (1 large block)	300
6	250
7	214
8	187
9	166
10 (2 large blocks)	150
11	136
12	125
13	115
14	107
15 (3 large blocks)	100
16	94
17	88
18	83
19	79
20 (4 large blocks)	75
21	71
22	68
23	65
24	63
25 (5 large blocks)	60
26	58
27	56
28	54
29	52
30 (6 large blocks)	50
31	48
32	47
33	45
34	44
35 (7 large blocks)	43
36	41
37	40
38	39
39	38
40 (8 large blocks)	37

termining heart rate are discussed below:

1. Count the number of QRS complexes in a 6-second strip segment and multiply by 10. The 6-second segment can be determined by counting vertical hash marks located at the upper portion of the tracing (the space between three vertical hash marks represents a 6-second segment). Alternatively, you can count the number of dark boxes. There are 15 dark boxes in a 3-second strip segment and 30 dark boxes in a 6-second strip segment. You can use this method to estimate ventricular rate in a patient with a regular or irregular rhythm.

2. If R-R and P-P intervals are irregular, use the following method: To determine ventricular rate, count the number of R waves occurring within the 6-second segment and multiply by 10; to determine atrial rate, count the number of P waves in a 6-second segment.

3. To determine ventricular rate, divide 300 by the number of dark boxes between R waves. (There are 300 0.20-second boxes in a 1-minute strip.) If a P wave falls on a dark line, you can use this method to estimate atrial rate.

4. If an R wave falls on one of the dark grid lines, estimate ventricular rate by counting the numbers 300, 150, 100, 75, 60, and 50 for each dark grid line that follows, until you see the next dark grid line with an R wave. The last number you count shows an estimated ventricular rate. This technique is called the sequence method. (See *Estimating heart rate quickly*.)

5. If an R wave doesn't fall on one of the dark grid lines, count the number of light grid lines between two R waves. Divide this number into 1,500 to obtain a precise ventricular rate.

Analyzing the ECG strip

After you determine the rate, analyze the ECG strip by answering the following questions:

• Is the patient's heart rate regular?

• Are P-P intervals (representing atrial rhythm) regular or irregular? Are R-R intervals (representing ventricular rhythm) regular or irregular? Consider a rhythm with only slight variations (up to 0.04 second) to be regular. If the patient's atrial or ventricular rhythm is irregular, is it markedly so? Does the irregular rhythm appear in a distinct pattern?

• Are P waves present? P waves indicate that the electrical impulse originated in the sinoatrial (SA) node, the atria, or the atrioventricular junctional tissue.

• If present, do the P waves appear normal? Are they upright and rounded? Abnormally shaped P waves suggest that the impulse originated in atrial or junctional tissue rather than in the SA node. Peaked P waves may occur with right atrial hypertrophy. Broad, notched P waves may appear in leads I, II, and aV_F and are associated with left atrial hypertrophy. Inverted P waves (in leads other than aV_R) may indicate that the SA node is not the pacemaker. Inverted P waves commonly occur in junctional arrhythmias.

• Does the P wave appear after the QRS complex? If so, it indicates retrograde conduction is occurring throughout the atria.

• Do shapes and sizes of P waves appear consistent or do they vary? Varied P waves may indicate irritability in the atrial tissue, damage near the SA node, or impulses originating at various sites.

• Does the PR interval fall within 0.12 and 0.20 second? If so, it indicates normal impulse conduction. PR intervals of more than 0.20 second indicate conduction delays from the atria to the ventricles. Associated conditions include first-degree AV block and digitalis toxicity. PR intervals of less than 0.12 second indicate that the impulse originated in an area other than the SA node. Shortened PR intervals may be caused by junctional arrhythmias.

• Does the QRS complex occur within normal time limits (0.06 and 0.10 second)? Wide QRS complexes can indicate conduction problems in the ventricles, such as bundle-branch block, or conditions in which the impulse is formed in the ventricles, such as premature ventricular contractions, idioventricular rhythms, and ventricular tachycardia.

• Does the QRS complex configuration appear normal? An altered QRS complex configuration may indicate an intraventricular conduction defect. For example, in bundle-branch block, you may see an extra R wave (R′) or an extra S wave (S′). If the sizes and shapes of the QRS complexes vary, an ectopic or aberrantly conducted impulse may have occurred. If ectopic impulses are present, determine if they are of ventricular or supraventricular origin. For example, the presence of an initial tall R wave (called a left-peak wave) in leads V_1 or MCL_1 usually indicates a ventricular ectopic beat. A taller right peak wave (rR′) in leads V_1 or MCL_1 usually indicates an aberrant supraventricular beat.

• Is the QRS complex absent? If a QRS complex doesn't appear after each P wave, suspect a condition in which the ventricles don't depolarize, such as AV block or complete ventricular standstill.

• Is the ST segment isoelectric with the baseline graph? ST segments that are elevated or depressed from the baseline may represent ischemia. ST-segment changes may also occur in patients taking digoxin. (See *Understanding ST-segment monitoring,* page 56.)

• Are T waves normal? Do they point in the same direction as the QRS complex? Do they have a normal shape? T waves represent electrical repolarization of the ventricles. A normal direc-

Understanding ST-segment monitoring

A new procedure, ST-segment monitoring is used to detect and monitor myocardial ischemia and infarction. In ST-segment monitoring, the computer records the heart's electrical activity and compares this information with baseline ST-segment data. Deviation from the baseline is an early indicator of insufficient myocardial oxygen supply.

ST-segment monitoring usually uses five electrodes to permit computer analysis of ST segments from several different angles. The resulting data can be displayed on the monitor continuously or on demand. In the electrocardiogram depicted below, leads I, II, and V₅ are recorded while a patient is being suctioned. Measuring ST-segment deviation provides information about the ischemic effects of suctioning on the patient. The ST segment is measured from the end of the S wave (at the J point) to the beginning of the T wave.

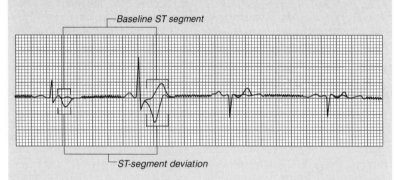

Baseline ST segment

ST-segment deviation

Indications

ST-segment monitoring is indicated for patients with known coronary artery disease. In patients with silent ischemia, ST-segment monitoring may help identify ischemic changes that might otherwise go undetected. ST-segment monitoring may also be used to:
• monitor reperfusion in patients undergoing thrombolytic therapy
• monitor patients during treatment with digoxin or a pacemaker or after percutaneous transluminal coronary angioplasty

• monitor high-risk surgical patients intraoperatively and postoperatively
• monitor patients with chest trauma, head injury, or vascular trauma who are at risk for cardiovascular complications
• monitor patients requiring significant electrolyte replacement
• obtain information about the myocardial effects of pericarditis, hyperthyroidism, pulmonary infarction, and hyperventilation.

tion and shape indicate normal repolarization.

If you note bumps in a T wave, a P wave may be hidden in it. If a P wave is hidden, atrial depolarization has occurred, so the impulse has originated in a site above the ventricles. An inverted T wave may indicate myocardial ischemia (inverted T waves occur normally in lead aV_R and may occur normally in the precordial leads V_1 and V_2). Peaked T waves commonly indicate hyperkalemia.

• Does the QT interval fall within normal limits (0.36 and 0.44 second)? QT intervals longer than 0.44 second indicate conduction or physiologic changes in the myocardial tissue. A QT interval shorter than 0.36 second may indicate hypercalcemia or digitalis toxicity.

• Does the rhythm strip show pronounced U waves? U waves represent repolarization of the Purkinje system and aren't always seen. If U waves are present, are they upright or inverted? A positively deflecting U wave may indicate hypokalemia. An inverted U wave may indicate heart disease.

Hemodynamic monitoring

Hemodynamic monitoring refers to noninvasive and invasive techniques to measure cardiovascular and pulmonary blood flow, resistance, and pressures. Noninvasive techniques include routine auscultation using a sphygmomanometer and automated systems for measuring and recording intermittent blood pressures.

Invasive hemodynamic monitoring techniques detect subtle changes in the heart's pumping ability that may lead to measurable changes in auscultated blood pressures or changes in the patient's condition.

Noninvasive blood pressure monitoring

Noninvasive systems automatically measure and record your patient's blood pressure at specific intervals. In this type of system, a cuff placed around the patient's arm automatically inflates at predetermined intervals to measure the patient's blood pressure. The measurement is displayed on a monitor until the cuff inflates for the next measurement. Generally, the readings are more accurate than readings obtained with a sphygmomanometer and less accurate than readings obtained by an intra-arterial line.

These systems have alarms that can be set to sound when the patient's blood pressure is above or below established limits.

Implementation

• When setting up the monitor, follow the manufacturer's instructions. Set the cuff pressure about 30 mm Hg higher than the patient's systolic pressure. Set the high and low systolic alarms. Apply the cuff and set the measurement interval.

• At the predetermined times, note and record the pressure reading on the display.

• Once per shift, or according to your hospital's policy, measure your patient's blood pressure with a sphygmomanometer and compare these results to the measurements recorded by the system.

• Periodically check to make sure the patient is comfortable. If the cuff is too tight, reset the cuff pressure mechanism.

• Be aware that pressure measurements may be inaccurate if the cuff is improperly secured, or is too large or too small for the patient's arm.

Intra-arterial blood pressure monitoring

This invasive procedure provides continuous information about your patient's arterial blood pressure. Readings obtained by intra-arterial pressure monitoring are more accurate than those obtained with a sphygmomanometer.

During intra-arterial blood pressure monitoring, a catheter with a disposable transducer is inserted through a large peripheral artery, typically the radial, brachial, or femoral artery. The transducer converts the blood pressure readings to an electrical impulse and data is then displayed on a monitor or recorded as a reference. The system also has an alarm that can be set to sound if the patient's blood pressure exceeds established limits.

The intra-arterial catheter system also provides direct access for drawing arterial blood to evaluate tissue perfusion and oxygenation.

Intra-arterial pressure monitoring allows ongoing evaluation of patients with unstable, dangerously high, or low blood pressure, and patients receiving drugs that profoundly affect blood pressure. In addition, intra-arterial monitoring may be ordered for a patient whose respiratory status requires frequent arterial blood gas analyses.

Anticipate using intra-arterial monitoring if your patient has experienced septic, cardiogenic, or hypovolemic shock; hypotension or severe hypertension; or is receiving I.V. dopamine, dobutamine, levophed, or nitroprusside. Intra-arterial monitoring may also be ordered if the patient's condition changes rapidly during mechanical ventilation or if he experiences ventilation and perfusion disturbances such as pulmonary embolism, infarction, pneumonia, or atelectasis.

Implementation
• Set up the line including the heparin flush solution, pressure infuser, tubing, continuous flush mechanism, transducer, stopcocks, and arterial pressure extension tubing.
• Before catheterization, perform Allen's test to assess circulation in the radial and ulnar arteries. (If the radial and ulnar arteries are functioning well, either one can supply the hand with ample perfusion if the other one becomes thrombosed.) Compress the patient's ulnar and radial arteries simultaneously for 60 seconds. Have the patient repeatedly clench his fist until the palm blanches. Remove pressure from the ulnar artery while maintaining pressure on the radial artery. If the palm becomes pink in 5 seconds, the ulnar artery is functioning well. Repeat the process, releasing pressure from the radial artery first, to assess the condition of the radial artery. Inform the doctor or technician if blood return is slow in either artery in either wrist.
• After the catheter is inserted and the arterial pressure line is attached, check to see that all connections are secure and that the line flushes easily using the flush mechanism. Be sure that the pressure bag over the flush solution is inflated to 300 mm Hg.
• Turn on the monitor and allow it to warm up. Adjust the transducer to the level of the patient's right atrium. Zero and calibrate the equipment. Observe the characteristics of the waveforms displayed on the monitor. (See *Recognizing common arterial waveforms,* pages 59 and 60.)
• Always use sterile technique when working with arterial lines.
• Level and zero the equipment at the beginning of each shift and any time the patient or equipment is moved.
• Change the dressing and tubing every 24 to 72 hours, and ensure that all connections are secure. If the system becomes disconnected, the patient will quickly lose a considerable amount of blood.
• Keep the pressure bag over the flush solution inflated to 300 mm Hg to en-

Interpretation

Recognizing common arterial waveforms

Normal arterial blood pressure waveform

In the arterial waveform illustrated below, note the rapid upstroke, clear dicrotic notch, and clear end diastole. Keep in mind the characteristics of this typical waveform to help you recognize and interpret other waveforms encountered in hemodynamic monitoring.

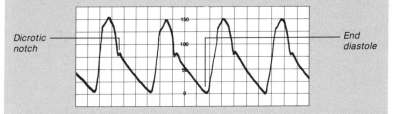

Alternating high and low waves

In the illustration below, alternating high and low waves occur in a regular pattern. This waveform may result from ventricular bigeminy. To confirm ventricular bigeminy, check the patient's electrocardiogram. It should show premature ventricular contractions every second beat.

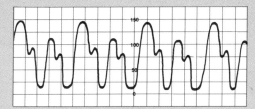

Flattened waveform

This pattern may appear as a result of waveform damping or hypotension. Check the patient's blood pressure with a sphygmomanometer. If pressure is very low or unobtainable, suspect hypotension. If you can obtain a blood pressure measurement, suspect damping. To eliminate damping, flush the line.

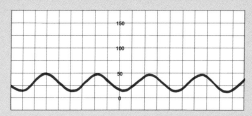

(continued)

Interpretation

Recognizing common arterial waveforms *(continued)*

Slightly rounded waveform with consistent variations in systolic height
This waveform may appear during mechanical ventilation, with positive end-expiratory pressure. Check the patient's systolic blood pressure regularly. The difference between the highest and lowest systolic pressure should be less than 10 mm Hg. If the difference is greater than 10 mm Hg, suspect pulsus paradoxus.

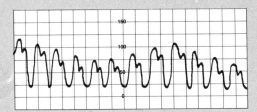

Erratic ragged waveform
This waveform may result from movement of the catheter tip in the artery. If it appears, stabilize the catheter by taping and splinting the insertion site. Notify the doctor; the catheter tip may need to be repositioned.

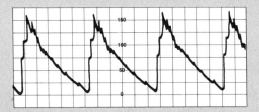

Slow upstroke
This waveform may occur secondary to aortic stenosis. If it appears, check the patient's heart sounds for signs of aortic stenosis.

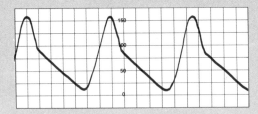

sure that blood does not flow back into the tubing. Be sure to flush the tubing after taking a blood sample to prevent clotting in the line or catheter.

• Keep alarms on at all times except when replacing tubing.

• At appropriate intervals, record the patient's blood pressure as displayed on the equipment, noting any changes. Verify the monitor's readings by auscultating the patient's blood pressure with a sphygmomanometer at least once each shift, or according to established procedures at your hospital. Be aware that there may be a discrepancy of 5 to 10 mm Hg between blood pressure readings obtained with an arterial catheter and those obtained using a sphygmomanometer.

Complications

Possible complications of intra-arterial monitoring include blood loss, hematoma, thrombosis, air embolism, arterial spasm, and systemic infection.

• Blood loss may be caused by a disconnected line or dislodged catheter. If the arterial line becomes dislodged or accidentally removed, immediately apply pressure at the insertion site for 5 to 10 minutes. After controlling the bleeding, apply a sterile occlusive bandage at the insertion site.

• Hematoma may be caused by leakage around the catheter resulting from a damaged artery.

• Thrombosis may result in a weak or absent pulse below the insertion site and a loss of warmth, sensation, and mobility below the insertion site. (The monitor may show a damped or straightened waveform.) Prevent thrombosis by flushing the catheter hourly and each time you draw a blood sample with heparin flush solution, or according to your hospital's established procedures. *Never irrigate an arterial catheter with a syringe — you may flush a thrombus into the bloodstream.*

• Air embolism may result in decreased blood pressure; a weak, rapid pulse; cyanosis; and loss of consciousness and may be caused by an empty I.V. container, air in the tubing, or loose connections. To prevent air embolism, expel all air from the line before starting the infusion, secure all connections and check them routinely, and change the I.V. container before it becomes empty.

• Arterial spasm, which may result in an intermittent loss or weakening of the pulse below the insertion site, may be caused by irritation of the artery by the catheter during or after insertion. The monitor may show an irregular waveform. Make sure you securely splint and tape the catheter at the insertion site to prevent it from moving within the artery.

• Systemic infection may result from poor aseptic technique or equipment contamination. To maintain asepsis, take care when bathing the patient and during routine dressing changes. Also, don't rejoin parts of the arterial line that become disconnected. Instead, replace them with sterile equipment.

In addition, inaccurate pressure readings and waveforms may result if air is in the tubing or transducer, the transducer is at the improper level, the system has loose connections or cracked or leaking tubing, a clot lodges in the catheter, or the catheter tip rests against the vessel wall. (See *Quick reference to troubleshooting hemodynamic monitoring systems,* pages 62 to 64.)

CVP monitoring

CVP monitoring measures the force of the blood flowing into the right atrium (right atrial pressure [RAP]), which reflects right ventricular pressure (RVP) and the pumping ability of the right side of the heart. CVP monitoring also

(Text continues on page 64)

Quick reference to troubleshooting hemodynamic monitoring systems

PROBLEM	POSSIBLE CAUSES	INTERVENTIONS
No waveform	• Power supply turned off	• Check power supply.
	• Monitor screen pressure range set too low	• Raise monitor screen pressure range, if necessary. • Rebalance and recalibrate equipment.
	• Loose connection in line	• Tighten loose connections.
	• Transducer not connected to amplifier	• Check and tighten connection.
	• Stopcock off to patient	• Position stopcock correctly.
	• Catheter occluded or out of blood vessel	• Use fast-flush valve to flush line, or try to aspirate blood from catheter. If the line remains blocked, notify the doctor and prepare to replace the line.
Drifting waveforms	• Improper warm-up	• Allow monitor and transducer to warm up for 10 to 15 minutes.
	• Electrical cable kinked or compressed	• Place monitor's cable where it can't be stepped on or compressed.
	• Temperature change in room air or I.V. flush solution	• Routinely zero and calibrate equipment 30 minutes after setting it up. This allows I.V. fluid to warm to room temperature.
Line fails to flush	• Stopcocks positioned incorrectly	• Make sure that stopcocks are positioned correctly.
	• Inadequate pressure from pressure bag	• Make sure that the pressure bag gauge reads 300 mm Hg.
	• Kink in pressure tubing	• Check pressure tubing for kinks.
	• Blood clot in catheter	• Try to aspirate the clot with a syringe. If the line still won't flush, notify the doctor and prepare to replace the line, if necessary. *Important:* Never use a syringe to flush a hemodynamic line.
Artifact (waveform interference)	• Patient movement	• Wait until the patient is quiet before taking a reading.
	• Electrical interference	• Make sure that electrical equipment is connected and grounded correctly.

Quick reference to troubleshooting hemodynamic monitoring systems *(continued)*

PROBLEM	POSSIBLE CAUSES	INTERVENTIONS
Artifact *(continued)*	• Catheter fling (tip of pulmonary artery catheter moving rapidly in large blood vessel or heart chamber)	• Notify the doctor. He may try to reposition the catheter.
False-high readings	• Transducer balancing port positioned below patient's right atrium	• Position balancing port level with the patient's right atrium.
	• Flush solution flow rate is too fast	• Check flush solution flow rate. Maintain it at 3 to 4 ml/hour.
	• Air in system	• Remove air from the lines and the transducer.
	• Catheter fling (tip of pulmonary artery catheter moving rapidly in large blood vessel or heart chamber)	• Notify the doctor, who may try to reposition the catheter.
False-low readings	• Transducer balancing port positioned above right atrium	• Position balancing port level with the patient's right atrium.
	• Transducer imbalance	• Make sure that the transducer's flow system isn't kinked or occluded and rebalance and recalibrate the equipment.
	• Loose connection	• Tighten loose connections.
Damped waveform	• Air bubbles	• Secure all connections. • Remove air from lines and transducer. • Check for and replace cracked equipment.
	• Blood clot in catheter	• Try to aspirate the clot with a syringe. If the line still won't flush, notify the doctor and prepare to replace the line, if necessary. *Important:* Never use a syringe to flush a hemodynamic line.
	• Blood flashback in line	• Make sure that stopcock positions are correct; tighten loose connections and replace cracked equipment; flush line with fast-flush valve; replace the transducer dome if blood backs up into it.

(continued)

Quick reference to troubleshooting hemodynamic monitoring systems *(continued)*

PROBLEM	POSSIBLE CAUSES	INTERVENTIONS
Damped waveform *(continued)*	• Transducer malpositioned	• Make sure that the transducer is level with the right atrium at all times. Improper levels give false-high or false-low pressure readings.
	• Arterial catheter out of blood vessel or pressed against vessel wall	• Reposition if the catheter is against the vessel wall. • Try to aspirate blood to confirm proper placement in the vessel. If you can't aspirate blood, notify the doctor and prepare to replace the line. *Note:* Bloody drainage at the insertion site may indicate catheter displacement. Notify the doctor immediately.
Pulmonary artery wedge pressure tracing unobtainable	• Ruptured balloon	• If you feel no resistance when injecting air, or if you see blood leaking from the balloon inflation lumen, stop injecting air and notify the doctor. If the catheter is left in, label the inflation lumen with a warning not to inflate.
	• Incorrect amount of air in balloon	• Deflate the balloon. Check the label on the catheter for the correct volume. Reinflate slowly with the correct amount. To avoid rupturing the balloon, never use more than the stated volume.
	• Catheter malpositioned	• Notify the doctor. Obtain a chest X-ray.

may be used to assess blood volume and vascular tone.

In CVP monitoring, a manometer is connected to a catheter that's threaded through the subclavian or jugular vein (or through the basilic, cephalic, or saphenous vein) and placed in or near the right atrium. The manometer measures CVP in centimeters of water pressure (cm H_2O). Normal values typically range from 3 to 15 cm H_2O but may vary with the patient's body size, position, and hydration status. In some systems, changes in CVP are measured in millimeters of mercury (mm Hg). A low CVP reading may indicate hypovolemia; a high CVP reading may indicate hypervolemia or ventricular contractility failure.

CVP monitoring is most often used if the patient has a condition that impairs the heart's pumping ability (especially the right side), such as congestive heart failure, hypervolemia, hypovolemia, constrictive pericarditis, pulmonary hypertension, cardiac tamponade, tricuspid valve dysfunction, right ventricular infarction, or peripheral vasoconstriction or vasodilation.

Because CVP monitoring detects increases only after significant changes have occurred in the left side of the heart or pulmonary venous system, PAP monitoring (which can detect changes in cardiovascular status earlier than CVP monitoring) may be used.

Implementation
After the CVP catheter is inserted, an X-ray must be taken to verify placement in the superior vena cava or right atrium.

• Inspect the CVP monitoring equipment to make sure it is properly set up. The manometer and three-way stopcock should be between the container of I.V. fluid and the catheter. All connections must be secure. Make sure that no air is in the tubing running from the I.V. container to the patient. Check to see that the manometer is aligned with the patient's right atrium.

To establish the position of the right atrium, identify the phlebostatic axis, which is the imaginary line located midway between the patient's anteroposterior chest wall and fourth intercostal space. (See *Locating the phlebostatic axis,* page 66.)

Timesaving tip: Mark the location of the phlebostatic axis on your patient's chest with a marking pen or piece of tape. This becomes the zero point for all future readings. It's also where the tip of the monitoring catheter should rest within the body.
• When taking a CVP reading, place the patient flat on his back without a pillow, if possible. The patient must be in the same position for each reading. Because a change in position can affect CVP readings, document the posi-

tion so other nurses will use the same position.
• Establish an initial baseline CVP range by taking readings at 15-, 30-, and 60-minute intervals. Thereafter, notify the doctor if a CVP reading varies by more than 2 cm H_2O (1 mm Hg) from the baseline.
• Check the patency of the line by briefly increasing the infusion rate. *Be sure to decrease the rate after you verify patency.* Never irrigate a clogged CVP line because doing so may release a thrombus into the patient's bloodstream.
• Turn the stopcock off to the patient and fill the manometer with I.V. solution.
• Open the stopcock to allow I.V. fluid from the manometer to flow to the patient. Expect the column to rise and fall slightly during breathing. The manometer's fluid level will react to normal changes in intrathoracic pressure that accompany respiration.
• Wait for the fluid column to stabilize before taking a reading. Then, tap the manometer lightly to dislodge any air bubbles that may distort pressure readings. Position yourself so the top of the fluid column is at eye level. As the patient exhales, take a reading when the base of the meniscus reaches its lowest level. When taking a reading, turn the stopcock off to the I.V. solution. The patient's CVP will be reflected on the manometer.
• Maintain catheter patency by promptly turning the stopcock open to the patient after each reading. Check the line for blood backflow.
• Compare each reading to previous readings. Report any deviations to the doctor. Correlate your measurements with clinical signs to ensure appropriate treatment. (See *CVP monitoring tips,* page 67.)

Locating the phlebostatic axis

The illustrations below show a nurse using a carpenter's level to locate the phlebostatic axis — the imaginary line located between the patient's anteroposterior chest wall and fourth intercostal space.

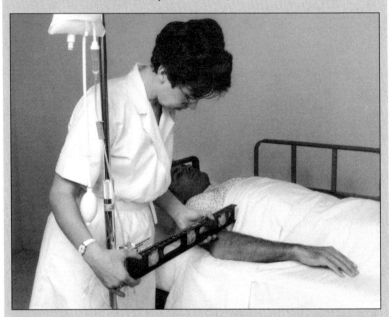

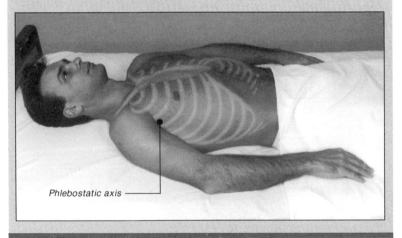

Phlebostatic axis —

Complications

Possible complications of CVP monitoring include infection, air embolus, and blood backflow.

• Avoid introducing infection by always using aseptic technique when caring for a patient with a CVP line. Maintain asepsis whenever you change the catheter dressing or I.V. lines.

• Keep the insertion site clean and dry to minimize the risk of infection. Replace the patient's dressing every 48 hours (or according to your hospital's policy) or whenever it becomes wet or soiled.

• Replace all components of the system every 48 hours, or according to your hospital's policy, to further reduce the risk of infection. If equipment becomes disconnected, immediately replace it with sterile parts—*never reconnect it.*

• During the insertion procedure, have the patient perform Valsalva's maneuver to increase intrathoracic pressure. This counteracts strong negative pressure from the vein and reduces the risk of introducing an air embolus.

• Periodically check the line to make sure all connections are secure. A loose connection may cause an air embolus or blood backflow, especially if CVP is high.

• When using bottles of I.V. solution, replace each one before it becomes empty. Negative venous pressure can pull air from the container into the vein, causing an air embolus.

PAP and PAWP monitoring

This procedure uses a pulmonary artery (PA) catheter (for example, a Swan-Ganz catheter) connected to a transducer and a monitor to measure PAP and PAWP. The multilumen, balloon-tipped, flow-directed PA catheter has evolved from a double-lumen monitoring device to the current six-lumen catheter. The six-lumen PA catheter includes the proximal and distal lumen,

---

CVP monitoring tips

• By itself, no single central venous pressure (CVP) reading is significant. When assessing response to therapy, look for trends in successive readings.

• Avoid taking pressure measurements while the patient is sitting up. Sitting causes false-low measurements, even if the patient has been in a sitting position within 3 minutes of your reading.

• Remember that a patient with chronic obstructive pulmonary disease usually has a high CVP.

• If your patient is connected to a ventilator and is receiving positive end-expiratory pressure, CVP readings may vary. To detect significant changes, record all pressure readings while the patient is connected to the ventilator, and take readings at end expiration before the next inspiration begins. If the patient's condition permits, and your hospital policy allows, disconnect the ventilator briefly for all CVP readings and then reconnect it immediately after the procedure. Be aware of the risk of hypoxia when removing the patient from the ventilator for the reading.

---

the balloon inflation lumen, the right ventricular lumen, the oximeter connector lumen, and the thermistor connector lumen complete with two intracardiac electrode lines.

The catheter is inserted by the doctor either percutaneously into the subclavian, jugular, or femoral vein or through a venous cutdown in the antecubital fossa and then threaded to the junction of the superior vena cava and right atrium.

Next, the balloon tip is inflated. Venous circulation carries the catheter through the right atrium and right ventricle into the pulmonary artery. The catheter is advanced in the pulmonary artery until the balloon tip is wedged in a small vessel of the artery. The balloon is deflated and the catheter remains in this position so that further wedge readings may be obtained. Catheter progress is usually evaluated by observing the changing waveforms on a cardiac monitor; however, progress can be tracked by fluoroscopy. (See *Monitoring PA catheter insertion*.)

The catheter is connected by tubing to a transducer and computer, which records pressures and graphically displays the data as waveforms on a monitor or a strip of paper. Once the catheter is in place, PAP can be monitored continuously and PAWP can be obtained as required. This system can also be used to monitor CVP, RAP, RVP, and cardiac output.

PAP and PAWP measurements are the most accurate methods of monitoring the function of the left side of the heart. They provide information about the heart's pumping ability, filling pressures, and vascular volume, which is used when assessing the effect of drug therapy and detecting complications of disorders such as acute MI.

Anticipate using PAP monitoring if your patient is experiencing left ventricular failure (because of MI or cardiomyopathy), pulmonary hypertension, hypervolemia, hypovolemia, mitral stenosis, or peripheral vasoconstriction caused by hypoxia.

Implementation

• Before catheter insertion, help set up the PAP monitoring system. The system includes an I.V. bag with heparin flush solution, which is placed inside an inflatable pressure bag unit; pressure tubing from the I.V. bag to the flush device; a connector with stopcocks; and a continuous flush device that connects the monitor, tubing system, and PAP line to the patient.

Because dextrose 5% in water (D_5W) isn't a plasma expander and therefore won't conduct electric current, it may be used as an I.V. solution. However, 0.9% sodium chloride solution is preferred because most transducers are made of disposable plastic, and dextrose adheres to the plastic.

• Take PAP and PAWP readings at the end of expiration. Watch the patient's chest and note the point at which he completely exhales. During expiration, intrathoracic pressure rises, causing a slight elevation of cardiac pressures. Therefore, the pressure at the end of expiration is the best indicator of normal cardiac pressures without respiratory interference.

• To measure PAWP, fill a small syringe with approximately 1.5 cc of air. Slowly inject the air from the syringe into the balloon while observing the monitor. Continue injecting the air until the PAP waveform changes to the PAWP waveform. The PAWP waveform often occurs before all of the air is injected.

Record the mean pressure. Remove the syringe, and then deflate the balloon passively by leaving the port lock open, which allows air to escape. Check the monitor to verify that the waveform has returned to a PAP waveform.

• To monitor CVP using this equipment, set the stopcocks to allow direct communication between the proximal lumen and the transducer. Set the monitor to the mean mode; then observe the waveform and record the CVP measurement. Return the stopcocks to their original positions. To monitor CVP continuously, attach a separate transducer system to the proximal lumen.

Complications of PAP monitoring

Possible complications include infection, air embolism, pulmonary artery perforation, ventricular arrhythmias, tricuspid or pulmonic valve damage,

Interpretation

Monitoring PA catheter insertion

When the pulmonary artery (PA) catheter passes through the heart, characteristic waveforms appear on the cardiac monitor.

Right atrial pressure

When the catheter tip reaches the right atrium from the superior vena cava, the waveform looks like the one shown below. The doctor then inflates the balloon. This carries the tip through the tricuspid valve and into the right ventricle.

Normal range
*Mean pressure:
3 to 6 mm Hg*

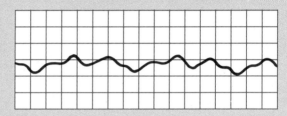

Right ventricular pressure

When the catheter tip reaches the right ventricle, the waveform illustrated below appears.

Normal range
*Systolic pressure:
17 to 22 mm Hg
Diastolic pressure:
1 to 7 mm Hg*

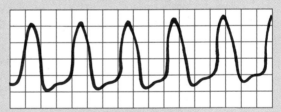

Pulmonary artery pressure

This waveform appears when the catheter tip has moved through the pulmonic valve and into the pulmonary artery.

Normal range
*Systolic pressure:
17 to 32 mm Hg
Diastolic pressure:
4 to 13 mm Hg
Mean pressure:
9 to 19 mm Hg*

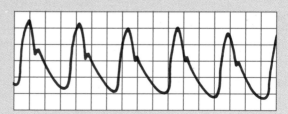

(continued)

Interpretation

Monitoring PA catheter insertion *(continued)*

Pulmonary artery wedge pressure
This waveform appears when the catheter's balloon, carried by the circulation, becomes wedged in a small vessel. At this point the doctor deflates the balloon, causing the catheter tip to slip back into the main branch of the pulmonary artery. The pulmonary artery pressure waveform then reappears.

Normal range
Mean pressure:
8 to 12 mm Hg

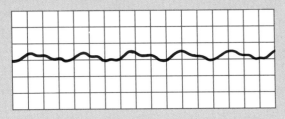

and, during insertion, tension pneumothorax.
• During catheter insertion, alert the doctor immediately if the patient experiences arrhythmias, dyspnea, tachypnea, hemoptysis, stridor, or drastic changes in vital signs or PAP readings. These signs may indicate cardiac perforation, pulmonary artery rupture, hemorrhage, pneumothorax, or hemothorax.
• Use aseptic technique to avoid infection. Change the tubing, stopcocks, continuous flush devices, and I.V. fluid every 24 to 72 hours, or according to your hospital's policy.
• Prevent exsanguination from a disconnection in the system by using luer locks or other positive locks at all connections.
• Make sure that the catheter and other parts of the system are visible at all times and observe electrical hazard precautions.
• Make sure that the monitor and alarms are on at all times.

• To prevent thrombus formation, activate the fast-flush device at the intervals specified by your hospital's policy.
• Check the extremity frequently for the presence of a pulse as well as pulse quality and rate, skin color and temperature, and sensation. Notify the doctor of any changes.
• Change the catheter dressing each time you change the tubing or when it becomes wet or soiled or at the intervals specified by your hospital's policy.
• Know the maximum volume of the balloon and avoid overinflating or aspirating from the balloon. During inflation, you should feel resistance. If you don't, notify the doctor immediately — the balloon may be ruptured. *Never introduce air into a balloon that you suspect is ruptured; this can cause an air embolus.* Air in the flush system can also cause an embolus.

Complications of PAWP monitoring
Possible complications include a catheter wedge, which may lead to pulmonary infarct and necrosis, ruptured

capillaries, and vessel spasm or rupture.

• Note the volume of air needed to obtain a PAWP reading. If the volume of air needed is significantly below that indicated on the catheter, notify the doctor because the catheter may have migrated distally.

• When taking PAWP, don't leave the balloon wedged for more than 15 to 30 seconds. If the waveform does not return to the PAP waveform, or if it is damping with low numbers and decreased pulmonary artery systolic-diastolic differential, check the equipment for problems. Then take the patient's blood pressure and pulse. If these values are unchanged, the catheter is probably wedged (a permanent wedge can cause pulmonary infarct and necrosis). Gently flush the PAP port to push the catheter tip away from a vessel wall. *Don't activate the fast-flush release; this can rupture capillaries.*

• Check for a slow drip rate and increased PAP readings — signs that the catheter is still wedged. If present, turn the patient on his right side and tell him to cough as you flush the line. If the PAP waveform doesn't return, turn the patient onto his left side and repeat the procedure. If the waveform and pressure remain unchanged, notify the doctor.

• Don't use the distal port to administer drugs or fluids other than the heparin flush solution because vessel spasm or rupture may result.

Cardiac output monitoring

Cardiac output (the amount of blood ejected by the heart each minute) is measured indirectly by the thermodilution method. In the thermodilution method, a balloon-tipped, flow-directed catheter is inserted into a large vein, advanced to the right side of the heart, and positioned in the pulmonary artery. A solution is injected into the proximal or right atrium port of the PA catheter. A computer then calculates cardiac output by monitoring temperature changes in the injected solution in the proximal lumen and the temperature of the pulmonary artery.

Normal cardiac output is between 4 and 8 liters/minute, although this measurement varies based on the patient's height, weight, and body surface area. By calculating the cardiac index you can arrive at a more accurate measurement of cardiac output. To calculate this value, divide the patient's cardiac output by his body surface area. The normal range is 2.5 to 4.2 liters/minute.

Cardiac output monitoring is used to evaluate fluid volume status, the heart's pumping ability, and signs of decompensation and to guide treatment with I.V. fluids and cardiac drugs. You may implement cardiac output monitoring if your patient has any of the following disorders: MI, hypertension, arteriosclerotic cardiovascular disease, valvular disorders, acidosis, hypoxia, intracardiac shunts (a complication of MI), or cardiogenic, septic, or hypovolemic shock.

Implementation

To measure cardiac output, you'll use the patient's PA catheter and a cardiac output computer.

• Use an iced or room-temperature dextrose or 0.9% sodium chloride solution. In most cases, you don't need to ice the solution before injection because there's usually a 20° F difference between the patient's core temperature and room air. However, the temperature of the injectant should be 32° to 39° F (0° to 4° C) to obtain the highest accuracy.

• If possible, use a closed system. In a closed system, the injectant and syringe are connected to the system through I.V. tubing and can be used repeatedly. This reduces the risk of infection and saves time by not requiring the preparation of individual syringes.

• When using a closed system, spike the 500-ml bag of injectant (D_5W) and prime the system.
• Connect the luer-lock end of the system to the proximal lumen of the PA catheter so that the syringe and the catheter lumen are in a straight line. One or more stopcocks may be used between the catheter and the closed system.
• Turn on the cardiac output computer and calibrate it, if necessary, according to the manufacturer's instructions.
• Open the clamp on the closed system and fill the syringe from the bag of injectant.
• Open the stopcock to the patient, and verify that the word READY appears on the computer display. Press the START button. Inject 5 to 10 ml of solution with one smooth, rapid motion within 4 seconds. The computer will display cardiac output values.
• Repeat the procedure two more times, waiting 1 minute between each injection.
• Calculate the average of the three measurements to determine cardiac output.

Complications
Possible complications of a cardiac output monitoring system include loss of patency, leaks, and contamination. You should also takes steps to prevent infection.
• Ensure patency by regularly flushing the PA line and closed cardiac output system.
• Check all connections for leaks or contamination.
• To reduce the risk of infection, change the tubing and catheter dressing according to your hospital's policy.
• If an iced injectant is used, you should keep a bucket of ice with sterile I.V. solution or individual syringes of solution at the patient's bedside.

CHAPTER 4

Caring for patients with coronary vascular disorders

Hypertension

Hypertension is marked by intermittent or sustained elevation of systolic pressure, diastolic pressure, or both. Generally, a sustained systolic pressure of 140 mm Hg or higher or a diastolic pressure of 90 mm Hg or higher constitutes hypertension.

Certain population groups have a higher risk for hypertension. For example, blacks are twice as likely as whites to be affected and four times as likely to die from the disorder. Also, hypertension occurs more commonly in groups with less formal education and lower socioeconomic status. For all population groups, incidence increases with age.

Hypertension represents a key risk factor for cardiovascular disorders, such as coronary artery disease (CAD) and cerebrovascular accident (CVA), and for renal disorders. The risk rises progressively with the extent of increase in systolic and diastolic pressures. (See *Classifying hypertension.*)

Causes

Essential hypertension, also called primary or idiopathic hypertension, accounts for 90% to 95% of all cases of hypertension. Its cause remains unknown. Family history, race, stress, obesity, a diet high in sodium or saturated fat, use of tobacco, sedentary life-style, and aging may contribute to its development.

Secondary hypertension results from an identifiable cause, such as renovascular disease; renal parenchymal disease; pheochromocytoma; primary hyperaldosteronism; Cushing's syndrome; diabetes mellitus; dysfunction of the thyroid, pituitary, or parathyroid gland; coarctation of the aorta; pregnancy; and neurologic disorders. Use of oral contraceptives may be the single most common cause of secondary hypertension. Hypertension is also associated with the use of cocaine, epoetin alfa (erythropoietin), or cyclosporine.

ASSESSMENT

Often times, the hypertensive patient has no symptoms and the disorder is revealed incidentally during evaluation for another disorder or during routine blood pressure screening. As a result, your assessment should include careful consideration of the patient's health history (including known risk factors), physical examination findings, and diagnostic test results.

Health history

When symptoms are present, they reflect the effect of hypertension on specific organ systems (target-organ disease). For example, the patient may report awakening with a headache in the occipital region that subsides spontaneously after a few hours. He may also complain of dizziness, palpitations, fatigue, and impotence. A patient with vascular involvement may complain of nosebleeds, bloody urine, weakness, and blurred vision. Complaints of chest pain and dyspnea may indicate cardiac involvement.

Find out if the patient has a history of dyslipidemia, diabetes mellitus, or cardiovascular, cerebrovascular, or renal disease. Assess the patient's life-style and environment for risk factors. Family history also provides indicators of hypertension risk. Find out if any members of the patient's family have a history of high blood pressure, premature CAD, CVA, cardiovascular disease, diabetes mellitus, or dyslipidemia.

Medication history

Find out if the patient is taking drugs that can raise blood pressure or that can interfere with the effectiveness of

Classifying hypertension

The National Institutes of Health recently developed a new blood pressure classification system. This system is designed for hypertensive adults who aren't currently on antihypertensive medication and aren't acutely ill. Staging of hypertension is based on an average of two or more readings taken during separate visits. When systolic and diastolic readings fall into different categories, the higher category is used to indicate the patient's status.

Category	Systolic (mm Hg)	Diastolic (mm Hg)
Normal	130 or below	85 or below
High normal	130 to 139	85 to 89
Stage 1 (mild hypertension)	140 to 159	90 to 99
Stage 2 (moderate hypertension)	160 to 179	100 to 109
Stage 3 (severe hypertension)	180 to 209	110 to 119
Stage 4 (very severe hypertension)	above 209	above 119

antihypertensives. Take note if the patient reports taking oral contraceptives, nonsteroidal anti-inflammatory drugs, corticosteroids, appetite suppressants, epoetin alfa, cold remedies, cyclosporine, tricyclic antidepressants, and monoamine oxidase inhibitors.

Physical examination
During the initial physical examination, establish baselines and assess for causes of secondary hypertension and the presence of target-organ disease. Record the patient's weight and height and note obesity, if present.

Blood pressure
Obtain two or more blood pressure measurements, allowing 2 or more minutes between readings. If the patient has been standing, have him sit or lie down for several minutes before obtaining a measurement. Make sure the patient has not smoked or had a caffeine-containing beverage within 30 minutes of the measurement. To ensure accuracy, choose a cuff size appropriate for the circumference of your patient's upper arm. The inflatable bladder should completely or nearly (80%) encircle the arm. Verify the reading by obtaining a measurement in the contralateral arm. If the values differ, make sure this information is documented in all patient records. Subsequent measurements should be taken on the side with the higher measurement.

Timesaving tip: To obtain an immediate blood pressure on a patient whose upper arm is too large for the available cuff, wrap the cuff around the patient's forearm and auscultate Korotkoff sounds over the patient's radial artery. Verify this measurement as soon as possible by using a proper size cuff on the upper arm.

Additional findings
• Inspection may reveal peripheral edema and distended neck veins, possibly indicating heart failure.
• Palpation of the peripheral arteries may reveal diminished or absent pulses; the carotid artery, stenosis or occlu-

sion; the neck, an enlarged thyroid gland. Palpation of the abdomen may reveal a pulsating mass, suggesting an abdominal aneurysm.

• Palpation may also reveal enlarged kidneys, suggesting polycystic disease, a cause of secondary hypertension.

• Auscultation may reveal an abdominal bruit auscultated to the right or left of the umbilicus midline, or in the flanks if renal artery stenosis is present. Bruits may also be heard over the abdominal aorta and femoral arteries.

• Auscultation of the heart may reveal an increased rate, clicks, murmurs, arrhythmias, and S_3 and S_4 heart sounds.

• Ophthalmoscopic evaluation may reveal arteriolar narrowing, arteriovenous nicking, hemorrhages, exudates, or papilledema.

• Neurologic examination may reveal effects of hypertension on the central nervous system, such as altered level of consciousness or retinal hemorrhage.

Diagnostic test results

The following tests may reveal predisposing factors and help identify causes of hypertension:

• Urinalysis may reveal protein, red blood cells, or white blood cells, suggesting renal disease; the presence of glucose suggests diabetes mellitus.

• Elevated blood glucose levels may indicate diabetes mellitus.

• Excretory urography may reveal renal atrophy, indicating chronic renal disease; if one kidney is more than 5/8″ (1.6 cm) shorter than the other, it suggests unilateral renal disease.

• Serum potassium levels below 3.5 mEq/liter may indicate adrenal dysfunction (primary hyperaldosteronism).

• Serum cholesterol (total and high-density lipoprotein) and triglyceride levels, when elevated, suggest increased risk for cardiovascular disease.

• Blood urea nitrogen levels above 20 mg/dl and serum creatinine levels above 1.5 mg/dl suggest renal disease.

• Electrocardiography may reveal cardiac abnormalities, such as left ventricular hypertrophy.

Other tests, which help determine the severity of cardiovascular or renal disease, include echocardiography, plasma renin and urinary sodium determination, and urinary microscopic albumin determination.

NURSING DIAGNOSIS

Common nursing diagnoses for a patient with hypertension include:

• High risk for injury related to complications of hypertension

• Knowledge deficit related to hypertension and its treatment

• Noncompliance related to the erroneous belief that therapy isn't needed because overt signs of ill health are absent.

PLANNING

Primary hypertension can't be cured; however, it can often be managed effectively through life-style modifications and drug therapy. Direct your nursing care toward controlling the patient's hypertension, avoiding complications, and teaching the patient about the disorder and its treatment.

Based on the nursing diagnosis *high risk for injury,* develop appropriate patient outcomes. For example, your patient will:

• state his intention to have his blood pressure monitored regularly to detect persistent and serious elevation

• agree to seek medical attention immediately if signs or symptoms of hypertension recur

• not show evidence of target-organ disease involving the retina or cardiac, renal, cerebrovascular, or peripheral vascular systems, as evidenced by physical examination or diagnostic tests.

Based on the nursing diagnosis *knowledge deficit,* develop appropriate patient outcomes. For example, your patient will:
• express a willingness to learn about hypertension and how to control it
• take advantage of opportunities to learn about hypertension and its treatment
• communicate an understanding of hypertension and its risks, and how to manage the disorder and prevent complications
• demonstrate an ability to measure blood pressure.

Based on the nursing diagnosis *noncompliance,* develop appropriate patient outcomes. For example, your patient will:
• communicate an understanding of the need for lifelong therapy despite absence of overt signs and symptoms
• comply with prescribed treatment, as evidenced by a normal blood pressure and absence of organ dysfunction caused by hypertension.

IMPLEMENTATION

A progressive program of antihypertensive therapy begins with life-style modifications. Modifications in diet, regular exercise, and other activities may help your patient achieve target blood pressure measurements and reduce his risk of cardiovascular disease and other complications.

If your patient requires more aggressive therapy, the doctor will prescribe appropriate antihypertensives. In such cases, life-style modifications can help reduce the number and dosage of medications. (See *Medical care of the patient with hypertension,* page 78.)

Nursing interventions
• Monitor the patient's blood pressure to detect persistent or serious elevations.
• Teach the patient or designated caregiver the proper method of monitoring blood pressure. Measurements should be recorded at least two times each week. Explain the blood pressure goal and the need to keep a journal of measurements that the doctor can review during follow-up visits. Explain the importance of taking measurements at approximately the same time of day and after the same type of activity.
• Explain to the patient the importance of seeking medical attention immediately if abnormal signs or symptoms occur.
• Teach the patient about hypertension and its treatment. Encourage the patient to articulate his understanding of the disease, its risks and management techniques, including the need for lifelong treatment, the therapeutic regimen, and life-style modifications.
• Encourage new dietary habits. If the patient is obese, provide teaching and referrals to help him achieve a desirable weight. Explain the importance of using less table salt and of eating fewer high-sodium foods (such as pickles, potato chips, canned soups, and cold cuts) and foods with high cholesterol or saturated fat content. Explain the importance of maintaining adequate levels of potassium, calcium, and magnesium in his diet.
• Explain that an aerobic exercise program improves cardiac status and can help reduce obesity and serum cholesterol levels.
• For patients who smoke tobacco, describe the effects of smoking and the importance of smoking cessation, or refer the patient to a smoking cessation program. Explain the proper use of nicotine patches or nicotine chewing gum.

Treatments

Medical care of the patient with hypertension

Treatment of primary hypertension usually includes life-style modification and drug therapy. Drug selection should take into consideration the cost of prescribed drugs, quality of life factors, age, race, presence and extent of existing cardiovascular disease, and potential drug interactions.

Primary hypertension
The National Institutes of Health suggests the following stepped-care approach.

Step 1
Help the patient initiate necessary life-style modifications, including:
- weight reduction
- moderation of alcohol intake
- regular physical exercise
- reduction of sodium intake
- smoking cessation.

Step 2
If the patient fails to achieve the desired blood pressure or make significant progress, continue life-style modifications and begin drug therapy. Preferred drugs include diuretics or beta blockers. These drugs have proved effective in reducing cardiovascular morbidity and mortality. If diuretics or beta blockers are ineffective or unacceptable, the doctor may prescribe angiotensin-converting enzyme inhibitors, calcium antagonists, alpha$_1$-receptor blockers, or an alpha-beta blocker. These drugs, while effective in reducing blood pressure, have yet to be proven effective in reducing morbidity and mortality.

Step 3
If the patient fails to achieve the desired blood pressure or make significant progress, increase the drug dosage, substitute a drug in the same class, or add a drug from a different class.

Step 4
If the patient fails to achieve the desired blood pressure or make significant progress, add a second or third agent or a diuretic (if one isn't already prescribed). Second or third agents may include direct-acting vasodilators, alpha$_1$-antagonists, and peripherally acting adrenergic neuron antagonists.

Secondary hypertension
Treatment of secondary hypertension focuses on correcting the underlying cause and controlling hypertensive effects.

Hypertensive emergencies
Examples of hypertensive emergencies include:
- hypertensive encephalopathy
- intracranial hemorrhage
- acute left ventricular failure with pulmonary edema
- dissecting aortic aneurysm
- eclampsia or severe hypertension associated with pregnancy
- unstable angina
- acute myocardial infarction.

Typically, hypertensive emergencies require parenteral administration of a vasodilator or adrenergic inhibitor or oral administration of a selected drug, such as nifedipine, captopril, clonidine, or labetalol, to rapidly reduce blood pressure.

Hypertension without accompanying symptoms or evident target-organ disease rarely requires emergency drug therapy.

Discharge TimeSaver

Ensuring continued care for the patient with hypertension

Review the following areas to ensure that your patient is adequately prepared for discharge.

Teaching topics
Make sure that the following topics have been covered and your patient's learning has been evaluated:
☐ an explanation of the disorder, its risk factors, and its complications
☐ self-monitoring
☐ target blood pressure
☐ prescribed medications
☐ life-style modifications, including weight control, dietary modifications, regular aerobic exercise, smoking cessation, and reduced intake of alcohol.

Referrals
Make sure that the patient has been provided with appropriate referrals to:
☐ dietitian
☐ social services
☐ smoking cessation program.

Follow-up appointments
Make sure that the patient has been provided with times and dates for these necessary follow-up appointments:
☐ doctor or clinic
☐ additional diagnostic tests, if necessary.

• Advise the patient to limit daily consumption of alcohol to 1 oz.

• Teach the patient that lifelong therapy is necessary, even when overt signs and symptoms of ill health are absent.

• If the patient expresses concern about the cost of treatment, explain that life-style modifications can reduce or eliminate the need for expensive drug therapy. If necessary, refer the patient to an appropriate social service agency.

• When drugs are prescribed, teach the patient about drug therapy. Explain that uncontrolled hypertension is a major risk factor for CVA and myocardial infarction.

• Encourage compliance by helping the patient establish a daily routine for taking medication. Tell the patient to keep a record of the drugs he takes and the effectiveness of each and to discuss this information with the doctor during follow-up visits.

• Explain that suddenly stopping drug therapy is dangerous and that any adverse effects should be reported immediately to the doctor.

• Advise the patient to avoid high-sodium antacids and over-the-counter cold and sinus medications, which may contain harmful vasoconstrictors.

• Schedule a follow-up appointment and explain the importance of keeping follow-up appointments.

• Continue to monitor the patient's blood pressure and compliance with treatment. Provide positive reinforcement and psychosocial support, as needed. (See *Ensuring continued care for the patient with hypertension*.)

EVALUATION

When evaluating a patient's response to your nursing care, gather reassessment data and compare this information with patient outcomes specified in your plan of care. (See *Assessing failure to respond to antihypertensive therapy*, page 80.)

Evaluation TimeSaver
Assessing failure to respond to antihypertensive therapy

If your patient fails to respond to nursing or medical interventions, this checklist can help you evaluate the reasons why. When performing evaluation, consult with the patient, the patient's family members, and members of the health care team. The doctor will evaluate drug therapy, if necessary.

Factors interfering with compliance
☐ Unclear instructions
☐ Failure to provide written instructions
☐ Inadequate patient teaching
☐ Organic mental syndrome (possibly causing a memory deficit)
☐ Inability to afford medication
☐ Inability to tolerate adverse effects of medication
☐ Inconvenient dosage form

Factors interfering with drug therapy
☐ Insufficient dosage
☐ Inappropriate drug combinations (for example, two centrally acting adrenergic inhibitors)
☐ Metabolic factors, such as genetic predisposition to rapid drug metabolism

Prescribed drugs or other substances causing hypertensive effects
☐ Nonsteroidal anti-inflammatory drugs
☐ Oral contraceptives
☐ Sympathomimetics
☐ Antidepressants

☐ Adrenal steroids
☐ Nasal decongestants
☐ Licorice-containing substances such as chewing tobacco
☐ Cocaine
☐ Cyclosporine
☐ Epoetin alfa (erythropoietin)

Conditions interfering with treatment
☐ Increasing obesity
☐ Daily alcohol consumption in excess of 1 oz

Disorders that may lead to secondary hypertension
☐ Renal insufficiency
☐ Renovascular hypertension
☐ Pheochromocytoma
☐ Primary aldosteronism

Indicators of possible volume overload
☐ Inadequate diuretic therapy
☐ Excessive sodium intake
☐ Fluid retention due to reduced blood pressure
☐ Progressive renal damage

Teaching and counseling
Begin by determining the effectiveness of teaching and counseling. Take note of statements by the patient indicating:
• an intention to monitor blood pressure regularly to detect persistent and serious elevations
• willingness to seek medical attention immediately if any abnormal signs or symptoms occur
• willingness to learn about hypertension and how to control it

• understanding of hypertension and its risks and how to manage the disorder and prevent complications
• understanding of the need for lifelong therapy even if overt signs and symptoms are absent.

During the course of evaluation, observe the patient's actions. Consider the following questions:
• Does the patient participate in opportunities to learn about hypertension and its treatment?

• Is the patient or caregiver able to demonstrate how to measure blood pressure?

Physical condition

Physical examination and diagnostic testing will also help to evaluate the effectiveness of care. If the patient complies with therapy and interventions are successful, reassessment should indicate an absence of target-organ disease involving the retina or cardiac, renal, cerebrovascular, or peripheral vascular systems. Blood pressure measurements should correspond to parameters specified in your patient outcomes.

Coronary artery disease

In coronary artery disease (CAD), fatty fibrous plaques or calcium-plaque deposits (or both) narrow the lumens of coronary arteries, thereby diminishing coronary perfusion. Acute occlusions usually contain thrombi, aggregates of fibrin, platelets, erythrocytes, and leukocytes that may cover or lie next to plaque.

Diminished coronary perfusion prevents oxygen and nutrients from reaching myocardial tissue. This deprivation causes angina pectoris and may eventually result in ischemia and myocardial infarction (MI).

CAD is more prevalent in men than women, strikes whites more than other racial groups, and typically affects middle-aged or older individuals. In fact, more than half of all men in North America ages 60 or older show signs of CAD on autopsy.

Causes

Atherosclerosis is the most common cause of CAD. Less common conditions that reduce coronary perfusion include dissecting aneurysms, infectious vasculitis, syphilis, congenital defects in the coronary vasculature, and coronary artery spasm.

ASSESSMENT

If the patient is experiencing angina, you'll need to perform a rapid assessment and intervene if necessary to prevent ischemia and MI. If the patient is stable, your assessment should include careful consideration of his health history (including risk factors), physical examination findings, and diagnostic test results.

Health history

Angina is the classic symptom of CAD. The patient may describe angina as a burning, squeezing, or crushing tightness in the substernal or precordial chest, which may radiate to the left arm, neck, jaw, or shoulder blade. These sensations may be accompanied by nausea, vomiting, fainting, sweating, or cool extremities. While describing the discomfort, the patient may clench his fist over his chest or rub his left arm. Often, the discomfort subsides within 10 minutes. Rest, stress reduction, or administration of nitroglycerin usually alleviates angina. In elderly patients, angina may lead to shortness of breath with exertion.

Angina may be precipitated or aggravated by physical exertion, emotional excitement, exposure to cold, or eating a large meal. However, angina occasionally occurs during periods of restful sleep, and pain may waken the patient. Angina that occurs without provocation while the patient is at rest is called variant, or Prinzmetal's, angina. This type of angina is due to coronary artery spasm. (See *Understanding coronary artery spasm*, page 82.)

Ask if the patient has a history of cardiovascular disease, including atherosclerosis, CAD, and hypertension. Has he ever had diabetes mellitus or

Understanding coronary artery spasm

Coronary artery spasm is a transient, abrupt, severe reduction in the diameter of a coronary artery that causes myocardial ischemia. Spasm may occur at one or more areas in one artery or in multiple arteries simultaneously. The coronary artery spasm leads to variant (Prinzmetal's) angina. Unlike classic angina, Prinzmetal's angina usually occurs spontaneously and is unrelated to physical exertion. The pain of Prinzmetal's angina is usually more severe than classic angina, lasts longer, and may be cyclic — recurring every day at the same time.

Coronary artery spasm may result in ischemic episodes leading to arrhythmias, altered heart rate, lower blood pressure, decreased cardiac output, fainting and, possibly, myocardial infarction.

Contributing factors
The cause of coronary artery spasm remains unknown, but contributing factors may include:
• endothelial injury
• hypercontractility of vascular smooth muscle
• hyperventilation
• elevated catecholamine levels
• fatty buildup in the arterial lumen.

Diagnosis and treatment
Diagnosis of coronary artery spasm usually requires coronary angiography with ergonovine, electrocardiography (ECG), and continuous ambulatory ECG (Holter monitoring). Treatment includes administration of calcium channel blockers (nifedipine or diltiazem) or nitrates (nitroglycerin or isosorbide dinitrate) to reduce coronary artery spasm, diminish vascular resistance, and relieve chest pain.

renal disease? Also ask if family members have a history of these disorders. Assess the patient's life-style and environment for risk factors. (See *Risk factors for atherosclerosis.*)

Physical examination
Assessment may reveal evidence of atherosclerotic disease. Inspection of the eyes may reveal a corneal arcus; of the skin, xanthomas. Also, a diagonal earlobe crease may be seen. Palpation may reveal diminished or absent peripheral pulses, signs of cardiac enlargement, and an abnormal cardiac impulse. A transient apical systolic murmur of mitral insufficiency may be heard during an episode of angina. Keep in mind, however, that assessment findings in CAD may be unremarkable.

Diagnostic test results
The following tests may confirm a diagnosis of CAD and reveal the extent of damage:

• *Electrocardiography (ECG).* During an anginal episode, ischemia is indicated by T-wave inversion or ST-segment displacement (elevation or depression). ECG readings may also indicate the presence of arrhythmias, such as premature ventricular contractions. Arrhythmias may occur without infarction, secondary to ischemia. During pain-free periods, the ECG tracing is normal unless there's an underlying disease, such as left ventricular hypertrophy.

• *Treadmill or bicycle exercise test.* Physical exertion may provoke chest pain and ECG signs of myocardial ischemia, including T-wave inversion or ST-segment depression in ischemic areas. Myocardial perfusion imaging with thallium-201 or technetium-99m Sestamibi (Cardiolite) during treadmill exercise may reveal ischemic areas of the myocardium, which appear as cold spots.

FactFinder
Risk factors for atherosclerosis

The most common cause of coronary artery disease (CAD), atherosclerosis is associated with numerous risk factors. Some are unavoidable, but others can be controlled with proper medical care and life-style modifications.

Unavoidable risk factors
• *Age.* Although atherosclerosis generally begins in childhood, it's a progressive disease that produces symptoms in middle to late adulthood.
• *Sex.* CAD is much less common in premenopausal women than in men of the same age. The incidence of CAD in women increases after menopause, however.
• *Heredity.* Patients with a family history of CAD have a higher risk.
• *Race.* White men are more susceptible than nonwhite men; nonwhite women are more susceptible than white women.

Controllable risk factors
• *Smoking.* Smokers have a much higher risk of atherosclerosis, myocardial infarction, and sudden death. These risks begin to drop dramatically as soon as smoking stops.
• *Hypertension.* Risk rises when systolic blood pressure exceeds 160 mm Hg or diastolic blood pressure exceeds 95 mm Hg.
• *Elevated serum cholesterol levels.* Risk increases with high levels of low-density lipoprotein or low levels of high-density lipoprotein.
• *Diabetes mellitus.* Diabetic patients have a higher risk, especially women. Proper management reduces the risk.
• *Oral contraceptives.* Using this form of birth control increases the risk of hypertension.
• *Obesity.* Obesity is associated with other cardiac risk factors, including diabetes mellitus, hypertension, and elevated serum lipid levels (which may increase the total risk).
• *Abdominal fat.* Increased waist-to-hip ratio is associated with increased risk of CAD in men and women.
• *Inactivity.* A lack of regular aerobic exercise increases the risk.
• *Stress.* Excessive emotional stress or type A behavior increases the risk.

• *Coronary angiography.* This test provides information about coronary artery stenosis or obstruction, the extent of collateral circulation, and the condition of the arteries beyond the narrowing. Also, it gives information about wall motion abnormalities and pressures inside the heart.

NURSING DIAGNOSIS

Common nursing diagnoses for patients with CAD include:
• Altered cardiopulmonary tissue perfusion related to reduced blood flow to the heart muscle caused by coronary artery narrowing or constriction
• Knowledge deficit related to CAD, its risk factors, and its treatment methods
• Pain related to an inadequate flow of oxygen to the myocardium resulting from a reduction in coronary artery blood flow
• Activity intolerance related to an imbalance between myocardial oxygen supply and demand, increased left ventricular pressure, and ineffectual myocardial contraction.

PLANNING

For a patient with angina, your immediate goal is to alleviate the patient's pain by reestablishing a balance between the myocardium's supply and demand for oxygen. After the patient is stable, direct your nursing care toward avoiding complications (such as arrhythmias and MI), controlling risk factors, and teaching the patient about CAD and its treatment.

Based on the nursing diagnosis *altered cardiopulmonary tissue perfusion,* develop appropriate patient outcomes. For example, your patient will:
• exhibit adequate myocardial tissue perfusion as demonstrated by a normal heart rate and rhythm and by an absence of ischemic changes on ECG readings.

Based on the nursing diagnosis *knowledge deficit,* develop appropriate patient outcomes. For example, your patient will:
• explain the causes and effects of CAD
• communicate an understanding of prescribed medical and surgical treatments and the importance of lifelong follow-up care
• identify personal risk factors for CAD
• agree to make the necessary changes in life-style to minimize the impact of CAD risk factors.

Based on the nursing diagnosis *pain,* develop appropriate patient outcomes. For example, your patient will:
• experience an absence or reduction in the occurrence and severity of anginal pain
• identify factors that precipitate angina and express an understanding of what to do during anginal episodes.

Based on the nursing diagnosis *activity intolerance,* develop appropriate patient outcomes. For example, your patient will:

• identify activities that must be avoided or modified or that require assistance
• demonstrate skill in conserving physical energy during approved daily activities
• engage in a medically supervised exercise program to improve his activity tolerance
• participate in activities without experiencing dyspnea.

IMPLEMENTATION

Prevention is an important aspect of CAD treatment. By reducing or eliminating risk factors, the patient reduces his risk of serious CAD complications. Risk reduction measures include dietary modifications, regular exercise, stress reduction and, if applicable, smoking cessation and control of diabetes and hypertension.

Activity restrictions may be required to prevent the onset of pain. In some instances, the patient may be able to prevent pain by performing activities slowly, rather than giving them up completely. For most patients, learning to use stress reduction techniques is essential. (See *Medical care of the patient with CAD.*)

Nursing interventions

If the patient is experiencing angina:
• Assess and document the patient's description of chest discomfort, including location, intensity, radiation, and duration of the pain and aggravating and alleviating factors.
• Assess the patient's vital signs, appearance, urine output, and mental status to determine the effect of myocardial ischemia on cardiovascular hemodynamics.
• Minimize the patient's physical activity.
• Administer antianginal medication as prescribed, and monitor the response. If a 12-lead ECG is readily

Treatments

Medical care of the patient with CAD

Therapy for coronary artery disease (CAD) may include drugs, surgery, or other procedures.

Drugs

Drug therapy for CAD consists primarily of nitrates, such as nitroglycerin, isosorbide dinitrate, beta-adrenergic blockers, or calcium channel blockers. Antilipemics, such as clofibrate, may be prescribed to control elevated serum cholesterol, triglyceride, or low-density-lipoprotein levels. And aspirin or sulfinpyrazone may be prescribed to minimize platelet aggregation.

Surgery

Obstructive lesions may require coronary artery bypass grafting (CABG). Complications to watch for after surgery include circulatory insufficiency, myocardial infarction, restenosis of the vessels, retroperitoneal bleeding, sudden coronary occlusions, or vasovagal response and arrhythmias.

Other procedures

Percutaneous transluminal coronary angioplasty (PTCA) may be performed to compress fatty deposits or fracture calcified obstructions. PTCA is less expensive than CABG and allows for a shorter hospital stay. Although PTCA has certain risks, it causes fewer complications than CABG. However, a patient with an unprotected left main coronary artery occlusion or a single vessel supplying all viable myocardium may not be able to undergo PTCA.

Laser angioplasty, which vaporizes fatty deposits with an excimer, or hot-tip laser device, may be used to correct an occlusion.

Atherectomy may be appropriate for certain patients. In this procedure, a special catheter is threaded into the artery that's narrowed by plaque and the plaque is cut away (directional atherectomy) or pulverized (rotational atherectomy).

---

available, obtain an ECG before administering nitroglycerin or other nitrates. However, *don't wait longer than 5 minutes* before administering the medication.

• Administer oxygen using a mask or nasal cannula to improve oxygen supply to myocardium when necessary.

• Provide a calm, supportive environment.

• If chest pain lasts more than 15 minutes or if prescribed medication fails to relieve pain, obtain a 12-lead ECG and prepare to draw blood for baseline and serial cardiac enzymes.

• Record the duration of pain and the amount of medication required to relieve it.

• Have your patient rank the severity of the pain on the *angina scale* described below:

1+ = Light, barely noticeable
2+ = Moderate, bothersome
3+ = Severe, very uncomfortable
4+ = Most severe pain ever experienced.

Using this scale helps the patient to assess the pain and the effectiveness of the medications needed to relieve it.

• Keep nitroglycerin tablets on the patient's bedside table, available for immediate use. Check to make sure this practice is permitted by hospital policy. Tell the patient to call before taking the nitroglycerin if he feels pain in his chest, arm, or neck or feels excessively short of breath.

Interventions for cardiac catheterization

• Before the procedure, describe cardiac catheterization to the patient and his family members. Explain the rationale for catheterization and risks involved. Explain that catheterization may indicate a need for additional therapies, such as percutaneous transluminal coronary angioplasty, coronary artery bypass grafting (CABG), atherectomy, or laser angioplasty.
• Give the patient and family members a tour of the catheterization laboratory, introduce them to the staff, and discuss postcatheterization care.
• After the procedure, monitor the catheter site for bleeding. Check for distal pulses.

Interventions for CABG

• Provide care for the I.V. set, pulmonary artery catheter, and endotracheal tube.
• Monitor blood pressure, intake and output, breath sounds, drainage from the chest tube, and cardiac rhythm. Watch for signs of ischemia and arrhythmias.
• Administer I.V. epinephrine, nitroprusside, dopamine, albumin, potassium, and blood products as ordered. The patient may need temporary epicardial pacing, especially if the aortic valve was replaced during surgery.
• If an intra-aortic balloon pump is inserted, observe the patient for chest pain and treat appropriately.

Patient teaching

• Explain CAD, its causes, and its complications.
• Help your patient identify activities that precipitate episodes of angina. Describe strategies that will allow your patient to eliminate or modify these activities.

• Help the patient identify effective mechanisms for coping with stress. For example, if work is a primary stressor, discuss whether the patient can change his occupation or change his position within the same company. Be aware, however, that these options aren't available to many patients.
• Teach your patient to respond to angina by slowing down activity, taking antianginal medication, and notifying the doctor immediately if the nature of the angina changes. Tell the patient to take sublingual nitroglycerin before performing activities known to produce angina.
• Explain the importance of following the prescribed drug regimen, which may include antihypertensives, nitrates, lipid-lowering preparations, calcium channel blockers, anticoagulants, and beta blockers.
• Teach your patient the proper method for taking nitroglycerin tablets: beginning with the onset of discomfort, take a maximum of three doses, one every 5 minutes. Tell your patient to get immediate emergency care if discomfort persists after three doses.
• Explain that an opened bottle of nitroglycerin may lose its potency in 3 to 6 months. When the patient first opens the bottle, have him mark the date on the bottle. Have him replace the bottle with a new one in 6 months.
• Teach your patient to prevent complications of angina, such as MI, by taking prophylactic nitroglycerin and reducing or eliminating physical activities and emotional stressors that provoke angina.
• Teach the patient the warning signs of serious complications, including angina, persistent fever, swelling or drainage at a surgical incision site (if present), dizziness, shortness of breath when resting, rapid or irregular pulse rate, and prolonged recovery time from exercise or sexual activity. Ex-

plain that any occurrence should be immediately reported to the doctor.

• Encourage the patient to adopt a diet that has less cholesterol, saturated fats, and sodium. If the patient is overweight, he'll need to cut down on calorie consumption as well. Enlist the help of a dietitian and family members when exploring ways to make dietary adjustments comfortable for your patient.

• Encourage regular, moderate exercise. Refer your patient to a cardiac rehabilitation center or cardiovascular fitness program for an appropriate exercise regimen. Encourage family members and close friends to exercise with the patient to help reinforce his commitment to the program.

• Reassure your patient that sexual activity can be resumed with some adjustments to alleviate his fear of overexertion, pain, or MI.

• If your patient smokes, refer him to a smoking cessation program. Acknowledge that quitting is difficult, but stress the importance of quitting immediately and permanently.

• Provide referrals for information and support to organizations, such as local chapters of the American Cancer Society, American Heart Association, and American Lung Association.

Timesaving tip: Consider providing group teaching for your patients with CAD. Not only will you save time, but you'll foster supportive relationships among patients.

• Schedule follow-up appointments. (See *Ensuring continued care for the patient with CAD.*)

Discharge TimeSaver

Ensuring continued care for the patient with CAD

Review the following areas to ensure that your CAD patient is prepared for discharge.

Teaching topics
Make sure that the following topics have been covered and your patient's learning has been evaluated:
□ cardiac physiology
□ an explanation of CAD, its risk factors, and its complications
□ medications
□ exercise program
□ dietary modifications
□ stress reduction techniques
□ weight reduction measures
□ warning signs and symptoms
□ modifications in activities of daily living.

Referrals
Make sure that the patient has been provided with appropriate referrals to:
□ social service specializing in financial assistance
□ dietary consultant
□ smoking cessation program
□ cardiac rehabilitation exercise program
□ organizations providing information and support.

Follow-up appointments
Be sure that appointments have been scheduled with:
□ doctor
□ surgeon, if necessary
□ laboratory for diagnostic tests.

EVALUATION

When evaluating the patient's response to your care, gather reassessment data and compare this to the outcomes specified in your plan of care.

Teaching and counseling

Document any statements made by the patient indicating:
• understanding of CAD and its treatment requirements
• willingness to comply with prescribed treatment.

Evaluation TimeSaver

Assessing failure to respond to CAD therapy

If your patient fails to respond to therapy for symptomatic coronary artery disease (CAD), evaluate whether you've established a realistic time frame for achieving patient outcomes. Consult with the patient and family members to determine factors that may be interfering with attaining desired outcomes. Then consult with members of the health care team, make necessary revisions in the plan, and set a target date for reevaluation.

Drug therapy
• Is the patient taking the prescribed medication?
• Does he understand the reasons for taking *all* prescribed drugs, including antihypertensives, nitrates, antilipemics, calcium channel blockers, and anticoagulants?
• Does he understand the proper method for taking nitroglycerin tablets?
• What factors — for example, lack of knowledge, lack of motivation, or financial constraints — are interfering with compliance with the drug regimen?

Life-style changes
• Has the patient made the necessary life-style modifications to reduce CAD risk? If not, why not?
• Which modifications — diet, regular exercise, stress reduction, or smoking cessation — are most problematic for the patient?
• Do family members support the patient's efforts to change habits that increase his risk?
• Are there alternative approaches to behavior modification that should be explored to help the patient make the needed life-style changes?
• Do the patient and family members make and keep follow-up appointments?
• Are they willing to make use of available sources of information and support?
• Has the patient's CAD progressed despite compliance with therapy, as evidenced by worsening symptoms and diagnostic test results?

During your evaluation, consider the following questions:
• Is the patient taking all prescribed medications?
• Has he made the necessary life-style modifications?
• Has he had further episodes of angina? If so, have the characteristics of the pain changed? (See *Assessing failure to respond to CAD therapy.*)

Physical condition
Physical assessment and diagnostic tests will also help you evaluate the effectiveness of your plan of care. If the patient complies with treatment, your ongoing assessment should indicate:
• adequate myocardial perfusion
• normal heart rate and rhythm
• absence of ischemia, as indicated by ECG readings
• absence of anginal pain or a reduction in its frequency and intensity
• improved activity tolerance.

Myocardial infarction

Myocardial infarction (MI), or heart attack, is one of the most common causes of death in developed nations. Mortality for MI patients is about 25%, usually the result of cardiac damage or complications. More than 50% of sudden deaths occur in the first hour after onset of symptoms, often before the patient reaches the hospital. Of those who recover from MI, up to 10% die within 1 year.

Males are more susceptible to MI than premenopausal females, although the incidence is rising among women who smoke or take oral contraceptives. The incidence in postmenopausal women is similar to that in men.

MI refers to necrosis of myocardial tissue caused by reduced or obstructed blood flow through one of the coronary arteries. The site of infarction depends on the vessel or vessels involved. Occlusion of the circumflex coronary artery causes a lateral wall infarction; occlusion of the left anterior coronary artery causes an anterior wall infarction. True posterior and inferior wall infarctions generally result from occlusion of the right coronary artery or one of its branches. Right ventricular infarctions also may result from occlusion of the right coronary artery or accompany inferior infarctions and cause right ventricular failure. In Q-wave (transmural) MI, tissue damage extends through all myocardial layers; non-Q-wave (subendocardial) MI typically involves only the innermost layer.

Causes
Usually, MI results from atherosclerosis of the coronary arteries with thrombosis.

ASSESSMENT

Prompt assessment of chest pain and immediate intervention to minimize myocardial damage is essential.

Health history
The patient may report a persistent, crushing substernal pain that radiates to the left arm, jaw, neck, or shoulder blades. The pain may be characterized as heavy, squeezing, or crushing and may persist for 12 hours or more. Some patients experience little pain, which may be misinterpreted as indigestion; others, particularly elderly or diabetic patients, may experience no pain.

Additional symptoms may include a feeling of impending doom, diaphoresis, fatigue, nausea, vomiting, and shortness of breath.

The patient with previous angina may report increasing frequency, severity, or duration of angina. Take note if anginal episodes have not been precipitated by exertion, a heavy meal, or cold. Sudden death may be the first and only indication of MI.

Additional findings
After the patient is stabilized, obtain further health history information, including a description of anginal episodes, if present, a patient and family history of cardiovascular disease, and the presence of risk factors. (See *Risk factors for MI,* page 90.)

Physical examination
Physical assessment of the patient is nonspecific for MI. Positive assessment findings generally indicate coexisting disease or related complications.

After MI, the patient may appear anxious and restless. You may note dyspnea and diaphoresis. Inspection may reveal jugular vein distention, suggesting right ventricular failure. Hyperactivity of the sympathetic nervous system (for example, tachycardia or hypertension) during the first hour after onset may indicate an anterior MI. Hyperactivity of the parasympathetic nervous system (for example, bradycardia or hypotension) during the same time may indicate an inferior MI.

If the patient develops ventricular dysfunction, auscultation may reveal an S_3 gallop, which is associated with a higher mortality rate if heard during the acute phase of MI. An S_4 gallop is commonly heard. A systolic murmur

FactFinder

Risk factors for MI

Various factors enhance a patient's risk of developing coronary artery disease (CAD). These factors, which also increase the risk of myocardial infarction (MI), include:
• a family history of CAD
• hypertension
• smoking
• elevated levels of serum triglycerides, low-density lipoproteins, and cholesterol; decreased levels of serum high-density lipoproteins
• diabetes mellitus
• obesity
• a sedentary life-style
• aging
• emotional stress or type A behavior (exemplified by aggressive, ambitious, or competitive behavior; an addiction to work; and chronic impatience).
    Also, MI may directly result from use of amphetamines, cocaine, and crack cocaine.

of mitral regurgitation may indicate papillary muscle dysfunction secondary to infarction. A pericardial friction rub may be evident in patients with pericarditis accompanying transmural MI and is most commonly heard 2 to 3 days after MI.

Temperature begins to rise 4 to 8 hours after the onset of MI, reaching 101° to 102° F (38.3° to 38.9° C). Fever usually resolves within 5 to 7 days.

Additional findings

Psychological complications after MI are common; they may result from the patient's fear of another MI or death or from an organic brain disorder caused by tissue hypoxia. For information about other complications associated with MI, see *Complications of MI*.

Diagnostic test results

Serial 12-lead electrocardiogram (ECG) readings may be used to detect and monitor MI. Serial T-wave inversion and ST-segment depression are characteristic of non-Q-wave MI. ST-segment elevation and Q waves, indicating scarring and necrosis, are characteristic of Q-wave MI. Note, however, that ECG readings may be normal or inconclusive for several hours after MI.

• Serum creatine kinase (CK) levels may be elevated, especially those of the CK-MB isoenzyme, the cardiac muscle fraction of CK. A ratio of CK-MB to CK exceeding 4% indicates MI.
• Echocardiography identifies regional wall motion abnormalities and allows evaluation of the ejection fraction.
• Nuclear imaging, such as thallium 201 scanning, technetium-99m Sestamibi scanning, positron emission tomography (PET), radionuclide angiography, or perfusion scintigraphy, helps assess the size and location of infarction.
• Cardiac catheterization may be performed to facilitate planning and implementation of treatment.

NURSING DIAGNOSIS

Common nursing diagnoses for MI patients include:
• Altered cardiopulmonary tissue perfusion related to imbalance between myocardial oxygen supply and demand
• Anxiety related to diagnosis, treatment, or prognosis of MI
• Decreased cardiac output related to complications of MI
• Pain related to myocardial tissue ischemia
• Knowledge deficit related to MI, its risk factors, and its treatment methods
• Activity intolerance related to an imbalance between myocardial oxygen supply and demand

Complications of MI

Complication	Assessment findings	Treatment
Arrhythmias	• Electrocardiogram (ECG) shows premature ventricular contractions, ventricular tachycardia, ventricular fibrillation, or atrial fibrillation; in inferior wall MI, bradycardia and junctional rhythms; in anterior wall MI, tachycardia or heart block.	• Antiarrhythmics such as atropine • Digoxin • Cardioversion • Defibrillation • Pacemaker
Heart failure	• In left ventricular failure, chest X-rays show venous congestion and possible cardiomegaly. • Pulmonary artery catheterization shows increases in pulmonary artery systolic and diastolic pressures, pulmonary artery wedge pressure (PAWP), central venous pressure, and systemic vascular resistance (SVR).	• Diuretics • Vasodilators • Inotropic agents
Cardiogenic shock	• Pulmonary artery catheterization shows decreased cardiac output, increased pulmonary artery systolic and diastolic pressures, decreased cardiac index, increased SVR, and increased PAWP. • Clinical signs include hypotension, tachycardia, decreased level of consciousness, decreased urine output, neck vein distention, S_3 and S_4, and cool, pale skin.	• I.V. fluids • Vasodilators • Cardiotonics • Digitalis glycosides • Intra-aortic balloon pump (IABP) • Vasopressors • Beta-adrenergic stimulants
Rupture of left ventricular papillary muscle	• Auscultation reveals apical holosystolic murmur. • Dyspnea is prominent. • Color-flow and Doppler echocardiogram show mitral insufficiency. • Pulmonary artery catheterization shows increased pulmonary artery pressure (PAP) and PAWP. • Inspection of jugular vein pulse or hemodynamic monitoring shows increased v waves.	• Nitroprusside • IABP • Surgical replacement of the mitral valve with possible concomitant myocardial revascularization (in patients with significant coronary artery disease)
Ventricular septal rupture	• In left-to-right shunt, auscultation reveals a harsh holosystolic murmur and thrill. • Pulmonary artery catheterization shows increased PAP and PAWP. • Increased oxygen saturation of right ventricle and pulmonary artery confirms the diagnosis.	• Surgical correction (may be postponed, but many patients have surgery immediately or up to 7 days after septal rupture) • IABP • Nitroglycerin • Nitroprusside • Low-dose inotropic agents (dopamine) • Cardiac pacing (if high-grade AV blocks occur)

(continued)

Complications of MI *(continued)*

Complication	Assessment findings	Treatment
Pericarditis or Dressler's syndrome	• Auscultation reveals a pericardial friction rub. • ECG may show ST-segment and T-wave elevation in all leads except aV$_R$ and V$_1$. • Symptoms include chest pain unlike previously experienced anginal pain; pain is relieved by moving to a sitting position but not by increasing nitrate dosage.	• Anti-inflammatory agents, such as aspirin
Ventricular aneurysm	• Chest X-rays may show cardiomegaly. • ECG may show arrhythmias and persistent ST-segment elevation. • Left ventriculography shows altered or paradoxical left ventricular motion. • Echocardiography shows regional dyskinesis.	• Cardioversion • Defibrillation (if ventricular tachycardia or fibrillation occurs) • Antiarrhythmics • Vasodilators • Anticoagulants • Digitalis glycosides • Diuretics • Possible surgery
Cerebral or pulmonary embolism	• Dyspnea and chest pain or neurologic changes occur • Nuclear scan shows ventilation-perfusion mismatch in pulmonary embolism • Angiography shows arterial blockage.	• Oxygen administration • Heparin • Cardiopulmonary resuscitation (CPR) • Possible cardiac pacing
Ventricular rupture	• Cardiac tamponade occurs. • Arrhythmias, such as ventricular tachycardia and ventricular fibrillation, or sudden death may occur.	• CPR and advanced cardiac life support • Possible emergency surgical repair if CPR is successful

• Altered sexuality patterns related to fear of causing heart damage or death.

PLANNING

Your nursing care should focus on preserving myocardial integrity, detecting complications, preventing further myocardial damage, and promoting patient comfort, rest, and emotional well-being.

Based on the nursing diagnosis *altered cardiopulmonary tissue perfusion,* develop appropriate patient outcomes. For example, your patient will:
• seek immediate emergency intervention to minimize myocardial tissue damage
• demonstrate adequate myocardial tissue perfusion
• not develop major complications, such as arrhythmias or heart failure.

Based on the nursing diagnosis *anxiety,* develop appropriate patient outcomes. For example, your patient will:
• express his feelings of anxiety about MI and death

• identify three or more effective coping mechanisms that will help him live with his diagnosis
• state that he feels less anxious
• identify three or more sources of support to help him cope during recovery from MI.

Based on the nursing diagnosis *decreased cardiac output,* develop appropriate patient outcomes. For example, your patient will:
• attain hemodynamic stability, as evidenced by blood pressure within normal limits, pulse rate under 100 beats/minute, oxygen saturation greater than 90%, and pulmonary artery pressure, pulmonary artery wedge pressure, cardiac index, and systemic vascular resistance within acceptable limits
• experience fewer dyspneic episodes
• not experience dizziness or syncope.

Based on the nursing diagnosis *pain,* develop appropriate patient outcomes. For example, your patient will:
• not experience new or worsening ischemic changes, as evidenced by ECG readings
• not report new episodes of chest pain
• demonstrate a return to baseline values for respiratory rate, pulse rate, and blood pressure.

Based on the nursing diagnosis *knowledge deficit,* develop appropriate patient outcomes. For example, your patient will:
• express knowledge about the normal heart and circulation and an understanding of the disease process
• express understanding of prescribed medical and surgical treatments, including drug therapy (name of drug, dosage, action, adverse effects, additional considerations where appropriate)
• acknowledge the importance of following the prescribed treatment plan and the need for lifelong care
• identify risk factors for complications or recurrence of MI

• express a willingness to initiate lifestyle changes to reduce his risk for complications or recurrence of MI
• identify appropriate actions to be taken if chest pain recurs.

Based on the nursing diagnosis *activity intolerance,* develop appropriate patient outcomes. For example, your patient will:
• demonstrate his ability to tolerate minimal activity, as evidenced by a respiratory rate under 16 breaths/minute, pulse rate under 100 beats/minute, blood pressure within normal limits, and warm, dry skin
• participate in a cardiac rehabilitation program.

Based on the nursing diagnosis *altered sexuality patterns,* develop appropriate patient outcomes. For example, your patient will:
• express his fears and concerns about resuming sexual activity
• express an understanding of how to resume sexual activity without increasing cardiac risk
• report resuming sexual activity 3 to 4 weeks after MI, or according to the doctor's recommendation.

IMPLEMENTATION

Most MI patients receive initial treatment in the intensive care unit (ICU) or coronary care unit (CCU), under constant observation for complications. Treatment focuses on preserving the myocardium, reducing the size of the infarction, increasing the myocardium's oxygen supply, and decreasing its demand for oxygen. This reduces the patient's chest pain, stabilizes his heart rhythm, and reduces the cardiac work load. Arrhythmias, the predominant problem during the first 48 hours, may be treated with antiarrhythmics, insertion of a pacemaker or, in some cases, cardioversion. (See *Medical care of the patient with MI*, page 94.)

Treatments

Medical care of the patient with MI

Medical treatment seeks to relieve chest pain, stabilize heart rhythm, and reduce cardiac work load. Other goals of treatment may include revascularization and preservation of myocardial tissue.

Drug therapy

Drug therapy for MI patients usually includes:
• lidocaine for ventricular arrhythmias or, if lidocaine is ineffective, other drugs (such as procainamide, quinidine, bretylium, or disopyramide)
• atropine I.V. for heart block or bradycardia
• nitroglycerin (sublingual, topical, transdermal, or I.V.); calcium channel blockers, such as nifedipine, verapamil, and diltiazem (P.O. or I.V.); or isosorbide dinitrate (sublingual, P.O., or I.V.) to relieve pain by redistributing blood to ischemic area of myocardium, increasing cardiac output and reducing myocardial work load
• morphine I.V. and, possibly, meperidine or hydromorphone for pain and sedation
• inotropic agents (such as dobutamine and amrinone), administered cautiously, to treat reduced myocardial contractility
• beta-adrenergic blockers (such as propranolol, timolol and metoprolol) and aspirin, to help prevent reinfarction after acute MI
• drugs that increase contractility (inotropic agents) or blood pressure (such as vasopressors or norepinephrine) for cardiogenic shock
• thrombolytic agents, such as alteplase (recombinant tissue plasminogen activator; rt-PA), anistreplase (anisoylated plasminogen-streptokinase activator complex; APSAC), or streptokinase, to promote revascularization through lysis of thrombi obstructing coronary arteries. The best response occurs when treatment is instituted within the first few hours after onset of symptoms.

Additional treatments

After MI, the doctor will probably order bed rest with a bedside commode to decrease cardiac work load. The patient may also receive oxygen (by face mask or nasal cannula) at a low flow rate for 24 to 48 hours; a lower concentration is necessary if the patient has chronic obstructive pulmonary disease.

A patient who experiences cardiogenic shock may require an intra-aortic balloon pump. Pulmonary artery catheterization may be performed to detect left or right ventricular failure and to monitor response to treatment, but it's not routinely done.

Arrhythmias are the predominant problem during the first 48 hours after the infarction. Besides antiarrhythmic drugs, the patient may require a pacemaker and, in some instances, cardioversion.

Nursing interventions

• On admission to the ICU, assess the patient's chest pain and record his description of the location, radiation, duration, and intensity of pain as well as aggravating and alleviating factors.
• Obtain baseline readings for a 12-lead ECG, blood pressure and, if available, pulmonary artery catheter measurements. After the baseline reading, obtain a 12-lead ECG daily for 3 days. Thereafter, obtain one if chest pain recurs or complications develop.
• Frequently assess the patient's vital signs, heart sounds, lung sounds, weight, and intake and output. Monitor

for complications. Crackles, cough, tachypnea, or edema may indicate impending left ventricular failure. Auscultate for S_3 or S_4 gallops.
• Initiate I.V. therapy with a catheter no smaller than 20G.
• Administer analgesics, as prescribed, and monitor the patient's response.
• Initiate ECG monitoring for changes in heart rate or arrhythmias. Analyze the strips frequently. A representative strip should be placed in the patient's chart when a new arrhythmia is noted or chest pain occurs, or at least once each shift, according to your hospital's protocol.
• Administer I.V. medications, as prescribed.

Timesaving tip: Avoid giving I.M. injections because of unpredictable absorption. I.V. administration provides more rapid relief of symptoms.
• Draw blood for serum enzyme measurements on admission, at ordered intervals thereafter, and with each recurrence of chest pain.
• Provide bed rest and a bedside commode for 24 hours.
• Provide psychological support to lessen the patient's anxiety. Answer questions posed by the patient and family members. Be aware that you may need to repeat information after the emergency is resolved. Administer tranquilizers as ordered.
• Administer oxygen as ordered.
• Provide a stool softener to prevent straining, which causes vagal stimulation and may slow heart rate. Provide the patient with as much privacy as possible when he's using the bedside commode.
• Provide a clear liquid diet with no caffeine-containing beverages. Progress to a low-cholesterol, low-saturated fat, low-sodium, caffeine-free diet as soon as the patient can tolerate it.
• Assist the patient with range-of-motion exercises. If the patient is com-

pletely immobilized by a severe MI, turn him often.
• Apply antiembolism stockings to help prevent venostasis and thrombophlebitis.
• Organize patient care and activities to maximize periods of uninterrupted rest.
• If the patient has undergone percutaneous transluminal coronary angioplasty (PTCA), provide sheath care. Keep the sheath line open with a heparin drip. Observe for generalized or site bleeding. Immobilize the leg containing the sheath insertion site. Maintain strict bed rest. Check peripheral pulses in the affected leg frequently. Provide analgesics for back pain, if needed.
• If the patient must undergo thrombolytic therapy, prepare him for the procedure. Afterwards, administer continuous heparin as ordered. Monitor the partial thromboplastin time every 6 hours and monitor the patient for evidence of bleeding. Monitor cardiac rhythm strips for reperfusion arrhythmias and treat according to your hospital's protocol. (See *Guidelines for administering thrombolytic therapy,* pages 96 and 97.)
• Have emergency equipment available at all times. A qualified nurse must be available to provide emergency resuscitation as needed. Follow your hospital's protocol for defibrillation and administration of emergency medications.

Patient teaching
The patient with MI has numerous teaching needs. Shortly after he's hospitalized, you'll need to explain the intensive care environment with its bewildering array of equipment. You'll also need to explain immediate treatment measures, such as PTCA or coronary artery bypass grafting (CABG). Be prepared to repeat your explanations after the patient stabilizes.

Guidelines for administering thrombolytic therapy

The thrombolytic enzymes streptokinase and alteplase (rt-PA) are used to manage acute myocardial infarction in adults. These drugs dissolve the thrombi obstructing the coronary arteries, thereby improving ventricular function and reducing the incidence of congestive heart failure.

Indications
Streptokinase or alteplase may be indicated when:
• the patient experiences chest pain characteristic of myocardial ischemia for at least 30 minutes.
• nitroglycerin or nifedipine fail to relieve chest pain.
• electrocardiogram (ECG) readings show ST-segment elevation of 0.2 mV or more in at least two adjacent leads.
• less than 8 hours have passed since onset of ischemic symptoms. (This criteria may be extended to 12 hours in certain cases.)
• the patient is age 75 or younger.

Contraindications
Both streptokinase and alteplase are contraindicated in:
• recent cerebrovascular event, intracranial neoplasm, arteriovenous malformation, or aneurysm
• past or current bleeding disorder
• intracranial or spinal surgery or trauma within the past 2 months
• severe, uncontrolled hypertension
• significant surgical procedure within the last 2 weeks
• serious terminal illness (such as cancer) with life expectancy of less than 1 year
• major surgery, obstetric delivery, or organ biopsy within the last 10 days
• pregnancy
• concurrent thrombolytic therapy.
Streptokinase is also contraindicated in:
• allergy to streptokinase
• prior streptokinase administration (within 6 months).

Cautions
Both streptokinase and alteplase should be administered cautiously in the following circumstances:
• puncture of a noncompressible vessel within the last 10 days
• diabetic hemorrhagic retinopathy or other hemorrhagic ophthalmic conditions
• concurrent anticoagulant therapy, if prothrombin time (PT) is greater than 15 seconds
• serious trauma within the last 10 days
• cardiopulmonary resuscitation within the last 10 days
• known or suspected left heart thrombus.
In addition, streptokinase should be administered cautiously to patients with:
• infectious endocarditis
• liver disease.

Administration
When administering streptokinase, take the following steps:
• Obtain baseline laboratory data.
• Establish two I.V. lines and reserve one port for streptokinase administration.
• Reconstitute streptokinase by injecting 5 ml of 0.9% sodium chloride solution. Further dilute to 100 ml.
• Administer streptokinase through designated I.V. sites. Usual dosage is 1.5 million units over 1 hour. Administer using an infusion pump or rate controller. Carefully monitor to ensure accuracy.
• Initiate heparin therapy 4 hours after start of streptokinase therapy.

Guidelines for administering thrombolytic therapy *(continued)*

When administering alteplase, take the following steps:
• Obtain baseline laboratory data.
• Insert two I.V. lines and reserve one port for alteplase administration.
• Reconstitute alteplase using sterile water for injection.
• Administer alteplase through the designated I.V. site. Standard dosage is 100 mg given as follows: 60 mg in the first hour, of which 6 to 10 mg is given as a bolus over the first 1 to 2 minutes. Then administer 20 mg/hour for 2 hours. Smaller adults (less than 143 lb [65 kg]) should receive a dose of 1.25 mg/kg in a similar fashion (60% in the first hour, with 10% as a bolus; then 20% of the total dose per hour for 2 hours).
• Administer alteplase through non-filtered I.V. tubing using an infusion pump or rate controller. Carefully monitor the infusion to ensure accuracy.
• At the beginning of the last hour of al-

teplase infusion, the I.V. container will be empty. Don't discontinue the drip because the remainder of the alteplase dose is still in the tubing. When the alarm sounds, inject 10 ml of 0.9% sodium chloride solution through the port and continue the infusion.
• Initiate heparin therapy within 1 hour after the initial alteplase bolus.

Aftercare
• Monitor the patient closely in the intensive care unit. Watch for evidence of hemorrhage.
• Monitor diagnostic studies, including PT, partial thromboplastin time, cardiac enzymes, complete blood count, and ECG.
• Assess for evidence of reperfusion, such as resolution of chest pain, resolution of ECG changes, appearance of reperfusion arrhythmias on ECG, and cardiac enzyme washout phenomena.

During recovery, you'll need to help the patient learn how to resume activities, make necessary diet modifications, follow the medication regimen, and recognize warning signs and symptoms of MI. The patient should also have an adequate understanding of the disease process in MI.

The patient may express anxiety about his ability to resume his normal life after discharge. Well-timed, sensitive teaching sessions help the patient understand that, with some guidelines to prevent overexertion, most activities can be resumed after MI. If the patient agrees, include family members in the teaching program. Whenever possible, provide written instructions and include illustrations.

Teaching about MI
Describe normal cardiac function and circulation. Explain how a blocked coronary artery reduces oxygen flow to the heart and causes the MI and associated pain. Tell the patient that necrosis occurs unless the blood supply is restored. Explain that MI is progressive and that the ultimate size of the infarct depends on collateral circulation, oxygen demand, and the degree of anaerobic metabolism.

Teach the patient ways to reduce his risk of extending the infarct or developing complications. For example, explain the importance of planning rest periods and of avoiding or modifying activities such as driving, returning to work, traveling, and heavy lifting and pushing. Explain the healing process and discuss MI causes and risk factors.

Teaching about tests
Describe the tests performed to confirm an MI and to determine the extent of myocardial damage, including serial blood studies, ECG, thallium and technetium scans, echocardiography, and cardiac catheterization. Describe tests that evaluate arrhythmias, assess perfusion and scarring, and evaluate drug therapy, including exercise ECG, continuous ambulatory ECG (Holter monitoring), and electrophysiologic studies. Tell the patient why each test is performed, where it is performed, who will perform the test, and how long it will take. Explain routine preparation, posttest care, and the risks involved.

Teaching about cardiac catheterization
Explain that cardiac catheterization evaluates the function of the heart and blood vessels and that the procedure takes less than 1 hour. Cardiac catheterization may be performed before CABG or PTCA to reveal coronary artery stenosis and to evaluate left ventricular function. Explain that the procedure involves injecting contrast dye through a catheter, which is threaded through an artery to the left side of the heart. Explain that a catheter may be inserted into a vein and to the right side of the heart to monitor pressures.

Tell the patient to follow all directions during the procedure, for example, coughing or breathing deeply when instructed. Explain that nitroglycerin may be administered to dilate coronary arteries. Describe the care that the patient will receive after cardiac catheterization and answer questions, especially those about risks.

Timesaving tip: Many hospitals have videotapes about cardiac catheterization. If your hospital does, have the patient and family mem-

bers watch the video, and then conduct a question-and-answer session.

Teaching about PTCA
Explain that PTCA involves threading a thin balloon-tipped catheter into the narrowed coronary artery and injecting a contrast dye to identify the exact site of arterial narrowing. Explain that the balloon catheter inflates to expand and reopen the artery.

Tell the patient that he'll receive a local anesthetic to numb the catheterization site, a sedative to promote relaxation, an anticoagulant to prevent embolism, and nitroglycerin to prevent coronary artery spasm. Warn the patient that he may feel flushed and experience brief chest pain as the contrast dye is infused.

Teaching about CABG
Explain that CABG restores normal blood flow to the heart. Tell the patient that a portion of healthy blood vessel, typically a saphenous vein or mammary artery, is removed or rerouted from one area of the body and then grafted to the affected coronary artery above and below the occlusion. Explain that coronary circulation is diverted through the grafts to the myocardium. Assure the patient that removing a healthy vein doesn't compromise circulation.

Describe preoperative care, including the endotracheal tube, pacing wires, and chest drains, and discuss long-term rehabilitation measures. Describe the equipment that will support the patient after surgery. This equipment can appear complex and frightening. Whenever possible, take the patient and family members on a tour of the ICU before surgery. Answer all questions.

Teaching about IABP insertion
Because intra-aortic balloon pump (IABP) insertion typically is an emergency procedure performed at the bedside or in the cardiac catheterization

laboratory, provide teaching at the earliest opportunity. If possible, explain that the doctor will place a special balloon catheter in the aorta to help the heart pump efficiently. Also explain that the catheter is inserted through the femoral artery and that it inflates and deflates with the heart. Inform the patient that the procedure conserves the heart's oxygen supply and reduces its oxygen demand. Mention that the catheter will be connected to an alarm system.

Tell the patient that his movement will be limited after the procedure; for example, the catheter will make it impossible to sit up, bend the knee, or flex the hip more than 30 degrees.

Teaching about diet
Explain that the patient's diet will consist of clear fluids until he can tolerate solid food. Caution the patient that caffeine-containing beverages stimulate the heart and, therefore, should be limited or avoided.

Teach the patient risk-reducing dietary modifications, such as reducing cholesterol, saturated fat, sodium and, if needed, caloric intake. Instruct him to limit his cholesterol intake to less than 300 mg/day and limit his fat intake to less than 30% of total calories. (See *Determining percentage of calories from fat*.) Explain the benefits of adding fiber, fish, and olive oil to the diet.

If the patient drinks alcoholic beverages, advise him to limit daily intake to no more than 1 oz of ethanol daily (equivalent to 2 oz of 100-proof whiskey, 8 oz of wine, or 24 oz of beer). Explain that alcohol can raise blood pressure and adversely affect his heart. Make sure the patient understands how his medications interact with alcohol.

Teaching about resuming daily activities
Explain the need for activity restrictions. The patient will require bed rest

---

Determining percentage of calories from fat

To help the patient recovering from MI limit his intake of fat, teach him how to determine the percentage of calories from fat in food items. Ideally, less than one-third of calories in the diet should be from fat, preferably in the form of unsaturated fat.

To determine the percentage of fat in a serving of food:
1. Determine the grams of fat per serving from the product label.
2. Multiply this number by 9 (9 calories per gram of fat) to determine total calories from fat per serving.
3. Divide calories from fat by total calories in the serving. Then multiply by 100.

An example
There are 130 calories and 6 g of fat in 1 oz of granola. To determine the percentage of calories from fat, multiply 6 by 9 to determine total calories from fat, which is 54. Then divide 54 by 130 (total calories), which equals 0.415, indicating about 42% of the calories in granola are from fat.

---

for 1 to 2 days after MI to reduce the demands on the heart. Describe the prescribed activity program and emphasize that activities should be resumed gradually. Teach the patient to plan daily activities so that he alternates between light and heavy tasks, and to plan rest periods between tasks. Encourage him to share tasks with family members.

Teaching about resuming sexual activity
Explain that sexual activity should be resumed progressively. Also explain that sexual intercourse is a moderate form of exercise, about as stressful as a brief walk. Advise the patient to choose relaxing positions that permit

unrestricted breathing. Caution the patient not to engage in sexual activity when he's tired or upset or immediately after a big meal. If the patient has experienced anginal pain during sexual intercourse, teach him to take nitroglycerin beforehand.

Teaching about drug therapy
Promote compliance by thoroughly explaining the dose, frequency, route, and purpose of each prescribed drug. Describe all possible adverse effects. Advise the patient to watch for, and report, signs of toxicity.

Teaching about exercise
Encourage the patient to join a cardiac rehabilitation program. Suggest a gradual, progressive program. Explain the dangers of exercising in extreme temperatures. Caution him to begin to cool down and discontinue exercising if he feels dizzy, faint, or short of breath or has chest pain.

Teaching about smoking cessation
If the patient smokes, stress the need to stop smoking. Explain that smoking reduces serum high-density lipoproteins, constricts arteries, and reduces the blood's ability to carry oxygen. Provide repetitive counseling and refer the patient to an effective smoking cessation program. Explain the use of the nicotine patch or nicotine gum. Refer the patient to local support and information groups, such as local branches of the American Cancer Society, American Heart Association, and American Lung Association.

Teaching about warning signs and symptoms
Teach your patient how to respond to new or recurrent symptoms. Tell him to notify the doctor if he experiences chest pain, persistent fever, dizziness, excessive shortness of breath, rapid or irregular pulse rate, or prolonged recovery time after exercise or sexual activity. If the patient has an incision, tell him to report redness, swelling, or drainage.

Describe postinfarction syndrome and its associated chest pain. Explain that this pain must be differentiated from the pain of recurrent MI, pulmonary infarction, and congestive heart failure. Schedule follow-up appointments and explain the importance of keeping them. (See *Ensuring continued care for the patient with MI.*)

Teaching about coping skills
Teach the patient techniques for coping with the emotional effects of an MI. Explain that depression and anxiety are common after an MI. Explore how the patient and family members are responding to anxiety, depression, and life-style changes. Encourage open expression of feelings to help the patient cope with depression. Teach relaxation exercises and other techniques for alleviating anxiety. Encourage the patient to focus on activities he will be able to participate in after recovery from MI.

EVALUATION

When evaluating the patient's response to your nursing care, gather reassessment data and compare this information to the patient outcomes specified in your plan of care. Consult with other members of the health care team, as necessary.

Teaching and counseling
Talk to the patient and family members to determine the effectiveness of teaching and counseling. Consider the following questions:
• Has the patient demonstrated adequate understanding of the normal heart and circulation and the disease process?

Discharge TimeSaver

Ensuring continued care for the patient with MI

Review the following areas to ensure that your patient is ready to leave the hospital.

Teaching topics
Make sure that the following topics have been covered and the patient's learning has been evaluated:
□ normal heart function, coronary arteries, and circulation
□ an explanation of myocardial infarction (MI), its complications, and risk factors for recurrence
□ healing process
□ activity restrictions
□ drug therapy
□ dietary modifications
□ resumption of sexual activity
□ smoking cessation
□ limits on alcohol intake
□ exercise program and precautions
□ how to take a pulse
□ warning signs and recommended actions
□ support groups and resources
□ preparation for diagnostic tests, if

scheduled
□ preparation for coronary artery bypass grafting or percutaneous transluminal coronary angioplasty, if scheduled.

Referrals
Make sure that the patient has been provided with all necessary referrals, including:
□ social services, if financial counseling is needed
□ cardiac rehabilitation program
□ dietitian
□ home health care agency, if needed.

Follow-up appointments
Make sure necessary follow-up appointments have been scheduled with:
□ doctor
□ diagnostic test center
□ surgeon, if necessary.

• Do his statements indicate an adequate understanding of prescribed medical and surgical treatments?
• Has he acknowledged the importance of following prescribed treatments and the need for lifelong care?
• Can he identify risk factors for complications or recurrence of MI?
• Does he appear willing to initiate life-style changes to reduce his risk of complications or recurrence of MI?
• Is he willing to participate in an exercise or cardiac rehabilitation program?

Emotional response to illness
Also evaluate the patient's emotional response to illness. Consider the following questions:
• Has the patient developed effective coping mechanisms to deal with the anxiety associated with MI diagnosis and fear of death?
• Has his anxiety diminished during the course of treatment?
• Has he expressed anxiety about resuming sexual activity or other aspects of life after MI?

Physical condition
Evaluate the patient's adherence to treatment and medication regimens, and consider the following questions:
• Has the patient experienced new or recurring symptoms, such as chest pain, dyspnea, dizziness, or syncope?
• Have his respiratory rate, pulse rate, and blood pressure returned to baseline levels?
• Is he able to tolerate gradual increases in activity?

• Do physical examination and diagnostic tests indicate adequate tissue perfusion, hemodynamic stability, and an absence of new or worsening ischemia?

• Are major complications, such as arrhythmias or heart failure, absent?

If specific patient outcomes aren't achieved, assess further to determine interfering factors. Discuss alternative approaches to adapting to the treatment regimen or life-style changes with the patient and family members, provide additional teaching or referrals, and set a date for reevaluation.

CHAPTER 5

Caring for patients with cardiac muscle disorders

Heart failure

In this condition, the heart fails to pump enough blood to meet the body's metabolic needs. Pump failure usually occurs in a damaged left ventricle (left ventricular failure). However, it may occur in the right ventricle, either as primary failure or as secondary failure brought on by left ventricular dysfunction. Left and right ventricular failure may also develop simultaneously. (See *Classifying heart failure.*)

Complications of heart failure include life-threatening pulmonary edema from congestion; brain, kidney, or other major organ failure from decreased perfusion; and myocardial infarction (MI) from insufficient oxygen.

Causes

Most patients with chronic heart failure have coronary artery disease (CAD), which may precipitate failure by causing MI. An infarction, depending on its size, can impair ventricular contractility and pump performance. Other causes of heart failure include:

• mechanical disturbances in ventricular filling during diastole, in which the ability of the ventricle to accept blood is impaired. Mechanical disturbances occur with hypertrophic cardiomyopathy or subendocardial fibrosis.

• systolic hemodynamic disturbances that increase cardiac work load and limit the heart's pumping ability. Such disturbances may result from mitral or aortic insufficiency, which cause high blood volume, and aortic stenosis or systemic hypertension, which increase resistance to ventricular emptying.

Other conditions may lead to heart failure, especially in patients with underlying heart disease. These include:

• arrhythmias, such as tachyarrhythmias, which reduce ventricular filling time; bradycardia, which reduces cardiac output; and arrhythmias that disrupt the synchrony of normal atrial and ventricular filling

• pregnancy or thyrotoxicosis, which increase cardiac output

• pulmonary embolism, which elevates arterial pressures

• infection, which increases the basal metabolic rate

• anemia, which increases oxygen demand by the tissues

• emotional stress

• increased physical activity

• increased sodium or water intake

• failure to follow treatment for underlying heart disease.

ASSESSMENT

Focus your initial assessment on the major signs of heart failure: increasing shortness of breath during exertion, orthopnea, and paroxysmal nocturnal dyspnea. Then consider associated symptoms. Carefully review the patient's health history, physical examination findings, and diagnostic test results.

Health history

The patient will likely complain of shortness of breath during exertion. He may also report having difficulty breathing when lying flat. For example, he may have to prop up his head with several pillows or sit in a chair to sleep comfortably. If heart failure has progressed, he may complain of waking shortly after falling asleep with a need to sit bolt upright to catch his breath.

In chronic heart failure, shortness of breath develops gradually over weeks or months and may be accompanied by a persistent cough. In acute heart failure, the patient may experience shortness of breath at rest.

Other complaints may include weakness, insomnia, anorexia, nausea, worsening fatigue, abdominal fullness or bloating, weight gain, and nocturia. Pe-

FactFinder

Classifying heart failure

Heart failure usually is classified by the site of failure (left or right ventricle, or both), but it may also be classified by level of cardiac output (high or low), stage (acute or chronic), and direction (forward or backward). These classifications represent different aspects of heart failure, not distinct diseases.

Site of failure

Left ventricular failure usually results from myocardial infarction (MI). Decreased left ventricular output causes fluid to accumulate in the lungs, which precipitates dyspnea, orthopnea, and paroxysmal nocturnal dyspnea. Other possible causes include high arterial blood pressure, myocardial ischemia, and aortic or mitral valve disease.

Right ventricular failure usually results from disorders that increase pulmonary vascular resistance, such as embolism, stenosis, or hypertension. Right ventricular failure produces congestive hepatomegaly, ascites, and subcutaneous edema.

Cardiac output

Heart failure with elevated cardiac output results from the heart's inability to keep pace with tissue demands for oxygenated blood. High-output failure occurs in arteriovenous fistula, hyperthyroidism, anemia, sickle cell anemia, beriberi, Paget's disease, and thyrotoxicosis.

Heart failure with reduced cardiac output results from diminished myocardial pumping ability. Low-output failure occurs in coronary artery disease, hypertension, primary myocardial disease, and valvular disease.

Stage

Acute failure occurs suddenly, for example, in an MI or when a cardiac valve ruptures. The sudden reduction in cardiac output causes systemic hypotension without peripheral edema. Acute failure may occur in any condition that causes stress in a diseased heart.

Chronic heart failure is gradual and sustained. Arterial blood pressure doesn't drop, but peripheral edema is present. Chronic failure may occur in cardiomyopathy or multivalvular disease or after healing in extensive MI.

Direction

In forward failure, the heart doesn't pump enough blood into the arterial system. The body retains sodium and water because of decreased renal perfusion and excessive proximal or distal tubular sodium reabsorption, caused by activation of the renin-angiotensin-aldosterone system.

In backward failure, one ventricle fails to empty normally, and end-diastolic ventricular pressures rise. This, in turn, increases pressure and volume in the atrium and venous system behind the affected ventricle. Elevated systemic venous and capillary pressures cause sodium and water retention and eventual transudation of fluid into the interstitial space.

ripheral edema may cause shoes and rings to fit tightly.

Medication history

Ask the patient what medications he's currently taking (over-the-counter and prescription). If he takes medication for chronic heart failure, find out if he has stopped taking his medication or altered the prescribed dosage.

Physical examination

During the initial examination, check for signs that reveal the duration and severity of heart failure. Patients with heart failure of recent onset appear acutely ill but are usually well nourished, whereas those with chronic heart failure often appear malnourished, even cachectic.

Observation may reveal dyspnea, anxiety, and respiratory distress. In mild heart failure, dyspnea may occur while the patient is lying down or active; in acute heart failure, it won't be affected by position or activity. If the patient has pulmonary edema, his cough will produce pink, frothy sputum.

Inspection may reveal cyanosis of the lips and nail beds, pale skin, diaphoresis, dependent peripheral and sacral edema, and jugular vein distention. Ascites may be present, especially in patients with right ventricular failure. In chronic heart failure, the patient may appear cachectic.

Palpation may reveal a rapid pulse and pulsus alternans. The skin may feel cool and clammy. Palpation and percussion of the abdomen may reveal hepatomegaly and splenomegaly. Percussion over the lung bases may reveal dullness if the lungs are filled with fluid.

Auscultation of blood pressure may reveal decreased pulse pressure, indicating reduced stroke volume. Auscultation may also disclose an S_3 gallop and a systolic murmur of mitral or tricuspid insufficiency. Auscultation of the lungs may reveal moist, bibasilar crackles. If pulmonary edema is present, typically you'll hear crackles accompanied by rhonchi and expiratory wheezing. However, if the patient has severe pulmonary edema, you may not be able to hear crackles, even if the lungs are filled with fluid, because air may not have sufficient space in which to move and thereby produce sounds.

Diagnostic test results

The following tests help identify heart failure:

• Electrocardiography (ECG) may show patterns of ventricular hypertrophy and myocardial ischemia, injury, or infarction. It may also reveal atrial enlargement and arrhythmias, especially atrial fibrillation and premature ventricular contractions.

• Chest X-ray may confirm the presence or absence of cardiomegaly and may show increased pulmonary vascular markings, interstitial edema, or pleural effusion.

• Pulmonary artery pressure monitoring may indicate elevated pulmonary artery diastolic pressure, pulmonary artery systolic pressure, and pulmonary artery wedge pressure (PAWP). In patients with left ventricular failure, it may disclose elevated left ventricular end-diastolic pressure; with right ventricular failure, elevated right atrial pressure or central venous pressure (CVP).

• Echocardiography may show ventricular hypertrophy, decreased contractility, and decreased ejection fraction and may identify valvular and other disorders causing heart failure.

• Arterial blood gas (ABG) values may show low partial pressure of oxygen in arterial blood (PaO_2) and low pH in patients with pulmonary edema. Because of decreased peripheral circulation, patients with pulmonary edema experience an accumulation of lactic acid and a corresponding decrease in pH and bicarbonate values (metabolic acidosis). Severely ill patients often show increased partial pressure of carbon dioxide in arterial blood ($PaCO_2$). However, with tachypnea, rapid breathing may cause a low $PaCO_2$.

NURSING DIAGNOSIS

Common nursing diagnoses for the patient with heart failure include:

• Decreased cardiac output related to reduced stroke volume resulting from mechanical, structural, or electrophysiologic cardiac problems

• Fluid volume excess related to pooling of blood in the pulmonary system, in the vena cava and systemic circulation, or in both

• Ineffective breathing pattern related to pulmonary congestion

• Activity intolerance related to impaired cardiac reserve

• Knowledge deficit related to the disorder and its treatment

• Sleep pattern disturbance related to anxiety, nocturia, orthopnea, and paroxysmal nocturnal dyspnea.

PLANNING

Based on the nursing diagnosis *decreased cardiac output,* develop the appropriate patient outcomes. For example, your patient will:

• regain hemodynamic stability as evidenced by vital signs, CVP, urine output, mental status, ABG levels, and PAWP, if warranted.

• exhibit warm, dry skin

• demonstrate clear or improved breath sounds during auscultation

• experience less frequent arrhythmias, as evidenced by ECG readings

• not experience dizziness, syncope, or chest pain, as indicated by verbal reports or behavior.

Based on the nursing diagnosis *fluid volume excess,* develop appropriate patient outcomes. For example, your patient will:

• exhibit absent or decreased distended neck veins, peripheral edema, or ascites

• indicate a willingness to maintain a fluid intake at the established daily limit

• maintain stable electrolyte values, as evidenced by laboratory tests

• maintain a stable weight.

Based on the nursing diagnosis *ineffective breathing pattern,* develop appropriate patient outcomes. For example, your patient will:

• maintain a stable baseline respiratory rate

• experience coughing, cyanosis, and dyspnea less frequently

• exhibit diminished cyanosis of the lips and nail beds.

Based on the nursing diagnosis *activity intolerance,* develop appropriate patient outcomes. For example, the patient will:

• help make decisions about the plan of care

• plan daily rest periods

• express a willingness to learn methods of conserving energy

• participate in prescribed physical activity.

Based on the nursing diagnosis *knowledge deficit,* develop appropriate patient outcomes. For example, your patient will:

• identify foods and medications containing sodium

• identify foods rich in potassium

• communicate an understanding of fluid restrictions

• demonstrate how to take his own pulse

• express a willingness to make necessary life-style changes

• list signs and symptoms that require immediate intervention

• communicate an understanding of the importance of following the prescribed treatment regimen and the need for keeping follow-up appointments.

Based on the nursing diagnosis *sleep pattern disturbance,* develop appropriate patient outcomes. For example, your patient will:

• communicate an understanding of his activity limitations

• manage his diuretic dosage to minimize sleep disturbance

• use effective relaxation techniques

• establish sleeping positions that minimize sleep disturbance

Treatments

Medical care of the patient with heart failure

Treatment for heart failure focuses on improving the heart's pumping ability. Heart failure can often be controlled quickly with medical interventions.

The doctor will probably place the patient on bed rest. Other measures include oxygen administration to increase oxygen supply to the myocardium and other vital organs and the use of antiembolism stockings to prevent venostasis and possible thromboembolism formation.

Drug therapy
Drugs used in the treatment of heart failure include:
• diuretics. Furosemide, hydrochlorothiazide, ethacrynic acid, bumetanide, spironolactone, or triamterene may be used to reduce total blood volume and circulatory congestion.
• aminophylline. This agent dilates bronchioles and promotes oxygenation.
• inotropic agents. Digoxin or other agents may be used to strengthen myocardial contractility. In acute heart failure, sympathomimetics, such as dopamine and dobutamine, are used. Amrinone, a powerful inotropic agent, may be used to increase contractility and cause arterial vasodilation.

• vasodilators. These drugs are used to decrease heart preload and work load. Nitroprusside, a balanced vasodilator, may be used to reduce preload and afterload.
• angiotensin-converting enzyme inhibitors. These agents decrease afterload.
• antiarrhythmics. Some of these agents, such as quinidine and amiodarone, are used to manage ventricular arrhythmias.
• potassium or magnesium supplements.

After recovery, most patients must continue to take digoxin and potassium supplements under medical supervision. If the patient has valvular dysfunction and recurrent acute heart failure, surgery may be necessary.

• report achieving undisturbed sleep for several hours.

IMPLEMENTATION

Treatment for heart failure seeks to minimize the patient's discomfort and prolong his life. It includes medical interventions, such as drug therapy, and life-style changes, such as modifications in diet, fluid intake, exercise, and sleep habits. (See *Medical care of the patient with heart failure.*)

Nursing interventions
Patients experiencing heart failure require immediate care to stabilize their condition, followed by measures to achieve relief of symptoms.

Initial care
• Place the patient in high Fowler's position. For severe symptoms, sit the patient upright with his legs dangling freely.
• Administer supplemental oxygen to help the patient breathe more easily.
• Draw arterial blood for ABG analysis and serum for other ordered studies, such as complete blood count, electrolyte levels, and enzyme levels.
• Obtain the patient's vital signs and reassess them frequently.

Timesaving tip: If possible, apply an automatic cuff to monitor the patient's blood pressure closely. For certain patients, the doctor may insert a catheter into the radial or femo-

artery to monitor blood pressure and obtain arterial samples.

• Start continuous cardiac monitoring, and check the patient's heart rate and rhythm for atrial fibrillation, which frequently accompanies heart failure.

• Insert an I.V. line. A central line may be used for monitoring cardiac status and for giving medications.

• Insert an indwelling urinary catheter if the patient is in acute heart failure or if aggressive diuresis is necessary.

• Obtain a baseline weight.

• Obtain a 12-lead ECG and assist with a chest X-ray.

• If echocardiography is scheduled, tell the patient what to expect and explain the test's purpose.

• Expect to assist with hemodynamic monitoring if the patient develops cardiogenic shock or responds poorly to treatment or if the cause of pulmonary edema is unclear. The doctor may insert a pulmonary artery (PA) catheter. Monitor cardiac output and PAWP. Seek to maintain cardiac output at 2.2 liters/minute/m^2 or higher and PAWP below 18 mm Hg.

Drug therapy

• Administer medications, as prescribed, and note the patient's responses. For example, 15 to 20 minutes after an I.V. bolus injection of furosemide (given over 1 to 2 minutes), tachypnea should decrease, and PaO$_2$ and urine output should increase. If, after aggressive therapy, the patient's PaO$_2$ falls below 50 mm Hg and his PaCO$_2$ rises above 50 mm Hg, intubation and mechanical ventilation may be warranted.

• If the patient receives morphine, monitor for hypoventilation. This drug is commonly used, especially in acute heart failure, to stimulate vasodilation, decrease preload, and reduce anxiety. However, some doctors reserve morphine for intubated patients.

• If the patient doesn't respond well to oxygen and the first dose of diuretic agents and his systolic pressure exceeds 100 mm Hg, administer a vasodilator. Monitor his pulse rate, respiratory rate, and blood pressure closely.

• If the patient's systolic pressure falls below 90 mm Hg, he may require inotropic drugs. In severe hypotension, expect to administer dobutamine and dopamine. Both of these drugs, however, can cause arrhythmias, so you'll need to monitor the patient closely. Correlate arterial blood pressure and other hemodynamic indices with assessment findings and titration of medications.

Alternatively, you may administer amrinone, possibly along with dopamine or dobutamine. If you do, watch for hypotension, arrhythmias, and thrombocytopenia.

If digoxin is administered, monitor its level and observe for signs of toxicity. Collect a blood sample for determining the drug's level 12 hours after an oral dose; note both the time the blood was obtained and the dose given on the laboratory slip. Also monitor serum potassium and magnesium levels because patients with hypokalemia and hypomagnesemia are more likely to develop digoxin toxicity. Once the crisis is over, digoxin may be used for long-term therapy.

Timesaving tip: If a patient has multiple I.V. and pressure-monitoring lines, color-code each one. For instance, label arterial lines with a piece of red tape, PA catheter lines with green tape, and central venous catheter lines with yellow tape.

• Monitor the patient for pulmonary edema, poor response to therapy, increasing acidosis, confusion, and a decreasing level of consciousness. Be prepared to assist with intubation and mechanical ventilation. Resuscitate the patient as needed.

Ongoing care
• Monitor the patient's ABG levels. Maintain his PaO_2 at 80 mm Hg and $PaCO_2$ at 30 to 40 mm Hg with a normal pH.
• Once the patient's condition has stabilized, monitor cardiopulmonary status at least every 4 hours. Assess blood pressure, apical and radial pulse rates and rhythm, respiratory rate, heart and breath sounds, and skin color. Keep in mind that arrhythmias, MI, and hypertensive crisis may accompany acute heart failure.
• If the patient is receiving nitroprusside, monitor his serum lactate and thiocyanate levels.
• Monitor intake and output. Weigh the patient daily, preferably before breakfast, to determine fluid retention. Measure the circumference of his feet and ankles and assess skin turgor.
• Assess the patient's ECG, serum electrolyte level, and digoxin level. Also monitor his blood urea nitrogen and creatinine levels. Impending renal shutdown may require emergency dialysis.
• Administer medications as prescribed and enforce fluid restrictions.
• Organize all activity to provide long rest periods.
• Assist the patient with range-of-motion exercises to prevent deep vein thrombosis from vascular congestion. Enforce bed rest and apply antiembolism stockings.
• Assist the patient with gradual increases in activity as his condition warrants.
• Report changes in the patient's condition immediately.

Patient teaching
The patient's compliance with treatment and his willingness to make lifestyle changes strongly influence the prognosis in heart failure. (See *Living with symptoms of heart failure.*) Therefore, effective patient teaching is essential. Use the following guidelines:

• Explain all diagnostic studies. Discuss the purpose of each study and explain the test procedure.
• Advise the patient to limit his sodium intake. Teach him which foods contain large amounts of sodium. Encourage him to read labels to spot high-sodium canned and commercially prepared foods.
• Instruct him to limit his fluid intake.
• Advise the patient to replace potassium and magnesium lost during diuretic therapy, if appropriate. He should take a prescribed potassium supplement and eat potassium-rich foods, such as bananas, apricots, orange juice, broccoli, raisins, and baked potatoes. Magnesium-rich foods include bran flakes, spinach, broccoli, bananas, peas, and skim milk.
• Stress the need for regular checkups.
• Teach the patient how to take his pulse.
• Advise the patient to weigh himself daily. Explain why this is important.
• Suggest ways the patient can stay active without exhausting himself. Encourage him to walk and to increase his distance gradually. Suggest that he plan most activities for the morning and rest periodically during the day. Discuss ways to simplify his routine and conserve energy. Help the patient delegate tasks.
• Stress the importance of taking medications as prescribed. Help the patient simplify his drug regimen and set up a medication schedule. Suggest he organize a week's worth of medication in a pillbox or empty egg carton and use an alarm clock to remind him when to take medication.
• Provide the patient with a wallet-size card listing medications and emergency phone numbers.
• If the patient is taking digoxin, teach him the signs of toxicity: anorexia, vomiting, confusion, a slow or irregular pulse rate, and blurred vision or visible yellow-green halos. An elderly pa-

Living with symptoms of heart failure

Explain to the patient that learning to recognize the common symptoms of heart failure helps prevent complications. Emphasize the importance of reporting his symptoms to the doctor.

Breathing difficulties
Explain to the patient that breathing difficulties occur when blood and fluids don't move fast enough through the lungs. Shortness of breath may occur with exertion, for example, when climbing stairs or lifting a small child. Teach the patient to stop what he's doing, steady himself, and rest until his shortness of breath passes. To increase activity tolerance, teach the patient to take sublingual nitroglycerin before the activity.

If the patient experiences shortness of breath while resting or lying down, tell him to try elevating the upper portion of the bed or raising his head with several pillows. If he's short of breath after a nap or a night's sleep, tell him to sit up, dangle his legs over the bedside, and wiggle his feet and ankles. Also suggest standing up and walking around to promote circulation.

Swelling
Explain to the patient that swelling occurs when the body fails to get rid of extra sodium and fluid. The patient may notice puffiness in his hands, ankles, or feet. Or he may see marks on

his skin from the elastic in his socks or rings on his fingers. Tell the patient he can test for swelling by pressing his finger against his skin and noting if a momentary impression remains.

To help reduce swelling, instruct the patient to elevate his hands or feet above the level of his heart. He should also weigh himself about the same time each day, using the same scale and wearing the same amount of clothing. Tell him to inform his doctor of any unexplainable gain of 2 lb (0.9 kg) or more.

Other symptoms
Instruct the patient to report the following symptoms to his doctor:
• a persistent dry cough
• frequent voiding during the night
• increased weakness and fatigue
• upper abdominal pain or a bloated feeling
• light-headedness, dizziness, or syncope.

Warn the patient to call the doctor immediately if he feels as if he can't breathe at all and his heart is pounding or if he coughs up pink, frothy sputum.

tient may also experience flulike symptoms. Tell him to report signs of toxicity immediately.
• If the patient is also taking cholestyramine (a lipid-lowering drug), tell him to take digoxin 2 to 3 hours before cholestyramine. That's because cholestyramine decreases digoxin levels or bioavailability.
• Tell the patient to take digoxin at least 1 to 2 hours before taking antacids

or eating high-bran foods. These can decrease the bioavailability of digoxin.
• Explain the importance of follow-up blood tests.
• Discuss any sleep pattern disturbances. If nocturia is a problem, help the patient adjust his diuretic schedule. For example, if he's taking a diuretic twice a day, advise him to take the second dose in the late afternoon or early evening. Otherwise, the drug's peak action will occur in the middle of the

Discharge TimeSaver

Ensuring continued care for the patient with heart failure

Review the following teaching topics, referrals, and follow-up appointments to ensure that your patient is adequately prepared for discharge.

Teaching topics
Make sure that patient teaching has been provided on the following topics and that the patient's learning has been evaluated:
☐ nature of heart failure, including compensation and decompensation
☐ self-monitoring
☐ activity limitations and energy conservation
☐ sodium and fluid restrictions
☐ medications, including dosage and possible adverse effects
☐ warning signs and symptoms of complications
☐ methods to relieve symptoms and minimize complications
☐ sources of additional information and support
☐ importance of learning cardiopulmonary resuscitation (for family members).

Referrals
Make sure that the patient has been provided with necessary referrals to:
☐ dietitian
☐ social services
☐ cardiac rehabilitation
☐ home health care agency
☐ medical equipment service for home oxygen.

Follow-up appointments
Make sure that the necessary follow-up appointments have been scheduled and that the patient has been notified:
☐ doctor
☐ surgeon
☐ additional laboratory tests.

night. If orthopnea is a problem, suggest that the patient elevate the head of his bed on blocks or sleep in a recliner. Raising the bed is more effective than piling up pillows. If dyspnea awakens the patient shortly after he goes to bed, encourage him to elevate his feet for an hour before lying down. Explain that his shortness of breath results from fluid in his legs returns to the circulation. By elevating his feet before retiring, he can prevent fluid accumulation in his lungs and allow his kidneys to clear excess fluid.

• Tell the patient to minimize edema in his legs and ankles by elevating his legs. (During an episode of acute heart failure, however, the patient should dangle his legs over the side of the bed to help drain fluid from his chest.)

• Instruct him to notify the doctor if he experiences dizziness, palpitations, blurred vision, an unusually irregular pulse rate, a pulse rate below 60 beats/minute, increased shortness of breath or fatigue during regular activities, a persistent dry cough, swelling in the legs or ankles that doesn't go away with elevation, decreased urine output, or a weight gain of 2 lb (about 0.9 kg) or more in 2 days.

• Teach relaxation techniques to reduce anxiety.

• Because the patient may be more susceptible to respiratory infections, suggest that he ask the doctor about pneumonia and influenza vaccinations. (See *Ensuring continued care for the patient with heart failure.*)

EVALUATION

When evaluating a patient's response to your nursing care, gather reassessment data and compare this information with patient outcomes specified in your plan of care.

Teaching and counseling
Begin by determining the effectiveness of patient teaching and counseling.
• Does the patient understand the nature of heart failure?
• Does he seem prepared to follow the treatment plan, adjust his activities, and restrict his sodium and fluid intake?
• Can he identify signs and symptoms that indicate a need for immediate medical attention?
• Can he identify foods and medications containing sodium and foods containing potassium?
• Can the patient or caregiver demonstrate how to take the patient's pulse?
• Does the patient understand the importance of following the prescribed treatment plan and the need for keeping follow-up appointments?
• Has the patient adjusted his medication schedule and taken other steps to minimize sleep disturbance?

Physical condition
Physical examination and diagnostic test results will also help to evaluate the effectiveness of care.
• Is the patient hemodynamically stable given your assessment of vital signs, CVP, PAWP (if warranted), urine output, mental status, and ABG levels?
• Does your inspection reveal an absence of distended neck veins, peripheral edema, or ascites?
• Does auscultation reveal clear breath sounds?
• Is the patient no longer experiencing dizziness, syncope, chest pain, or rapid pulse rate?
• Do ECG readings demonstrate an absence of arrhythmias?

• Are the patient's weight and baseline respiratory rate stable?
• Are his electrolyte levels normal?
• Have his cough, cyanosis, and dyspnea diminished?

Dilated cardiomyopathy

Formerly called congestive cardiomyopathy, dilated cardiomyopathy occurs when myocardial fibers sustain extensive damage. This disorder interferes with myocardial metabolism and grossly dilates the ventricles without proportional compensatory hypertrophy, thereby causing the heart to develop a globular shape. (See *How dilated cardiomyopathy affects the heart*, page 114.)

The heart contracts poorly during systole and ejects blood inefficiently. Consequently, a large volume of blood remains in the left ventricle after systole, causing signs of heart failure.

Dilated cardiomyopathy is most common in middle-aged men and is usually diagnosed in advanced stages. The prognosis is generally poor. Most patients, especially those past age 55, die within 2 years of onset of symptoms. Complications include intractable heart failure, arrhythmias (ventricular arrhythmias may lead to syncope and sudden death), and emboli.

Causes
The cause of most cardiomyopathies is unknown. It can result from myocardial destruction by toxic, infectious, or metabolic agents, such as viruses; endocrine or electrolyte disorders; and nutritional deficiencies. Other causes include sarcoidosis; muscle disorders, such as myasthenia gravis and progressive muscular dystrophy; and infiltrative disorders, such as hemochromatosis and amyloidosis.

How dilated cardiomyopathy affects the heart

In this disorder, gross dilation causes the heart to assume a globular shape. Because of ineffective ventricular contraction, a large volume of blood collects in the heart and the ventricular walls become chronically stretched and thinned.

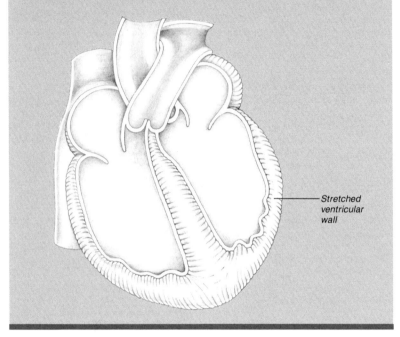

Stretched ventricular wall

Cardiomyopathy may be a complication of alcoholism. If so, cardiomyopathy may improve with abstinence but may recur if the patient resumes drinking. Cardiomyopathy may also result from rheumatic fever, especially among children with myocarditis.

Antepartum or postpartum cardiomyopathy may develop during the last trimester of pregnancy or within months after delivery. The cause of this cardiomyopathy is unknown. It occurs most frequently in multiparous women over age 30 with malnutrition or preeclampsia. In these patients, treatment may reverse the progression of cardiomyopathy and congestive heart failure and allow a normal pregnancy. However, if cardiomyopathy persists despite treatment, the prognosis is poor.

Specific drugs, including doxorubicin, cyclophosphamide, cocaine, and fluorouracil (rare), have been linked to dilated cardiomyopathy. In addition, familial forms may exist, possibly with an X-linked inheritance pattern.

ASSESSMENT

Clinical signs of this disorder closely resemble heart failure. The patient's medical and social histories may provide insight into factors contributing to development of dilated cardiomyopathy. You may also need to assess the patient's life-style to recommend an appropriate home health care program. Consider his age, occupation, family status, motivation to learn, and financial status.

Health history
The patient may complain of a gradual onset of shortness of breath. He may also report orthopnea, dyspnea on exertion, paroxysmal nocturnal dyspnea, fatigue, an irritating dry cough at night, heart palpitations, and vague chest pain.

Physical examination
Inspection may reveal peripheral edema, jugular vein distention, ascites, and peripheral cyanosis.

Palpation of peripheral pulses may reveal tachycardia (even at rest) and pulsus alternans in late stages; palpation of the abdomen may indicate hepatomegaly and splenomegaly.

Percussion may reveal hepatomegaly. Dullness is heard over lung areas that are filled with fluid. Auscultation of blood pressure may reveal a narrow pulse pressure. Cardiac auscultation may reveal irregular rhythms, diffuse apical impulses, pansystolic murmur (mitral and tricuspid insufficiency secondary to cardiomegaly, dilated chambers, and papillary muscle dysfunction), and S_3 and S_4 gallops. Lung auscultation may reveal crackles and rhonchi.

Diagnostic test results
No single test confirms dilated cardiomyopathy. The following tests help determine the presence and severity of complications:
• Electrocardiography (ECG) and angiography may rule out ischemic heart disease; ECG readings may also show biventricular hypertrophy, sinus tachy-cardia, atrial enlargement, ST-segment and T-wave abnormalities and, in 20% of patients, atrial fibrillation or left bundle-branch block. QRS complexes may show decreased voltage and poor R-wave progression.
• Chest X-ray may show moderate to marked cardiomegaly, usually in all chambers. It may also reveal pulmonary congestion, pulmonary venous hypertension, or pleural effusion. Pericardial effusion may be visible as a "hot water bottle" shape.
• Echocardiography may identify ventricular thrombi, global hypokinesia, and the degree of left ventricular dilation and dysfunction.
• Cardiac catheterization may show left ventricular dilation and dysfunction, elevated left ventricular and right ventricular end-diastolic pressure, diminished cardiac output, and normal coronary arteries.
• Gallium scans may help identify dilated cardiomyopathy and myocarditis.

NURSING DIAGNOSIS

Common nursing diagnoses for a patient with dilated cardiomyopathy include:
• Decreased cardiac output related to impaired cardiac contractility
• Fluid volume excess related to pooling of blood in the pulmonary system or in both the vena cava and systemic circulation
• Ineffective breathing pattern related to impaired gas exchange caused by pulmonary congestion
• Activity intolerance related to fatigue and shortness of breath caused by impaired cardiac reserve
• Altered nutrition: Less than body requirements, related to chronic fatigue and impaired absorption and transportation of nutrients caused by reduced cardiac output
• Knowledge deficit related to the disease process and methods of treatment

• Sleep pattern disturbance related to anxiety, nocturia, orthopnea, and paroxysmal nocturnal dyspnea
• Anxiety related to the need for significant changes in life-style and to the uncertainty of prognosis.

PLANNING

Based on the nursing diagnosis *decreased cardiac output,* develop appropriate patient outcomes. For example, your patient will:
• maintain or regain hemodynamic stability as shown by vital signs, central venous pressure (CVP), pulmonary artery wedge pressure (PAWP), urine output, arterial blood gas (ABG) levels, and mental status
• maintain clear breath sounds
• demonstrate a decrease in arrhythmias, as evidenced by ECG readings
• report that dizziness, syncope, and chest pain are absent
• exhibit warm, dry skin.

Based on the nursing diagnosis *fluid volume excess,* develop appropriate patient outcomes. For example, your patient will:
• maintain fluid intake at an established daily limit, with intake not exceeding output
• exhibit an absence or a decrease in peripheral edema and ascites
• return to his baseline weight and maintain a stable baseline weight for an extended period.

Based on the nursing diagnosis *ineffective breathing pattern,* develop appropriate patient outcomes. For example, your patient will:
• demonstrate a stable, baseline respiratory rate
• experience coughing and dyspnea less frequently.

Based on the nursing diagnosis *activity intolerance,* develop appropriate patient outcomes. For example, your patient will:

• demonstrate an understanding of activity limitations and express a willingness to comply with them
• plan daily rest periods
• demonstrate skill in conserving energy during activities.

Based on the nursing diagnosis *altered nutrition,* develop appropriate patient outcomes. For example, your patient will:
• communicate an understanding of the need for adequate nutrition
• express an understanding of the need for adequate protein intake.

Based on the nursing diagnosis *knowledge deficit,* develop appropriate patient outcomes. For example, your patient will:
• communicate an understanding of dilated cardiomyopathy, its symptoms, and its complications.
• describe sodium restrictions and identify high-sodium foods and medications.
• list signs and symptoms that indicate a need for immediate intervention
• demonstrate the ability to take his pulse
• express an understanding of the medical regimen, especially prescribed medications and their possible adverse effects
• communicate an understanding of the need for life-style changes and enhanced coping skills
• express an understanding of the importance of complying with lifelong treatment, including follow-up appointments.
• communicate an understanding of the preoperative, postoperative, and long-term care associated with heart transplantation.

Based on the nursing diagnosis *sleep pattern disturbance,* develop appropriate patient outcomes. For example, your patient will:
• manage his diuretic dosage so that it doesn't interfere with his sleep

• express an understanding of effective relaxation techniques

• report establishing comfortable sleeping positions

• report achieving undisturbed sleep for several hours.

Based on the nursing diagnosis *anxiety,* develop appropriate patient outcomes. For example, your patient will:

• express feelings of anxiety

• show fewer signs of anxiety and report diminishing feelings of anxiety

• help make decisions about the plan of care

• report using stress reduction techniques

• express a willingness to seek support from others.

IMPLEMENTATION

The prognosis for a patient with dilated cardiomyopathy depends on the cause and severity of the disorder, adherence to the treatment plan, and enactment of life-style changes. Drug therapy along with modifications in diet, fluid intake, exercise, and sleep positions may prolong the patient's life and help reduce his discomfort. (See *Medical care of the patient with dilated cardiomyopathy,* page 118.)

Nursing interventions

• Provide bed rest. Alternate rest with required activities and treatments. Provide personal care as needed to prevent fatigue.

• Administer oxygen as needed.

• Prepare the patient for diagnostic studies and assist as needed.

• Obtain a 12-lead ECG.

• Obtain a baseline weight.

• If the patient is receiving vasodilators, check his blood pressure and heart rate frequently. If he develops hypotension, decrease or stop the infusion, place him in the supine position, and elevate his legs to increase venous return and ensure cerebral perfusion.

• If the patient is receiving diuretics, monitor for increased urine output and resolving congestion (decreased crackles and dyspnea).

• If the patient is receiving digoxin, monitor for signs of hypokalemia, a precursor of digoxin toxicity, and toxicity.

• Monitor cardiopulmonary status closely. Assess the patient's blood pressure, apical and radial pulse rates and rhythms, respiratory rate, heart and breath sounds, and skin color. Watch for signs of worsening heart failure. Also, monitor for signs of pulmonary, cerebral, or peripheral thromboemboli.

• Monitor intake and output. Weigh the patient daily, ideally before breakfast and after voiding. Measure the circumference of the patient's feet and ankles and assess his skin turgor. Apply antiembolism stockings if necessary.

• Assess the patient's ECG, serum electrolyte level, and digoxin level daily. Also, monitor his blood urea nitrogen and creatinine levels.

• Provide range-of-motion exercises to prevent muscle atrophy while the patient is on bed rest.

• Consult with the dietitian to provide a diet that meets the patient's need for sodium and fluid restrictions.

• Therapeutic restrictions and an uncertain prognosis usually cause profound anxiety and depression. Encourage the patient and family members to express their feelings and help them identify effective coping strategies. Be flexible with visiting hours. If hospitalization is prolonged, seek permission for the patient to spend time away from the hospital. Make referrals for psychological counseling as needed. If the patient has a history of alcohol abuse, refer him to an alcohol counseling service and a support group, such as Alcoholics Anonymous.

Patient teaching

• Explain cardiomyopathy, including its causes, symptoms, and complications.

Treatments

Medical care of the patient with dilated cardiomyopathy

Treatment for dilated cardiomyopathy focuses on correcting the underlying causes and improving the heart's pumping ability. To help the patient conserve energy, the doctor may order bed rest and the administration of supplemental oxygen.

Often, fluid overload can be controlled with a diet that restricts sodium and fluid intake. Vitamins are recommended. In addition, the patient should not drink alcohol, and female patients should avoid pregnancy.

Drug therapy
Drugs used in the treatment of dilated cardiomyopathy include:
• inotropic agents. Digoxin or other agents may help strengthen myocardial contractility. During the acute stage, the doctor may order dobutamine or amrinone. In addition, the patient may receive outpatient dobutamine therapy two or three times each week.
• diuretics. These drugs reduce circulating blood volume and circulatory congestion.
• vasodilators. These drugs reduce preload and afterload, thereby decreasing congestion and increasing cardiac output. An angiotensin-converting enzyme inhibitor, such as captopril, may be used to reduce afterload and increase cardiac output. In acute heart failure, the doctor may order nitropruss-

ide I.V. or nitroglycerin I.V. to promote vasodilation. Oral vasodilators may be used thereafter.
• antiarrhythmics. These drugs may be administered if the patient develops arrhythmias.
• anticoagulants. Because patients with dilated cardiomyopathy commonly develop atrial and ventricular thrombi, they may require long-term anticoagulant therapy.
• corticosteroids. Administered selectively in patients with dilated cardiomyopathy, corticosteroids are likely to be used if myocardial inflammation is present.

Surgery
If the treatment regimen fails, surgery may be necessary and may include heart transplantation.

• Teach the patient or his caregiver how to take pulse rate and blood pressure. Tell the patient to weigh himself daily, preferably before breakfast. He should weigh himself at the same time each day, using the same scale and wearing the same amount of clothing.
• Emphasize the importance of lifelong follow-up care.
• Stress the importance of adhering to activity restrictions. Encourage frequent rest periods and explain the proper use of supplemental oxygen at home.
• Emphasize the importance of adhering to dietary modifications, which typically include sodium and fluid restric-

tions. Suggest seasoning food with spices and herbs or using a salt substitute.

Timesaving tip: Ask the dietitian to talk to the patient about reducing sodium and fluid intake. Then, assess the patient's understanding and answer any remaining questions about diet and vitamin supplements.
• Explain all medications and stress the importance of taking them according to the doctor's orders to prevent serious complications. Suggest ways that the patient can simplify his drug regimen and maintain a medication schedule. For example, suggest using a pill-

box to organize medications and an alarm clock to keep him on schedule.

• If the patient is taking digoxin, tell him to immediately report any signs of toxicity, such as anorexia, vomiting, confusion, a slow or irregular pulse rate, and blurred vision or visible yellow-green halos. Also, in elderly patients, flulike symptoms may indicate toxicity.

Timesaving tip: Provide the patient with printed instructions about each drug in his regimen. Give him a wallet-size card listing the names of his drugs, the doctor's phone number, and other emergency numbers.

• Discuss any sleep pattern disturbances. If nocturia is a problem, help the patient manage his diuretic schedule. For example, if he's taking a diuretic twice a day, advise him to take the second dose in the late afternoon or early evening. Otherwise, the drug's peak action will occur in the middle of the night. If orthopnea is a problem, recommend elevating the head of the bed or sleeping in a recliner. If the patient experiences shortness of breath soon after bedtime, suggest that he sit with his feet elevated for about an hour before going to bed. Explain that, when he lies down, the accumulated fluid in his legs reenters his circulation. Shortness of breath is caused by this fluid, which must be oxygenated by the lungs or cleared by the kidneys. Elevating his feet before retiring gives his lungs and kidneys a chance to adjust.

• Teach the patient relaxation techniques to help reduce his anxiety.

• Discuss the signs and symptoms that the patient must report immediately to the doctor, including an unusually irregular pulse or a pulse rate of less than 60 beats/minute; episodes of dizziness, blurred vision, increasing shortness of breath or fatigue; a persistent dry cough; palpitations; swelling in the legs or ankles that doesn't go away when his feet are elevated; decreased

urine output; or a weight gain of 2 lb (0.9 kg) or more in 2 days.

• Explain that the patient may be more susceptible to respiratory infection and suggest that he discuss pneumonia and influenza vaccinations with the doctor.

• Urge family members to learn cardiopulmonary resuscitation.

• Help the patient and family members cope with changes in life-style. Provide names of counselors, support groups, and other community resources, such as the local chapter of the American Heart Association. (See *Ensuring continued care for the patient with dilated cardiomyopathy,* page 120.)

• If the patient is scheduled for heart transplantation, describe preoperative and postoperative care, and explain long-term care requirements.

EVALUATION

When evaluating a patient's response to your care, gather reassessment data and compare this information with the patient outcomes specified in your plan of care.

Teaching and counseling

Determine the effectiveness of teaching and counseling.

• Does the patient understand the nature of dilated cardiomyopathy?

• Does he seem prepared to follow the medical treatment plan, adjust his activities, and restrict his sodium and fluid intake?

• Does he understand the importance of adequate nutrition?

• Can he identify signs and symptoms that indicate a need for immediate medical attention? Can he demonstrate how to take his pulse?

• Has he taken steps to minimize sleep disturbances?

• Does he fully understand the need for lifelong treatment?

• Is he willing to comply with activity limitations? Can he successfully demon-

Discharge TimeSaver
Ensuring continued care for the patient with dilated cardiomyopathy

Review the following teaching topics, referrals, and follow-up appointments to ensure that your patient is adequately prepared for discharge.

Teaching topics
Make sure that patient teaching has been provided on the following topics and that the patient's learning has been evaluated:
☐ the nature of dilated cardiomyopathy, including its signs and symptoms and complications
☐ techniques for self-monitoring blood pressure and pulse rate
☐ activity limitations and energy conservation techniques
☐ sodium and fluid restrictions
☐ medications, including dosage and possible adverse effects
☐ methods to relieve symptoms and minimize complications
☐ warning signs and symptoms of complications
☐ benefits of pneumonia and influenza vaccinations
☐ importance of learning cardiopulmonary resuscitation (for family members)

☐ preoperative and postoperative procedures and long-term care for patients undergoing heart transplantation.

Referrals
Make sure that the patient has been provided with appropriate referrals to:
☐ dietitian
☐ social services
☐ home health care agency
☐ medical equipment service for home oxygen
☐ psychological counseling
☐ support groups, such as Alcoholics Anonymous.

Follow-up appointments
Make sure that the necessary follow-up appointments have been scheduled and that the patient has been notified:
☐ doctor
☐ surgeon, if necessary
☐ additional laboratory tests.

strate energy conservation techniques? Is he willing to plan daily rest periods?
• Does his behavior suggest that he's less anxious? Has he told you that his feelings of anxiety have lessened? Is he willing to help plan his care? Does he accept support from others?

Physical condition
Physical examination and diagnostic test results will also help to evaluate the effectiveness of care.
• Is the patient hemodynamically stable given your assessment of vital signs, CVP, PAWP (if warranted), urine output, mental status, and ABG levels?
• Does your inspection indicate a decrease in peripheral edema and ascites? Is his skin warm and dry?

• Does auscultation reveal clear breath sounds?
• Is the patient no longer experiencing dizziness, syncope, chest pain, or rapid respirations?
• Do ECG readings demonstrate an absence of arrhythmias or a decrease in their frequency?
• Is the patient's weight stable?
• Has his cough and dyspnea diminished?

Hypertrophic cardiomyopathy

Also called idiopathic hypertrophic subaortic stenosis, hypertrophic car-

How hypertrophic cardiomyopathy affects the heart

Hypertrophic cardiomyopathy is characterized by a thickening and enlargement of the heart muscle. The heart muscle becomes less flexible and ventricular contraction is weakened. This decreases the amount of blood that circulates with each heartbeat.

In the illustration below, note how the septum has thickened and bulges into the left ventricle. The thickened septum partially blocks the aortic valve, diminishing blood flow from the left ventricle.

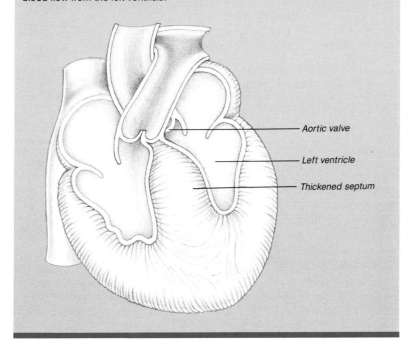

Aortic valve

Left ventricle

Thickened septum

diomyopathy is a primary disorder of cardiac muscle. In this disorder, the left ventricle becomes thickened, enlarged, and inflexible, which hinders normal expansion and contraction. This causes less blood to circulate with each heartbeat.

In the obstructive form of the disorder, the interventricular septum becomes thickened and bulges into the ventricle, partially blocking the aortic valve and hindering blood flow from the left ventricle, further decreasing circulatory volume. Cardiac output may be further compromised if the anterior leaflet of the mitral valve moves into the outflow tract during ventricular contraction. (See *How hypertrophic cardiomyopathy affects the heart.*)

In the nonobstructive form of the disorder, left ventricular hypertrophy occurs in the midventricular apex, or the lower portion of the septum.

Depending on whether hypertrophic cardiomyopathy is obstructive or non-obstructive, cardiac output may be low, normal, or high. Eventually, however, left ventricular dysfunction caused by rigidity and decreased compliance results in pump failure. When cardiac output is normal or high, hypertrophic cardiomyopathy may go undetected for years. Low cardiac output may lead to pulmonary hypertension and congestive heart failure.

The course of hypertrophic cardiomyopathy varies. The patient may deteriorate or remain stable for several years. Hypertrophic cardiomyopathy may lead to sudden death, usually in asymptomatic children and young adults after physical exertion. In most cases, sudden death results from ventricular arrhythmias, such as ventricular tachycardia or premature ventricular contractions.

Causes

About half of all hypertrophic cardiomyopathies are transmitted as an autosomal dominant trait. No other causes are known.

ASSESSMENT

In most cases, symptoms don't occur until the disease is advanced. In an asymptomatic patient, a family history may provide the most important diagnostic clues. In your nursing assessment, carefully consider the patient's health history, physical examination findings, and diagnostic test results.

Health history

The patient may complain of dyspnea on exertion and orthopnea. He may report fatigue, chest pain similar to angina (pain may occur when resting), and syncope (when resting or during exercise). Usually, symptoms occur in adult patients after physical exertion or emotional stress.

Physical examination

• Inspection of the carotid artery may show a rapidly rising carotid arterial pulse, followed by a secondary rise.
• Palpation of peripheral arteries may reveal a double impulse (pulsus biferiens). Palpation of the chest may reveal a double or triple apical impulse displaced laterally from the fifth intercostal space at the midclavicular line; a systolic thrill may be present. Palpation of the ankle and other extremities may reveal edema.
• Percussion may reveal bibasilar crackles if heart failure is present.
• Auscultation may reveal a harsh crescendo-decrescendo systolic murmur, heard after S_1 at the apex near the left sternal border. This pathognomonic murmur intensifies with Valsalva's maneuver or when the patient stands suddenly and decreases when the patient squats. The murmur also diminishes or disappears if heart failure develops. An S_4 may be audible.

Diagnostic test results

The following diagnostic test findings may help identify hypertrophic cardiomyopathy:
• Echocardiography may reveal ventricular hypertrophy. In the obstructive form of the disorder, findings may indicate a thickened asymmetrical interventricular septum. The septum may have a ground-glass appearance. Other findings in obstructive hypertrophic cardiomyopathy include poor septal contraction, abnormal motion of the anterior leaflet of the mitral valve during systole, and narrowing or occlusion of the left ventricular outflow tract. The left ventricular cavity appears small, with vigorous posterior wall motion but reduced septal excursion. If the disease is nonobstructive, echocardiography may reveal hypertrophy in various areas of the left ventricle.

• Cardiac catheterization may indicate elevated left ventricular end-diastolic pressure and mitral insufficiency.

• Electrocardiography (ECG) may show left ventricular hypertrophy, left anterior hemiblock, left axis deviation, and ventricular and atrial arrhythmias. In leads II, III, aV_F, or V_4 to V_6, ST-segment and T-wave abnormalities and Q waves may appear; these changes are caused by hypertrophy (rather than infarction).

• Chest X-ray may show a mild-to-moderate increase in heart size.

• Thallium scan may reveal defects in myocardial perfusion.

NURSING DIAGNOSIS

Common nursing diagnoses for a patient with hypertrophic cardiomyopathy include:

• Activity intolerance related to an imbalance between oxygen supply and demand

• Decreased cardiac output related to ventricular dysfunction

• Pain related to an imbalance between oxygen supply and demand resulting from outflow tract obstruction

• Fluid volume excess related to left ventricular rigidity caused by hypertrophic cardiomyopathy

• Anxiety related to the need for major changes in life-style and an uncertain prognosis.

PLANNING

Based on the nursing diagnosis *activity intolerance,* develop appropriate patient outcomes. For example, your patient will:

• express satisfaction with the prescribed activity level

• maintain his blood pressure and pulse and respiratory rates within prescribed limits during activity

• demonstrate skill in conserving energy while carrying out activities to tolerance level

• communicate an understanding of the relationship between hypertrophic cardiomyopathy and symptoms of activity intolerance.

Based on the nursing diagnosis *decreased cardiac output,* develop appropriate patient outcomes. For example, your patient will:

• maintain his blood pressure and pulse and respiratory rates within acceptable limits

• maintain adequate urine output

• demonstrate a decrease or absence of cardiac arrhythmias, as evidenced by ECG readings

• remain alert and oriented.

Based on the nursing diagnosis *pain,* develop appropriate patient outcomes. For example, your patient will:

• restrict his physical activity to the prescribed level

• comply with his medication regimen

• maintain an optimal weight

• report an absence of chest pain

• not experience ischemic changes, as evidenced by ECG findings.

Based on the nursing diagnosis *fluid volume excess,* develop appropriate patient outcomes. For example, your patient will:

• not report physical or emotional discomfort when adjusting to restrictions on fluid and sodium intake

• demonstrate an understanding of the signs and symptoms of acute fluid volume excess

• comply with the prescribed treatment regimen to minimize fluid retention

• demonstrate intact skin and the absence of infection.

Based on the nursing diagnosis *anxiety,* develop appropriate patient outcomes. For example, your patient will:

• express feelings of anxiety

• demonstrate fewer symptoms of anxiety and express that he feels less anxious

• participate in decisions about his care

• use stress reduction techniques to help alleviate anxiety

• seek support from others as needed.

IMPLEMENTATION

Treatment for hypertrophic cardiomyopathy seeks to reduce the patient's discomfort and prolong his life. Both medical interventions and life-style changes are necessary. (See *Medical care of the patient with hypertrophic cardiomyopathy*.)

Nursing interventions
• Monitor the patient frequently for signs of decreased cardiac output. Assess his blood pressure, pulse rate, respiratory rate, urine output, skin temperature, and mental status. Weigh the patient daily.
• If the patient is undergoing hemodynamic monitoring, assess pulmonary artery wedge pressure for evidence of increased ventricular pressure and volumes.
• Help the patient avoid fatigue. Explain the importance of bed rest in the acute stage. Provide personal care as needed. Schedule required activities and treatments to allow for periods of rest.
• Encourage exercise. If the patient is confined to bed, provide passive range-of-motion exercises to prevent muscle atrophy.
• Administer medications, such as propranolol, a beta-adrenergic blocker. When increasing the dosage of this drug, you may need to assess the patient's tolerance level. To do so, take his pulse to check for bradycardia, and have him stand and walk around slowly to check for orthostatic hypotension.

When discontinuing propranolol, don't stop abruptly; doing so may cause rebound effects that result in myocardial infarction or sudden death.
• Therapeutic restrictions and an uncertain prognosis usually cause profound anxiety and depression. Provide the patient and family members with support. Help them express their feelings and identify effective coping strategies. Provide diversional therapy by encouraging activities such as reading, listening to a portable radio or radio headset, or watching television, home movies, or videos (if equipment is available). Refer the patient or family members for psychological counseling, if warranted. Be flexible with visiting hours. If hospitalization is prolonged, try to obtain permission for the patient to spend time away from the hospital.

Patient teaching
• Teach the patient about hypertrophic cardiomyopathy, including its signs and symptoms and complications.
• Emphasize the importance of lifelong treatment.
• Describe the diagnostic workup.
• Emphasize the importance of following the doctor's orders regarding exercise. Explain that the type and amount of exercise allowed will depend on the severity of his disease. Tell the patient that he must avoid strenuous activities, such as running, and that he shouldn't exercise alone. Encourage frequent rest periods. Reinforce the doctor's restrictions on activities such as lifting, working, or driving.
• Teach the patient how to avoid Valsalva's maneuver. Also, instruct the patient to move slowly when sitting or standing up, as these movements can increase obstruction if performed suddenly.

Timesaving tip: Ask the dietitian to talk with the patient about dietary modifications for weight loss and reduced sodium and fluid intake. Then assess the patient's understanding and answer any remaining questions.
• Explain drug therapy and stress the importance of taking drugs as ordered. Provide the patient with printed information about his prescribed drugs.

Treatments

Medical care of the patient with hypertrophic cardiomyopathy

Treatment in hypertrophic cardiomyopathy focuses on relaxing the ventricle and relieving outflow tract obstruction.

Drug therapy
The drug of choice for treating hypertrophic cardiomyopathy is propranolol, a beta-adrenergic blocker, which slows the heart rate and increases ventricular filling by relaxing the obstructing muscle. These actions reduce the patient's angina, syncope, dyspnea, and arrhythmias. However, propranolol can aggravate symptoms of cardiac decompensation.

The doctor may order calcium channel blockers to reduce diastolic pressure and the severity of outflow tract gradients, and to increase exercise tolerance. Disopyramide may be used to reduce left ventricular contractility and the outflow tract gradient.

If heart failure occurs, the doctor may order amiodarone to reduce ventricular or supraventricular arrhythmias. If the patient has an atrioventricular block, amiodarone is contraindicated.

Vasodilators (such as nitroglycerin) and sympathetic stimulators (such as isoproterenol) are contraindicated in patients with hypertrophic cardiomyopathy because they may worsen outflow tract obstruction. Also, nitrates for chest pain are contraindicated, as they can cause syncope or sudden death.

Cardioversion
A patient who develops atrial fibrillation will require cardioversion. Because of the high risk of systemic embolism, expect to administer heparin before cardioversion and then to continue administration until converted to sinus rhythm. Also, the patient may receive anticoagulant therapy to reduce the incidence of emboli.

Activity and diet restrictions
Treatment usually includes restrictions on physical activity because exercise stimulates the release of catecholamines, which intensify outflow tract obstruction. If the patient is overweight, treatment also includes dietary modifications to help the patient lose weight, thus reducing the heart's work load.

Surgery
If drug therapy fails, surgery is indicated. Ventriculomyotomy (resection of the hypertrophied septum) alone or in combination with mitral valve replacement may ease outflow tract obstruction and relieve symptoms. However, ventriculomyotomy may cause complications, such as complete heart block and a ventricular septal defect.

• Tell the patient and family members that propranolol may cause depression, insomnia, and impotency and that they should notify the doctor if any of these adverse effects occur.

• Explain the importance of receiving antibiotic prophylaxis for subacute bacterial endocarditis before any dental work or surgery.

• Urge family members to learn cardiopulmonary resuscitation.

• If the patient is scheduled for cardiac surgery, provide preoperative and postoperative teaching.

• Hypertrophic cardiomyopathy is often inherited; therefore, advise couples of childbearing age to seek genetic counseling. If the patient has children, suggest that the children be evaluated for heart abnormalities.

• Help the patient and family members cope with the necessary changes in

Ensuring continued care for the patient with hypertrophic cardiomyopathy

Review the following teaching topics, referrals, and follow-up appointments to ensure that your patient is adequately prepared for discharge.

Teaching topics
Make sure that patient teaching has been provided on the following topics and that the patient's learning has been evaluated:
☐ the effect of hypertrophic cardiomyopathy on the heart muscle and circulation
☐ signs and symptoms of hypertrophic cardiomyopathy
☐ potential complications, such as heart failure
☐ need for lifelong treatment and follow-up
☐ activity restrictions
☐ dietary restrictions
☐ the actions and adverse effects of medications, including beta-adrenergic blockers, calcium channel blockers, and anticoagulants, if the patient has experienced atrial fibrillation
☐ preoperative care, postoperative care, and long-term care (for patients undergoing ventriculomyotomy)

☐ need for genetic counseling
☐ importance of learning cardiopulmonary resuscitation (for family members)
☐ need for antibiotic prophylaxis before dental work or surgery
☐ sources of additional information and support.

Referrals
Make sure that the patient has been provided with appropriate referrals to:
☐ dietitian
☐ home health care agency
☐ psychological counseling
☐ social services.

Follow-up appointments
Make sure that the appropriate follow-up appointments have been scheduled and that the patient has been notified:
☐ doctor
☐ surgeon
☐ additional laboratory tests.

life-style. Provide names of counselors, support groups, and other community resources, such as the local chapter of the American Heart Association. (See *Ensuring continued care for the patient with hypertrophic cardiomyopathy.*)

EVALUATION

When evaluating the patient's response to your nursing care, gather reassessment data and compare this information to the patient outcomes specified in your plan of care.

Teaching and counseling
Determine the effectiveness of teaching and counseling.
• Does the patient understand the nature of hypertrophic cardiomyopathy?
• Is he willing to adhere to the treatment plan and follow recommendations concerning modifications in diet and activity level?
• Does he understand why he tires so easily? Does he demonstrate energy conservation skills?
• Does he understand the signs and symptoms of acute fluid volume excess? Does he seem willing to comply with prescribed treatment to minimize fluid retention?

• Does he seem able to handle the stress associated with alterations in life-style and a poor prognosis? Has he expressed feelings of anxiety? Have symptoms of anxiety increased or diminished? Does he participate in decisions about his care? Has he learned to use stress reduction techniques?

Physical condition
Physical examination and diagnostic tests will help evaluate the effectiveness of care. Consider the following questions:
• Is the patient alert and oriented?
• Do ECG readings indicate an absence or decrease in arrhythmias? Do they indicate an absence of ischemic changes?
• Are blood pressure and pulse and respiratory rates within acceptable limits, both during activity and when at rest?
• Is the patient's urine output greater than 250 ml in an 8-hour period?
• Has his weight remained within the targeted range?
• Does he report continued chest pain?
• Is his skin intact and are signs of infection absent?

Restrictive cardiomyopathy

A less common disorder of the myocardial musculature (the least common in Western countries), restrictive cardiomyopathy is characterized by endocardial fibrosis and thickening. As the disease progresses, increasing myocardial rigidity leads to poor distention during diastole and incomplete ventricular filling, causing a low cardiac output. Decreased output leads to pulmonary and systemic congestion and decreased perfusion. The patient may also develop insufficiency in the atrioventricular valves. Severe cases of restrictive cardiomyopathy are irreversible.

Causes
Precisely what causes primary restrictive cardiomyopathy is unknown. However, restrictive cardiomyopathy syndrome, a manifestation of amyloidosis, results from infiltration of amyloid into the intracellular spaces in the myocardium, endocardium, and subendocardium. This syndrome may be seen in sarcoidosis, neoplasms, endomyocardial fibrosis, radiation sickness, and scleredema.

ASSESSMENT

Besides reviewing the patient's health history, physical examination findings, and diagnostic test results, check his medical records for a history of amyloidosis.

Health history
The patient may complain of dyspnea on exertion, which may progress to paroxysmal nocturnal dyspnea, and orthopnea. He may also report fatigue, chest pain, and weight gain.

Physical examination
Throughout the examination, check for signs of fluid retention.

Inspection may reveal peripheral edema, jugular vein distention, tachypnea, ascites, and peripheral cyanosis.

Palpation of peripheral pulses may reveal tachycardia. Palpation of the carotid artery may reveal rapid pulsations with a biphasic upstroke. Irregular pulses may be due to the presence of heart block, atrial arrhythmias, or tachycardia-bradycardia syndrome. Palpation also may reveal peripheral edema, hepatomegaly and splenomegaly, and ascites.

Percussion may detect dullness over lung areas that are fluid filled, indicating pulmonary congestion and hepatomegaly.

Cardiac auscultation may reveal S_3 and S_4 gallops; lung auscultation may reveal crackles and rhonchi.

Diagnostic test results

The following test results may help detect restrictive cardiomyopathy:

• Chest X-ray may show massive cardiomegaly, affecting all four heart chambers, indicating the disease is in an advanced stage.

• Echocardiography helps rule out constrictive pericarditis as the cause of restricted filling by revealing increased left ventricular muscle mass and differences in end-diastolic pressures between the ventricles. Echocardiography may also show narrowed chambers, atrial enlargement, and thickening of the left ventricular wall, with resulting poor contractility.

• Electrocardiography (ECG) may show low-voltage complexes, hypertrophy, or atrioventricular conduction defects.

• Cardiac catheterization demonstrates increased left ventricular end-diastolic pressure and helps rules out constrictive pericarditis as the cause of restricted filling.

• Transvenous endomyocardial biopsy may indicate an underlying cause, such as amyloidosis or endomyocardial fibrosis.

NURSING DIAGNOSIS

Common nursing diagnoses for a patient with restrictive cardiomyopathy include:

• Decreased cardiac output related to restricted ventricular filling

• Fluid volume excess related to medical condition, diuretic therapy, or both

• Ineffective breathing pattern related to pulmonary congestion

• Activity intolerance related to imbalance between oxygen supply and demand

• Knowledge deficit related to disease process and treatment

• Sleep pattern disturbance related to anxiety, nocturia, orthopnea, and paroxysmal nocturnal dyspnea

• Anxiety related to necessity for significant life-style changes and to an uncertain prognosis.

PLANNING

Based on the nursing diagnosis *decreased cardiac output,* develop appropriate patient outcomes. For example, your patient will:

• maintain or regain hemodynamic stability as evidenced by his vital signs, urine output, mental status, and arterial blood gas (ABG) levels

• maintain clear breath sounds, as demonstrated during auscultation

• experience fewer arrhythmias or none at all, as evidenced by his ECG readings

• not experience dizziness, syncope, or chest pain

• exhibit warm, dry skin.

Based on the nursing diagnosis *fluid volume excess,* develop appropriate patient outcomes. For example, your patient will:

• maintain fluid intake at established daily limits; intake shouldn't exceed output

• return to his baseline weight and maintain this weight

• exhibit intact skin, free from infection

• maintain stable electrolyte levels within established parameters

• not experience electrolyte imbalances secondary to the use of diuretics.

Based on the nursing diagnosis *ineffective breathing pattern,* develop appropriate patient outcomes. For example, your patient will:

• demonstrate a return to his baseline respiratory rate and maintain this rate

• maintain ABG levels within established limits

• demonstrate adequate oxygenation, evidenced by an alert mental status and the absence of cyanosis
• demonstrate an absence or decrease in coughing and dyspnea.

Based on the nursing diagnosis *activity intolerance,* develop appropriate patient outcomes. For example, your patient will:
• identify and comply with activity limitations
• plan daily rest periods
• demonstrate skill in conserving energy while carrying out activities.

Based on the nursing diagnosis *knowledge deficit,* develop appropriate patient outcomes. For example, your patient will:
• express an understanding of the disorder and its symptoms and complications
• communicate an understanding of sodium and fluid restrictions
• demonstrate how to take his pulse
• communicate an understanding of the medical regimen, especially prescribed medications and their adverse effects
• express an understanding of necessary life-style changes and techniques to enhance coping
• communicate an understanding of signs and symptoms that require immediate intervention
• agree to the importance of following lifelong treatment and keeping follow-up appointments.

Based on the nursing diagnosis *sleep pattern disturbance,* develop appropriate patient outcomes. For example, your patient will:
• manage his diuretic dosage to minimize sleep disturbances
• demonstrate effective relaxation techniques
• establish sleeping positions that minimize sleep disturbances
• report undisturbed sleep for the specified number of hours.

Based on the nursing diagnosis *anxiety,* develop appropriate patient outcomes. For example, your patient will:
• express feelings of anxiety
• participate in decisions related to his care
• perform stress reduction techniques to help alleviate anxiety
• seek help from appropriate agencies or individuals
• exhibit fewer symptoms of anxiety
• report that he feels less anxious.

IMPLEMENTATION

Treatment for restrictive cardiomyopathy combines medical interventions with life-style changes with the goals of reducing the patient's discomfort and prolonging his life. (See *Medical care of the patient with restrictive cardiomyopathy,* page 130.)

Nursing interventions
• Provide bed rest.
• Perform personal care as needed to prevent undue fatigue.
• Alternate required activities and treatments with periods of rest.
• Administer oxygen as needed.
• Obtain a 12-lead ECG.
• Obtain baseline vital signs and weight.
• Prepare the patient for diagnostic studies and assist as needed.
• Administer medications, as prescribed, and monitor their effects.

If the patient is receiving digoxin, monitor for indications of toxicity, such as ventricular arrhythmias. Observe for signs of hypokalemia, which may predispose the patient to digoxin toxicity. Digoxin should be used with caution in these patients because of their sensitivity to the drug. Customary doses may lead to serious arrhythmias. If the patient is receiving dobutamine I.V., monitor his ECG for arrhythmias and frequently assess his vital signs.
• Monitor the patient's cardiopulmonary status closely. Assess his blood

Treatments

Medical care of the patient with restrictive cardiomyopathy

Because no cure currently exists for restricted ventricular filling, treatment focuses on easing symptoms of congestive heart failure (CHF). It may include digitalis glycosides, diuretics, and a restricted sodium diet. The doctor may order bed rest and oxygen to help the patient conserve energy.

Oral vasodilators, such as isosorbide dinitrate, prazosin, and hydralazine, may be used to help control intractable CHF. Patients with atrial fibrillation or those on prolonged bed rest may require anticoagulants to prevent thrombophlebitis. Antiarrhythmics or emergency treatment for acute pulmonary edema may be necessary as well.

pressure, apical and radial pulse rates and rhythms, respiratory rate, heart and breath sounds, and skin color. Watch for signs of worsening heart failure.
• Monitor intake and output. Weigh the patient daily, ideally before breakfast. Measure the circumference of his feet and ankles and assess his skin turgor.
• Assess the patient's ECG, serum electrolyte level, and digoxin level daily. Also monitor his blood urea nitrogen and creatinine levels.
• Provide active or encourage passive range-of-motion exercises to prevent muscle atrophy while the patient is on bed rest.
• Consult with the dietitian to provide a diet that includes sodium and fluid restrictions and that's acceptable to the patient.
• Therapeutic restrictions and an uncertain prognosis usually cause profound anxiety and depression. Encourage the patient and family members to express their feelings, and help them identify coping strategies. Be flexible with visiting hours. If hospitalization is prolonged, obtain permission for the patient to spend time away from the hospital. Refer the patient for psychological counseling, if needed.

Patient teaching
• Teach the patient about restrictive cardiomyopathy and its symptoms and potential complications.
• Teach the patient or his caregiver how to take a pulse and blood pressure reading. Advise the patient to weigh himself daily, preferably before breakfast. He should weigh himself at the same time each day, using the same scale and wearing the same amount of clothing.
• Discuss activity restrictions and encourage frequent rest periods. Explain the use of home oxygen, if warranted.
• Advise the patient to follow a sodium-restricted diet. Suggest the use of herbs, spices, or a salt substitute when seasoning food. Teach the patient about fluid restrictions and explain the need to eat potassium-rich foods to replace potassium lost because of diuretic therapy.
• Explain the patient's drug therapy, and stress the importance of taking medications exactly as prescribed to prevent serious complications. If he's taking digoxin, explain the signs of toxicity, such as anorexia, vomiting, confusion, a slow or irregular pulse rate, and blurred vision or yellow-green halos. Also, flulike symptoms may be a sign of toxicity in elderly patients. Tell the patient to immediately

Discharge TimeSaver

Ensuring continued care for the patient with restrictive cardiomyopathy

Review the following teaching topics, referrals, and follow-up appointments to ensure that your patient is adequately prepared for discharge.

Teaching topics

Make sure that patient teaching has been provided on the following topics and that the patient's learning has been evaluated:
☐ explanation of the disorder and its symptoms and complications
☐ pulse-taking techniques
☐ activity restrictions and energy conservation techniques
☐ sodium restrictions
☐ fluid restrictions, when appropriate
☐ medications, including their purpose, dosage, and adverse effects
☐ measures to relieve symptoms and minimize complications
☐ warning signs and symptoms of complications
☐ benefits of pneumonia and influenza vaccinations
☐ importance of learning cardiopulmo-

nary resuscitation (for family members)
☐ sources of additional information and support.

Referrals

Make sure that the patient has been provided with appropriate referrals to:
☐ dietitian
☐ social services
☐ home health care agency
☐ medical equipment service for home oxygen
☐ psychological counseling.

Follow-up appointments

Make sure that the necessary follow-up appointments have been scheduled and that the patient has been notified:
☐ doctor
☐ additional laboratory tests.

---

report signs of toxicity to the doctor. Provide the patient with printed information for each medication.

• Help the patient determine why he can't sleep. If nocturia is a problem, advise the patient on managing his diuretic schedule. If orthopnea is a problem, suggest he try different sleep positions. Teach relaxation techniques to help reduce anxiety.

• Explain the symptoms that must be reported to the doctor: an unusually irregular pulse rate or a pulse rate of less than 60 beats/minute; blurred vision; dizziness; increases in shortness of breath, fatigue, or chest pain; a persistent dry cough; heart palpitations; swelling in the legs or ankles that doesn't go away when his legs are elevated; decreased urine output; or a weight gain of 2 lb (0.9 kg) or more in 2 days.

• Because the patient may be susceptible to respiratory infections, suggest that he talk to the doctor about pneumonia and influenza vaccinations.

• Urge family members to learn cardiopulmonary resuscitation.

• Help the patient and family members cope with changes in life-style. Provide them with names of counselors, support groups, and other community resources, for example, the local chapter of the American Heart Association. (See *Ensuring continued care for the patient with restrictive cardiomyopathy.*)

EVALUATION

When evaluating a patient's response to your nursing care, gather reassessment data and compare this information with the patient outcomes specified in your plan of care.

Teaching and counseling
Begin by determining the effectiveness of teaching and counseling.

• Does the patient express an understanding of the disorder?

• Is he willing to follow the treatment plan? Does he understand the rationales for activity and diet restrictions?

• Can he identify signs and symptoms that indicate a need for immediate attention?

• Can the patient or his caregiver demonstrate the proper method for taking a pulse?

• Has the patient taken steps to minimize any sleep disturbances?

• Does he plan daily rest periods? Does he demonstrate skill in conserving energy while carrying out activities?

• Does his behavior suggest that he's less anxious? Has he told you that his feelings of anxiety have lessened? Is he willing to help plan his care? Does he accept support from others?

Physical condition
Physical examination and diagnostic tests will help evaluate the effectiveness of care.

• Is the patient hemodynamically stable given your assessment of vital signs, urine output, mental status, and ABG levels?

• Is his skin intact and of normal temperature?

• Is the patient no longer experiencing dizziness, syncope, chest pain, or rapid respirations?

• Do ECG readings demonstrate an absence of arrhythmias or a decrease in their frequency?

• Are electrolyte levels within normal limits?

• Is the patient's weight stable?

• Are his intake and output equal?

Caring for patients with inflammatory disorders

Myocarditis

Myocarditis refers to a focal or diffuse inflammation of the myocardium. Usually uncomplicated and self-limiting, this disorder may be acute or chronic and can occur at any age. In many patients, myocarditis doesn't produce specific cardiovascular symptoms or electrocardiogram (ECG) abnormalities.

Recovery is usually spontaneous and without residual defects. Myocarditis may become severe and induce myofibril degeneration, right and left ventricular failure with cardiomegaly, and arrhythmias. Rarely, it may lead to cardiomyopathy. Myocarditis may also recur or produce chronic valvulitis (when it results from rheumatic fever) or thromboembolism. (See *Complications of myocarditis.*)

Causes

Myocarditis may result from any of the following causes:
• viral infections (the most common cause of myocarditis in North America and western Europe), including coxsackievirus A and B and, possibly, poliomyelitis, influenza, rubeola, rubella, human immunodeficiency virus, adenoviruses, and echoviruses
• bacterial infections — including diphtheria, tuberculosis, typhoid fever, tetanus, and Lyme disease — and staphylococcal, pneumococcal, and gonococcal bacterial infections
• hypersensitive immune reactions, such as acute rheumatic fever and postcardiotomy syndrome
• radiation therapy, especially large doses to the chest during treatment of lung or breast cancer
• exposure to toxic substances, which may occur in chronic alcoholism
• parasitic infections, especially toxoplasmosis and South American trypanosomiasis (Chagas' disease) in infants and immunosuppressed adults
• helminthic infections, such as trichinosis.

A rare type, giant cell myocarditis, is of unknown cause.

ASSESSMENT

Because myocarditis is difficult to diagnose, obtain a thorough medical history. Be especially alert to a possible cause of the disorder. For example, the patient may report a recent upper respiratory tract infection with fever, viral pharyngitis, or tonsillitis. This information may suggest a viral infection that could lead to myocarditis.

Health history

The patient may complain of nonspecific symptoms, such as fatigue, dyspnea, palpitations, persistent tachycardia, and persistent fever. Occasionally, the patient may complain of a mild, continuous pressure or soreness in the chest. This pain is unlike the recurring, stress-related pain of angina pectoris.

Physical examination

Findings vary depending on the nature of the illness and the presence or absence of complications.

Inspection may reveal a flushed appearance if fever is present. The patient may appear tired and dyspneic. If myocarditis has resulted in heart failure, you may notice jugular vein distention. Fever may be present.

Palpation of the patient's pulse reveals resting or exertional tachycardia, which may be disproportionate to the degree of fever.

Auscultation usually reveals S_3 and S_4 gallops, a muffled S_1, possibly a murmur of mitral insufficiency (from papillary muscle dysfunction) and, if the patient has pericarditis, a pericardial friction rub.

Complications of myocarditis

Use the diagram below to quickly note how delayed or inadequate treatment of myocarditis can result in severe complications.

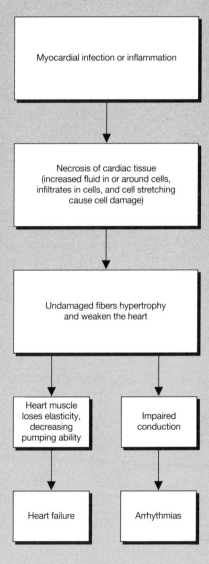

Diagnostic test results

Endomyocardial biopsy confirms a diagnosis of myocarditis. The following test results can support the diagnosis:

• Cardiac enzyme levels, including creatine kinase (CK), MB isoenzyme of CK (CK-MB), serum aspartate aminotransferase (formerly SGOT), and lactate dehydrogenase, are elevated.

• White blood cell count and erythrocyte sedimentation rate are elevated.

• Antibody titers are elevated, such as antistreptolysin-O titer, when myocarditis results from rheumatic fever.

• ECG may show diffuse ST-segment and T-wave abnormalities (similar to pericarditis), conduction defects (a prolonged PR interval), and other ventricular and supraventricular ectopic arrhythmias.

• Cultures of stool, throat, pharyngeal washing, or other body fluids may identify the causative bacteria or virus.

NURSING DIAGNOSIS

Common nursing diagnoses for a patient with myocarditis include:

• Activity intolerance related to fatigue, dyspnea, and palpitations

• Hyperthermia related to inflammatory process

• Altered nutrition: Less than body requirements, related to poor cardiac output

• Decreased cardiac output related to decreased myocardial contractility resulting from inflammatory process

• Diversional activity deficit related to activity restrictions.

PLANNING

Based on the nursing diagnosis *activity intolerance,* develop appropriate patient outcomes. For example, your patient will:

• continue bed rest as prescribed

• seek assistance when performing activities of daily living

• tolerate usual activity level once myocarditis is resolved.

Based on the nursing diagnosis *hyperthermia,* develop appropriate patient outcomes. For example, your patient will:

• experience a reduction in fever

• not experience dehydration, seizures, or other complications associated with hyperthermia

• maintain a normal temperature without the use of antipyretics, once myocarditis is resolved.

Based on the nursing diagnosis *altered nutrition,* develop appropriate patient outcomes. For example, your patient will:

• maintain adequate nutrition as evidenced by normal weight and normal fluid volume status

• demonstrate improved strength and activity tolerance

• maintain caloric and protein intake adequate for metabolic needs

• maintain serum albumin, blood urea nitrogen (BUN), and creatinine levels within established limits.

Based on the nursing diagnosis *decreased cardiac output,* develop appropriate patient outcomes. For example, your patient will:

• maintain hemodynamic stability as evidenced by vital signs, urine output, and mental status

• not experience severe chest pain related to myocardial ischemia

• not experience cardiac arrhythmias, as evidenced by his ECG readings

• not experience fluid retention, as evidenced by his intake and output measurements and the absence of dyspnea and peripheral edema.

Based on the nursing diagnosis *diversional activity deficit,* develop appropriate patient outcomes. For example, your patient will:

• communicate a willingness to participate in quiet activity

• choose from available activities

Treatments

Medical care of the patient with myocarditis

Treatment for myocarditis usually consists of anti-infective drugs to combat the underlying causative infection, modified bed rest to decrease the heart's work load, and careful management of complications.

Treating complications
Complications of myocarditis include left ventricular failure and arrhythmias.

Left ventricular failure
The patient with left ventricular failure may require:
• activity restriction to minimize myocardial oxygen consumption
• supplemental oxygen therapy to increase oxygen supply to the myocardium and other tissues
• sodium-restricted diet to decrease fluid retention
• diuretics to decrease fluid retention
• a digitalis glycoside to increase myocardial contractility
   Note that the digitalis glycoside must be administered carefully because patients with myocarditis may be sensitive even to small doses and should be watched for signs of toxicity.

Arrhythmias
Arrhythmias necessitate prompt administration of antiarrhythmics, such as quinidine or procainamide. Drugs that depress myocardial contractility, such as beta blockers, are usually avoided. Thromboembolism requires anticoagulant therapy.

Other complications
The doctor may order corticosteroids or other immunosuppressants. However, use of these agents is controversial and usually limited to combating life-threatening complications, such as intractable heart failure. Nonsteroidal anti-inflammatory drugs, such as ibuprofen and aspirin, are contraindicated during the acute phase (first 2 weeks) of viral myocarditis because they can increase myocardial damage. They may be prescribed later in the course of therapy.

• participate in chosen activities that conform to prescribed physical restrictions
• report feeling less bored.

IMPLEMENTATION

Treatment for myocarditis usually includes drug therapy along with measures to encourage rest and decrease the heart's work load. (See *Medical care of the patient with myocarditis.*)

Nursing interventions
• In acute situations, stress the importance of bed rest. Assist the patient with bathing, if necessary. Provide a bedside commode because its use places less stress on the heart than a bedpan.

Timesaving tip: If the patient uses a bedside commode, make sure that toilet tissue isn't out of reach. Suggest that the maintenance department install a toilet tissue holder on an arm of each bedside commode. Also, attach a plastic bag containing moist towelettes for hand washing. This will save you the time and trouble of searching for toilet supplies.
• Promote participation in activities that aren't physically demanding. Find out the patient's interests and hobbies. If possible, ask family members to bring items from home that may stimulate the patient's interests.

• Engage the patient in conversation while carrying out procedures. To help reduce anxiety, let the patient express any concerns about the effects of activity restrictions on his responsibilities and routines. Reassure the patient that the restrictions are temporary.
• Administer oxygen as needed.
• Administer parenteral anti-infectives, as prescribed. Also administer antipyretics as warranted.
• Monitor the patient for indications of impending complications. Watch for signs of heart failure, such as increasing dyspnea, tachycardia, persistent cough, and jugular vein distention. Check the patient's pulse rate, cardiac monitor, or ECG for signs of arrhythmias. Be prepared to take immediate action if a life-threatening arrhythmia occurs. Also observe for indications of thrombophlebitis, such as complaints of calf pain or tenderness. Monitor the patient's temperature.
• Evaluate arterial blood gas values regularly to monitor oxygenation.
• Look for signs of digitalis toxicity (anorexia, nausea, vomiting, blurred vision, cardiac arrhythmias) and for complicating factors that may potentiate toxicity, such as electrolyte imbalance, hyperkalemia, and hypoxia.

Patient teaching
Include the following in your patient-teaching program:
• Explain the disorder and its causes and complications.
• If an endomyocardial biopsy is scheduled, explain that it can confirm myocarditis. Describe the procedure and point out that it will be performed in the cardiac catheterization laboratory or in the operating room. Tell the patient he'll be sedated but awake. Explain other diagnostic tests as well.
• Teach the patient to take medications exactly as prescribed and not to discontinue them because he feels better. Teach the patient that nonsteroidal anti-inflammatory drugs, such as ibuprofen and aspirin, relieve inflammation, whereas antibiotics combat specific microorganisms. If the patient is to take a digitalis glycoside at home, teach him to time his pulse rate for a full minute before taking each dose. Tell him that if his heart rate falls below the predetermined rate (usually 60 beats/minute) he shouldn't take the dose and should notify the doctor. Describe other signs of digitalis toxicity, such as anorexia, nausea, confusion, and flulike symptoms in elderly people.
• Stress the importance of restricting activities for as long as the doctor orders. During recovery, recommend that the patient resume normal activities gradually and avoid competitive sports. Offer advice on ways to save energy, such as by alternating light and heavy tasks and by resting frequently.
• Advise the patient to notify the doctor of any chest pain, increasing shortness of breath, unusual fatigue, swelling, and weight gain. He should also report a sore throat, flulike symptoms, or a recurrent fever immediately.
• As needed, inform the patient about local sources of information and support, including the local chapter of the American Heart Association. (See *Ensuring continued care for the patient with myocarditis.*)

EVALUATION

During your evaluation, compare patient outcomes with reassessment findings. Consider the patient's overall health, activity level, nutritional status, cardiac status, and ability to adjust to activity restrictions.

Overall health
When assessing the patient's health status, measure his vital signs. The following should occur:

Discharge TimeSaver

Ensuring continued care for the patient with myocarditis

Review the following teaching topics, referrals, and follow-up appointments to ensure that your patient is adequately prepared for discharge.

Teaching topics
Make sure that the following topics have been covered and that your patient's learning has been evaluated:
□ explanation of myocarditis, including its causes and potential complications
□ activity restrictions
□ drug therapy, including antibiotic and anti-inflammatory agents
□ signs and symptoms to report to the doctor
□ sources of information and support.

Referrals
Make sure that the patient has been provided with necessary referrals to:
□ home health care agency
□ social services
□ dietitian, if necessary.

Follow-up appointments
Make sure that the necessary follow-up appointments have been scheduled and that the patient has been notified:
□ doctor
□ additional diagnostic tests.

• The patient's fever should be reduced.

• You should note the presence or absence of complications of hyperthermia, such as dehydration or seizures.

• The patient should maintain a normal temperature without the use of antipyretics once myocarditis is resolved.

Cardiac status
Assess for hemodynamic stability by noting the patient's vital signs, urine output, and mental status. Take note of:
• the presence or absence of chest pain
• the presence or absence of fluid retention as determined by checking the patient's intake and output measurements and assessing for dyspnea and peripheral edema.

Activity level
Consider whether the patient has adhered to a schedule of bed rest. Consider the following questions:
• Does the patient seek assistance when performing common everyday activities?

• Has his activity tolerance returned to normal?

Adjustment to restrictions
Assess the patient's adjustment to activity restrictions. Consider the following questions:
• Has the patient selected and participated in activities that conform to prescribed physical restrictions?
• If the patient reported feelings of boredom, is there any indication that these feelings have diminished?

Nutritional status
To evaluate the patient's nutritional status, assess his weight and fluid volume status. The following should occur:
• If nutrition intake is adequate, the patient should demonstrate improved strength and activity tolerance.
• Serum albumin, BUN, and creatinine levels should remain within established limits.

Pericarditis

Pericarditis refers to an inflammation of the fibroserous sac that envelops, supports, and protects the heart. It occurs in acute and chronic forms. The acute form can be fibrinous or effusive, with serous, purulent, or hemorrhagic exudate. The chronic form (called constrictive pericarditis) is characterized by dense fibrous pericardial thickening. (See *Key points about pericarditis*.)

Causes
Possible causes of pericarditis include:
• bacterial, fungal, viral (infectious pericarditis), tuberculous, and protozoal infections
• neoplasms (primary or metastatic from lungs, breasts, or other organs)
• high-dose radiation to the chest
• uremia
• hypersensitivity or autoimmune disease, such as acute rheumatic fever (the most common cause of pericarditis in children), systemic lupus erythematosus, and rheumatoid arthritis
• drugs, such as hydralazine or procainamide
• idiopathic factors (most common in acute pericarditis)
• cardiac injury — such as myocardial infarction (MI) — which later causes Dressler's syndrome (an autoimmune reaction) in the pericardium. Other types of cardiac injury include trauma or surgery (postpericardiotomy syndrome) that leaves the pericardium intact but allows blood to leak into the pericardial cavity.

Less common causes of pericarditis include aortic aneurysm with pericardial leakage, and myxedema with cholesterol deposits in the pericardium.

ASSESSMENT

If you suspect pericarditis, carefully consider the patient's medical history. Look for possible causes of pericarditis, such as chest trauma, MI, or a recent bacterial infection.

Health history
The patient with acute pericarditis may complain of sharp, sudden chest pain, usually starting above the sternum and radiating to the neck, shoulders, back, and arms. Ask about aggravating and alleviating factors.

With acute pericarditis, the pain is frequently pleuritic and increases with deep inspiration and coughing. Also, the pain is often aggravated by turning over in bed and assuming the supine position. However, pain may be steady and constrictive, resembling MI.

Pericardial pain is usually relieved when the patient sits up and leans forward. Dyspnea often accompanies chest pain. The patient may report other signs and symptoms that may relate to the underlying cause of pericarditis. In addition, the patient may not experience pain if he has slowly developing tuberculous pericarditis or postirradiation, neoplastic, or uremic pericarditis.

Physical examination
With pericarditis, auscultation almost always reveals a pericardial friction rub (a scratchy or grating sound produced when the pericardial surfaces have lost their lubricating fluid because of inflammation, causing them to rub against each other). (See *Auscultating a pericardial friction rub,* page 142.)

The patient with acute pericarditis may develop a fever and tachycardia. Constrictive pericarditis causes the membrane to calcify and become rigid. The patient may experience a gradual increase in systemic venous pressure and signs similar to those of chronic right ventricular failure, including fluid retention, ascites, and hepatomegaly. Limited cardiac output may lead to dyspnea and activity intolerance.

Diagnostic test results
Laboratory test results suggest inflammation and may help identify the cause of pericarditis. Common findings include:
• a normal or elevated white blood cell count, especially in infectious pericarditis
• an elevated erythrocyte sedimentation rate
• slightly elevated level of MB isoenzyme of creatine kinase with associated myocarditis.

A culture of pericardial fluid may be obtained by open surgical drainage or pericardiocentesis. In bacterial or fungal pericarditis, this culture may help identify a causative organism.

Other laboratory studies may include blood urea nitrogen levels to check for uremia, antistreptolysin-O titers to detect rheumatic fever, and a purified protein derivative test to check for tuberculosis.

In acute pericarditis, electrocardiogram (ECG) readings usually show diffuse elevated ST segments in all leads except aV_R and V_1. They occur without the significant changes in QRS morphology that accompany MI. ECG readings may also show atrial ectopic rhythms, such as those that occur in atrial fibrillation. In pericardial effusion, you may note diminished QRS voltage.

Echocardiography may suggest pericardial effusion if an echo-free space between the ventricular wall and the pericardium is noted.

FactFinder
Key points about pericarditis

• *Chief complaint:* Pain is present in approximately 60% of cases. The patient may describe a stabbing pain that is aggravated by respiration, coughing, body movement, and swallowing. Intensity and quality may vary from a dull ache to agonizing, severe pain simulating a myocardial infarction. Pain may be accompanied by dyspnea and fever.
• *Complications:* Pericardial effusion is the major complication of acute pericarditis. Fluid may accumulate slowly in the pericardium with minimal hemodynamic disturbance or change in intrapericardial pressure. However, if fluid accumulates rapidly, cardiac tamponade may occur, resulting in shock, cardiovascular collapse, and eventual death.
• *Chief physical sign:* A pericardial friction rub results from the loss of fluid in the pericardial sac that normally separates the layers of the pericardium. The rub is a scratchy sound heard best along the left sternal border and the xiphoid area during forced expiration with the patient leaning forward.
• *Prognosis:* The prognosis depends on the underlying cause and the degree of complications. Patients with acute pericarditis who don't develop constriction tend to have a more favorable prognosis.

NURSING DIAGNOSIS

Common nursing diagnoses for a patient with pericarditis include:
• Decreased cardiac output related to development of thickening of the pericardial membrane or pericardial effusion constricting the movement of the heart
• Ineffective breathing pattern related to pain
• Diversional activity deficit related to prescribed bed rest
• Pain related to inflammation of the pericardial sac.

Assessment TimeSaver

Auscultating a pericardial friction rub

Keep the following points in mind when auscultating for a pericardial friction rub.

• You can hear the rub best with the stethoscope diaphragm and usually in the third intercostal space to the left of the sternum or along the lower left sternal border.
• You can usually hear the rub best when the patient leans forward and exhales.
• The rub may have up to three components that correspond to atrial systole, ventricular systole, and the rapid-filling phase of ventricular diastole.

• Occasionally, the rub is heard only briefly or not at all.
• If acute pericarditis has caused large pericardial effusions, heart sounds may be distant.
• Have the patient hold his breath for a few seconds while you auscultate for the rub. If you note the rub while the patient holds his breath, you can rule out extraneous pleural or respiratory noises as the source of the rub.

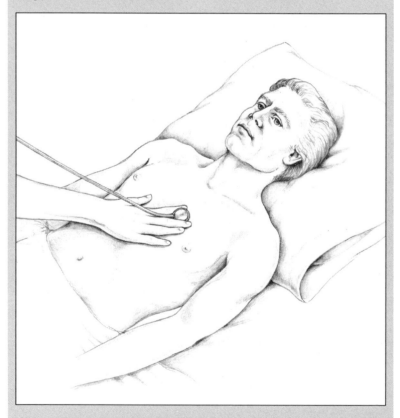

PLANNING

Based on the nursing diagnosis *decreased cardiac output,* develop appropriate patient outcomes. For example, your patient will:

• maintain hemodynamic stability as evidenced by stable vital signs

• not exhibit signs of impaired tissue perfusion, such as mental status changes or decreased urine output

• not exhibit or report clinical signs of increased central venous pressure (CVP), such as jugular vein distention or fullness in chest.

Based on the nursing diagnosis *ineffective breathing pattern,* develop appropriate patient outcomes. For example, your patient will:

• maintain a respiratory rate within 5 breaths/minute of baseline

• demonstrate normal arterial blood gas (ABG) levels

• achieve comfort without depressing respirations

• report being able to breathe comfortably.

Based on the nursing diagnosis *diversional activity deficit,* develop appropriate patient outcomes. For example, your patient will:

• express a willingness to participate in quiet activities

• select and participate in activities that conform to the prescribed restrictions

• report satisfaction with his use of time while on bed rest.

Based on the nursing diagnosis *pain,* develop appropriate patient outcomes. For example, your patient will:

• express feelings of comfort after analgesic administration

• maintain vital signs within an acceptable range

• establish positions for sitting and resting that help to minimize pain

• report an end to pain once the inflammation subsides.

IMPLEMENTATION

Focus your nursing care on teaching the patient about pericarditis, enforcing bed rest, alleviating pain, and preventing complications. (See *Medical care of the patient with pericarditis,* page 144.)

Nursing interventions

• Emphasize the importance of bed rest to the patient with acute pericarditis. Assist with bathing, if necessary. Provide the patient with a bedside commode because using it places less stress on the heart than using a bedpan.

• Place the patient in an upright position to relieve dyspnea and chest pain.

• Provide analgesics to relieve pain, and monitor their effectiveness.

• Administer oxygen, if needed, to prevent tissue hypoxia.

• Monitor the patient closely for complications. Faint heart sounds, tachycardia, and a feeling of fullness in the chest may occur with pericardial effusion. If fluid accumulates in the pericardial cavity, restricting diastolic ventricular filling, cardiac tamponade may occur. Signs will vary, depending on how fast the tamponade develops, but may include pallor, clammy skin, hypotension, neck vein distention, orthopnea, hepatic engorgement, or dyspnea. Notify the doctor at once if signs of cardiac tamponade are present. Because cardiac tamponade requires immediate treatment, keep a pericardiocentesis tray handy whenever you suspect pericardial effusion.

Timesaving tip: When you don't have time for a complete assessment, check for a paradoxical pulse, an important (although not foolproof) indicator of cardiac tamponade. To detect this sign, use a sphygmomanometer. Deflate the cuff as the patient slowly breathes until you hear the first Korotkoff sound during expiration. Note the systolic pressure. Continue to

Treatments

Medical care of the patient with pericarditis

Appropriate treatment aims to relieve symptoms, manage underlying systemic disease, and prevent or treat pericardial effusion and cardiac tamponade.

Idiopathic pericarditis
In idiopathic pericarditis, treatment consists of bed rest as long as fever and pain persist and the administration of nonsteroidal anti-inflammatory drugs, such as aspirin, indomethacin, and ibuprofen, to relieve pain and reduce inflammation. If symptoms continue, the doctor may prescribe corticosteroids. Although they provide rapid and effective relief, corticosteroids must be used cautiously because pericarditis may recur when drug therapy ends. Similar treatment is recommended for postthoracotomy pericarditis.

Drugs such as indomethacin, ibuprofen, and large doses of corticosteroids may lead to thinning of the myocardium and possible myocardial rupture. They should be used very cautiously in patients with acute myocardial infarction.

Infectious pericarditis
If pericarditis results from disease of the left pleural space, mediastinal abscesses, or septicemia, the patient will require antibiotics, surgical drainage, or both. If cardiac tamponade develops, the doctor may perform emergency pericardiocentesis and may inject antibiotics directly into the pericardial sac.

Recurrent pericarditis
Recurrent pericarditis may require partial pericardiectomy, which creates a window that allows fluid to drain into the pleural space where it's gradually drained by the lymphatic system. In constrictive pericarditis, total pericardiectomy may be necessary to permit the heart to fill and contract adequately. Treatment must also include management of rheumatic fever, uremia, tuberculosis, and other underlying disorders.

---

deflate the pressure cuff until Korotkoff sounds are heard continuously during inspiration and expiration. Again, note the systolic pressure. If the difference between the first and second systolic measurements exceeds 10 mm Hg, suspect a paradoxical pulse.

• During the time the patient is confined to bed rest, promote activities that are physically undemanding. Seek out the patient's interests and enlist the support of family members.

• Engage the patient in conversation while you're carrying out treatments. To reduce anxiety, allow the patient to express his concerns about the diagnosis. Reassure him that the activity restrictions are temporary. Explain that an analgesic will help alleviate pain.

• Before giving antibiotics, obtain a patient history of allergies. Administer antibiotics on time to maintain consistent drug levels in the blood.

• For patients undergoing surgery for constrictive pericarditis, provide appropriate preoperative and postoperative care.

• If pericardial fluid accumulation threatens heart function, prepare the patient for pericardiocentesis. (See *Understanding pericardiocentesis.*)

Understanding pericardiocentesis

If your patient is undergoing pericardiocentesis, explain that the procedure relieves the pressure and discomfort caused by fluid that collects in the pericardium and restricts heart function. In this procedure, the doctor aspirates fluid through a needle inserted into the pericardial cavity.

Tell the patient that his chest will be cleaned and draped, to prevent infection, and numbed with an anesthetic, to prevent pain. Reassure him that he won't feel pain, only possibly some pressure. Then describe the monitors and devices, such as an electrocardiograph (ECG), that will monitor his heart's activity.

The procedure may be performed in the cardiac catheterization laboratory, in a special procedures room, or at the patient's bedside. Tell the patient that a sedative will be given to decrease his anxiety. Mention that the doctor may leave a flexible pericardial catheter in place temporarily so that excess fluid can be drained later, if necessary.

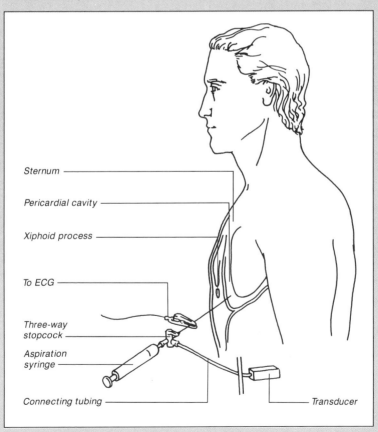

Ensuring continued care for the patient with pericarditis

Review the following teaching topics, referrals, and follow-up appointments to make sure that your patient is adequately prepared for discharge.

Teaching topics
Make sure that the following topics have been covered and that your patient's learning has been evaluated:
□ explanation of pericarditis, including its causes and potential complications
□ activity restrictions
□ drug therapy, including antibiotic and anti-inflammatory agents
□ explanation of the pericardiocentesis procedure, if applicable
□ signs and symptoms to report to the doctor
□ preoperative and postoperative care, if a pericardiectomy is scheduled.

Referrals
Make sure that the patient has been provided with necessary referrals to:
□ home health care agency
□ social services.

Follow-up appointments
Make sure that the necessary follow-up appointments have been scheduled and that the patient has been notified:
□ doctor
□ surgeon
□ additional diagnostic tests, if applicable.

Patient teaching
• Explain the nature of the disorder, its symptoms, causes, and complications.
• Explain all diagnostic tests.
• Teach the patient about prescribed medications. Tell him that nonsteroidal anti-inflammatory drugs, such as indomethacin, aspirin, and ibuprofen, help relieve pain and reduce inflammation. If these drugs aren't effective and corticosteroids are prescribed, explain their use and potential adverse effects. You may need to explain antibiotic therapy as well.
• When fever, pain, and malaise resolve, tell the patient with acute pericarditis to resume his daily activities slowly and to schedule rest periods into his daily routine for a while. If he develops chronic pericarditis, advise him to limit strenuous activities, such as running or contact sports.
• If surgery is necessary, help clarify the doctor's explanation of the procedure and teach the patient about preoperative and postoperative care.

• Explain the importance of keeping follow-up appointments. Tell the patient to immediately report any recurrence or change in the nature of his chest pain, increasing shortness of breath or fatigue, or swelling and weight gain. (See *Ensuring continued care for the patient with pericarditis*.)

EVALUATION

When evaluating a patient's response to your nursing care, gather reassessment data and compare this information with the patient outcomes specified in your plan of care.

Cardiopulmonary status
Reassess the patient's vital signs. Consider the following questions:
• Do vital signs indicate hemodynamic stability?
• Are there signs of adequate tissue perfusion, such as an absence of mental status changes and adequate urine output?

• Are clinical signs of increased CVP, such as jugular vein distention or reports of fullness in the chest, present or absent?

Reassess the patient's breathing pattern. Consider the following questions:
• Does the patient maintain a respiratory rate within 5 breaths/minute of baseline?
• Are ABG levels within an appropriate range?
• Does the patient report being able to breathe comfortably?

Adjustment to restrictions

Evaluate the patient's ability to adjust to activity restrictions. Consider the following questions:
• Is the patient willing to participate in quiet activities?
• Does the patient participate in activities that conform to prescribed physical restrictions?

Take note of any statements made by the patient that indicate he's satisfied with his use of time while on bed rest.

Pain relief

Evaluate the patient's response to pain. Consider the following questions:
• After analgesic administration, did the patient report pain relief?
• Was he able to establish positions for sitting and resting that help to minimize pain?

When inflammation subsides, note whether the patient reports a presence or an absence of continued pain.

Infective endocarditis

Infective endocarditis refers to a bacterial or fungal infection of the heart valves, endocardium, or cardiac prosthesis. In this disorder, fibrin and platelets cluster on valve tissue and engulf circulating bacteria or fungi. This produces vegetation that can cover the valve surfaces, causing deformities or destruction of valve tissue. Vegetation may also extend to the chordae tendineae and cause them to rupture, leading to valvular insufficiency. Occasionally, vegetation forms on the endocardium, usually in areas altered by rheumatic, congenital, or syphilitic heart disease. It also may form on healthy tissue.

In patients with subacute infective endocarditis, the heart may compensate for the malfunctioning valves for years until the onset of left ventricular failure, valve stenosis or insufficiency, or myocardial erosion. In addition, vegetation on the heart valves or on the endocardial lining of a heart chamber can embolize to the spleen, kidneys, central nervous system, lungs, and coronary arteries. (See *Classifying endocarditis*, page 148.)

Untreated infective endocarditis is usually fatal. With proper treatment, however, about 70% of patients recover. The prognosis is worse when the endocarditis causes severe valvular damage or when it involves a prosthetic valve.

Causes

The most common causative organisms of this disorder are group A nonhemolytic streptococci, staphylococci, and enterococci. However, almost any organism can cause endocarditis.

Acute bacterial endocarditis usually results from bacteremia that follows septic thrombophlebitis; open-heart surgery involving prosthetic valves; or infections of the skin, bone, or lungs. The causative organism, most often *Staphylococcus aureus,* is extremely virulent.

Subacute bacterial endocarditis usually occurs in patients with acquired valvular or congenital cardiac lesions. It may also occur after dental, genitourinary, gynecologic, or GI procedures. The causative organism is usually low in virulence and is normally present in the body — for example, *Streptococcus*

FactFinder

Classifying endocarditis

In the course of your practice, you may see several types of endocarditis. The following are among the most common.

Infective endocarditis
This term refers to forms of the disorder that result from microbial infections. Types of infective endocarditis include acute bacterial endocarditis, subacute bacterial endocarditis, prosthetic valve endocarditis, and right-sided endocarditis.

Acute bacterial endocarditis
The acute form of the disorder is usually caused by *Staphylococcus aureus.*

Subacute bacterial endocarditis
The subacute form of the disorder is usually caused by *Streptococcus viridans.*

Prosthetic valve endocarditis
This term refers to infective endocarditis that develops in patients in the year after prosthetic valve replacement.

Right-sided endocarditis
This type of endocarditis usually involves the tricuspid valve and occurs in patients who use illicit I.V. drugs or have central venous lines.

Noninfective endocarditis
Also called nonbacterial thrombotic endocarditis, noninfective endocarditis occurs when platelets and fibrin thrombi form on cardiac valves and the adjacent endocardium in response to trauma, local turbulence, circulating immune complexes, vasculitis, and hypercoagulable states.

viridans, which normally inhabits the upper respiratory tract, and *Enterococcus faecalis,* which is typically found in GI and perineal flora.

Certain preexisting conditions may predispose a patient to infective endocarditis. They include rheumatic valvular disease, congenital heart disease, mitral valve prolapse, degenerative heart disease, calcific aortic stenosis (in elderly people), asymmetrical septal hypertrophy, Marfan syndrome, and syphilitic aortic valve. However, many patients have no underlying heart disease. Patients with arteriovenous shunts or fistulas who are on long-term hemodialysis are also at risk for the disorder.

ASSESSMENT

Note any preexisting condition that could place the patient at risk for endocarditis. In many cases, symptoms of the disorder appear within 2 weeks of the precipitating event.

Health history
The patient may report nonspecific symptoms, such as weakness, fatigue, weight loss, anorexia, arthralgia, night sweats, visual deficits, or a fever that recurs for weeks. With an acute form of the disorder, there may be an abrupt onset of fever. Fever is almost always present except in elderly patients, patients with renal failure or congestive heart failure, or those who have been previously treated with antibiotics.

Physical examination
When measuring vital signs, you may detect a fever. Usually, a low-grade fever accompanies subacute bacterial endocarditis; the fever may be higher in the acute form.

Inspection may reveal petechiae of the skin (especially common on the upper anterior trunk) and the buccal, pharyngeal, or conjunctival mucosa, and splinter hemorrhages under the nails.

You may observe Osler's nodes (tender, raised, subcutaneous lesions on the fingers or toes) and Janeway lesions (purplish macules on the palms or soles). Patients with long-standing disease may exhibit finger clubbing.

Ophthalmoscopic examination may reveal Roth's spots (hemorrhagic areas with white centers the retina).

Auscultation usually reveals a murmur, except in patients with early acute endocarditis and I.V. drug users with tricuspid valve infection. Percussion and palpation may reveal splenomegaly in long-standing disease.

Timesaving tip: If the patient exhibits an unexplained fever and a heart murmur, question him about the presence of preexisting conditions that increase the risk for endocarditis. Be prepared to obtain blood cultures.

Detecting complications
During your physical examination, you may detect evidence of complications. Embolization from vegetating lesions or diseased valve tissue is a frequent complication of subacute bacterial endocarditis. (See *How embolism occurs,* page 150.) Embolization may produce signs of splenic, renal, cerebral, or pulmonary infarction or peripheral vascular occlusion.
• Signs of splenic infarction include pain in the left upper quadrant, radiating to the left shoulder, and abdominal rigidity.
• Signs of renal infarction include hematuria, pyuria, flank pain, and decreased urine output.
• Signs of cerebral infarction include an altered level of consciousness (LOC), hemiparesis, aphasia, and other neurologic deficits.
• Signs of pulmonary infarction include a cough, pleuritic pain, a pleural friction rub, dyspnea, and hemoptysis. These signs are most common in right-sided endocarditis, which typically oc-

curs among I.V. drug abusers and after cardiac surgery.
• Signs of peripheral vascular occlusion include numbness and tingling in an arm, leg, finger, or toe, or gangrene.

The patient may also exhibit signs of congestive heart failure (CHF). Renal disease caused by glomerulonephritis is present in about 80% of cases, while infarction affects approximately 50% of patients.

Diagnostic test results
In up to 95% of patients, three or more blood cultures taken during a 24- to 48-hour period can identify the causative organism. Other patients may have negative blood cultures, possibly suggesting fungal or difficult-to-diagnose infections, such as *Haemophilus parainfluenzae.* Nonspecific laboratory findings in infective endocarditis may include:
• a normal or elevated white blood cell count and differential
• abnormal histiocytes (macrophages)
• normocytic, normochromic anemia (in subacute bacterial endocarditis)
• elevated erythrocyte sedimentation rate and serum creatinine levels
• a positive serum rheumatoid factor (occurs in about half of patients who have had the disorder for at least 6 weeks)
• proteinuria and microscopic hematuria.

Ultrasonography
In a patient with native valve disease, echocardiography (cardiac ultrasound) may reveal valvular damage. It also may show atrial fibrillation and other arrhythmias that accompany valvular disease.

In transesophageal echocardiography, a more specific form of cardiac ultrasound, the ultrasound transducer is placed in the esophagus next to the heart, allowing for better visualization of the anatomic features of the heart.

How embolism occurs

Besides impairing heart valves, infective endocarditis causes further complications when valve vegetations break away as emboli, travel through the bloodstream, and lodge in other organs, causing infarction. This flowchart shows the domino-like effect of infective endocarditis from infection to embolism.

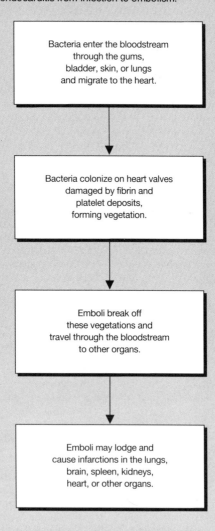

Bacteria enter the bloodstream
through the gums,
bladder, skin, or lungs
and migrate to the heart.

Bacteria colonize on heart valves
damaged by fibrin and
platelet deposits,
forming vegetation.

Emboli break off
these vegetations and
travel through the bloodstream
to other organs.

Emboli may lodge and
cause infarctions in the lungs,
brain, spleen, kidneys,
heart, or other organs.

Transesophageal echocardiography is especially useful for obese patients and patients with chronic lung disease.

NURSING DIAGNOSIS

Common nursing diagnoses for a patient with infective endocarditis include:
• Activity intolerance related to infectious process, decreased cardiac output, or both
• Decreased cardiac output related to valvular dysfunction, CHF, or both
• Hyperthermia related to systemic infection
• High risk for injury related to effects of vegetating lesions or diseased valve tissue
• Diversional activity deficit related to prescribed bed rest.

PLANNING

Based on the nursing diagnosis *activity intolerance,* develop appropriate patient outcomes. For example, your patient will:
• maintain blood pressure and pulse and respiratory rates within prescribed limits during restricted activity
• demonstrate skill in conserving energy within levels of tolerance while carrying out daily activities
• express an understanding of why symptoms of activity intolerance occur
• express satisfaction with a gradual increase in activity level, either verbally or through his behavior.

Based on the nursing diagnosis decreased cardiac output, develop appropriate patient outcomes. For example, your patient will:
• maintain hemodynamic stability reflected by stable vital signs
• not exhibit signs of impaired tissue perfusion, such as a change in mental status or decreased urine output
• not experience chest pain, dizziness, or arrhythmias, as indicated by a physical examination or by verbal reports

• maintain warm, dry skin.

Based on the nursing diagnosis *hyperthermia,* develop appropriate patient outcomes. For example, your patient will:
• exhibit a reduced temperature with administered antipyretics and antibiotics
• not develop complications associated with hyperthermia, such as dehydration and seizures
• regain normal laboratory values and vegetative blood cultures
• regain and maintain a normal temperature without the use of antipyretics when endocarditis is resolved.

Based on the nursing diagnosis *high risk for injury,* develop appropriate patient outcomes. For example, your patient will:
• not experience flank pain
• maintain an adequate voiding pattern with his urine remaining clear
• not demonstrate signs and symptoms associated with neurologic dysfunction, such as a decreased LOC, visual changes, aphasia, or hemiparesis
• not demonstrate peripheral numbness, tingling, or discoloration of limbs or digits or a change in peripheral pulses
• not demonstrate dyspnea, hemoptysis, a cough, pleuritic pain, or abnormal breath sounds
• not experience chest pain or changes in apical pulse and blood pressure, as indicated by verbal reports or by a physical examination
• not experience left upper quadrant pain or abdominal rigidity
• maintain normal organ function in all body systems.

Based on the nursing diagnosis *diversional activity deficit,* develop appropriate patient outcomes. For example, your patient will:
• express a desire to participate in quiet activities
• select and participate in activities that conform to prescribed physical restrictions

Medical care of the patient with infective endocarditis

The goal of treatment is to eradicate all the infecting organisms from the vegetation. Therapy usually continues over several weeks. Selection of an anti-infective drug is based on the infecting organism and sensitivity studies. Parenteral administration is preferred to ensure satisfactory drug absorption. I.V. antibiotic therapy usually lasts about 4 to 6 weeks.

Supportive treatment
Supportive treatment includes bed rest, aspirin for fever and body aches, and sufficient fluid intake. Severe valvular damage, especially aortic regurgitation or infection of a cardiac prosthesis, may require corrective surgery if refractory heart failure develops or if an infected prosthetic valve must be replaced.

• report satisfaction with his use of time while on bed rest.

IMPLEMENTATION

Focus your nursing care on teaching the patient about infective endocarditis, enforcing bed rest, reducing anxiety, and monitoring the patient's status. You will also implement medical therapies aimed at eradicating the infecting organism. (See *Medical care of the patient with infective endocarditis.*)

Nursing interventions
• Stress the importance of bed rest. Assist the patient with bathing, if necessary. Provide a bedside commode because using it places less stress on the patient's heart than using a bedpan.
• During the time the patient is on bed rest, promote activities that aren't physically demanding. Enlist the support of family members. Seek out the patient's interests.
• Engage the patient in conversation while you're carrying out treatments. To reduce anxiety, allow the patient to express concerns. Reassure him that activity restrictions are temporary.
• Administer oxygen if needed and monitor his arterial blood gas levels.

• Before giving antibiotics, obtain a patient history of allergies. Administer antibiotics on time to maintain consistent drug levels in the blood. Observe for signs of infiltration or inflammation at the venipuncture site, a possible complication of long-term I.V. administration. Rotate venous access sites. Provide meticulous care at the I.V. site.
• Encourage passive range-of-motion exercises and assist with frequent position changes. Apply antiembolism stockings.
• Administer antipyretics as needed and monitor the patient's response. Check his temperature every 4 hours. Monitor the results of blood cultures.
• Monitor for signs of embolization, a common occurrence during the first 3 months of treatment. Be sure to assess urine color and output, LOC, breath sounds, vital signs, peripheral sensations, pulses, and pain (especially splenic or pulmonary related).
• Monitor the patient's renal status (including blood urea nitrogen levels, creatinine clearance, and urine output) to check for signs of renal emboli and drug toxicity.
• Assess cardiovascular status frequently. Watch for signs of left ventricular failure, such as dyspnea, hypotension, tachycardia, tachypnea, crackles,

Teaching the patient about antibiotic therapy

Teach the patient recovering from infective endocarditis the importance of antibiotic therapy. Emphasize the importance of taking antibiotics exactly as prescribed. Explain that if the patient is exposed to an infection, an antibiotic can help the body defend itself by killing bacteria before they multiply and cause illness.

Communicating with the doctor
Explain to the patient that he will need to take antibiotics before dental work or some kinds of surgery. Dental work, for example, may allow germs to enter the bloodstream through the gums. Encourage the patient to let his dentist or any other doctor know about his disorder before undergoing treatment.

Tell the patient to immediately let the doctor know if he forgets to finish or renew his prescription. He should also inform his doctor if he notices a break in his skin or feels sick. Explain that a cut, puncture, rash, or abscess can introduce germs. A sore throat, fever, cold, or flu means that germs are already at work.

Tell the patient to immediately call his doctor or go to the nearest emergency department if he has any signs and symptoms that suggest reinfection of the heart valves, such as:
• shortness of breath
• fever
• fatigue
• weakness
• swollen ankles
• a sudden weight gain, such as 5 lb (2.3 kg) in a week or 1 lb (0.5 kg) overnight.

An important reminder
Tell the patient to get a card from his doctor or from the local chapter of the American Heart Association that lists antibiotics taken to prevent heart valve infection. Tell him to always carry the card and to present it to dentists and other health care providers when appropriate. Each year, he should have the card checked to make sure the information is up-to-date.

neck vein distention, edema, and weight gain. Check for changes in cardiac rhythm or conduction.

Patient teaching
• Explain the nature of the disorder and its symptoms, causes, and complications.
• Explain all diagnostic tests.
• Teach the patient about long-term, prescribed anti-infectives. Stress the importance of taking the medication and restricting activities for as long as the doctor prescribes.
• Tell the patient to watch closely for fever, anorexia, and other signs of relapse about 2 weeks after treatment ends. Tell him to notify the doctor immediately if such signs occur and to immediately report any sign of infection, such as a sore throat.
• Advise the patient to immediately report indications of complications, especially heart failure or embolization. They may occur at any time, even weeks or months after treatment.
• Make sure that the patient understands the need for prophylactic antibiotics before and after invasive procedures, such as dental work, cystoscopy, incision, and drainage of infected tissue. (See *Teaching the patient about antibiotic therapy.*)
• Encourage good daily oral hygiene.
• As needed, inform the patient about local resources and sources of support,

Ensuring continued care for the patient with infective endocarditis

Review the following teaching topics, referrals, and follow-up appointments to ensure that your patient is adequately prepared for discharge.

Teaching topics
Make sure that the following topics have been covered and that your patient's learning has been evaluated:
□ explanation of endocarditis, including its causes, symptoms, and potential complications
□ activity restrictions
□ use of an oral thermometer and how to record the findings
□ drug therapy, including antibiotic and antipyretic agents
□ signs and symptoms to report to the doctor
□ sources of information and support

□ need for prophylactic antibiotic therapy before invasive procedures.

Referrals
Make sure that the patient has been provided with necessary referrals to:
□ social services
□ home health care agency.

Follow-up appointments
Make sure that the necessary follow-up appointments have been scheduled and that the patient has been notified:
□ doctor
□ additional diagnostic tests, if necessary.

including the local chapter of the American Heart Association. (See *Ensuring continued care for the patient with infective endocarditis*.)

EVALUATION

When evaluating the patient's response to your nursing care, gather reassessment data and compare this information with the patient outcomes specified in your plan of care.

Coping with activity intolerance
Evaluate your patient's ability to cope with activity intolerance. Consider the following questions:
• Has your patient maintained his blood pressure and pulse and respiratory rates within prescribed limits during activity?
• Does he communicate an understanding of why symptoms of activity intolerance occur? Does he demonstrate skill in conserving energy?

• Has the patient selected and participated in activities that conform to prescribed physical restrictions?
Note the patient's response as his activity tolerance gradually increases.

Cardiac output
Reassess your patient's cardiac output. Look for indications of hemodynamic stability.
• Note the presence or absence of signs of impaired tissue perfusion, such as a change in mental status or decreased urine output.
• Also note the presence or absence of chest pain, dizziness, or arrhythmias, as indicated by a physical examination or verbal reports.
• Check whether the patient's skin is warm and dry.

Fever
Consider the following for the patient with fever:

• Note whether administration of anti-pyretics and antibiotics reduced his temperature.

• Document the presence or absence of complications associated with fever, such as dehydration and seizures, and current laboratory values and the results of vegetative blood cultures.

• Following treatment, evaluate whether the patient can maintain a normal temperature without the use of antipy-retics.

Complications

If treatment for infective endocarditis is successful, evaluation should indicate normal organ function in all body systems. Note the presence of any complications, including:

• flank pain
• altered elimination pattern
• decreased LOC or visual changes
• aphasia
• hemiparesis or paresthesias
• discoloration of limbs or digits
• altered peripheral pulses
• dyspnea
• cough or hemoptysis
• pleuritic or chest pain
• abnormal breath sounds
• changes in apical pulse or blood pressure
• left upper quadrant pain
• abdominal rigidity.

Rheumatic fever and rheumatic heart disease

A systemic inflammatory disease of childhood, acute rheumatic fever develops after an infection of the upper respiratory tract with group A beta-hemolytic streptococci. It principally involves the heart, joints, central nervous system, skin, and subcutaneous tissues. Recurrence is common.

The term *rheumatic heart disease* refers to the cardiac involvement of rheu-matic fever — its most destructive effect. Cardiac involvement develops in up to 50% of patients and may affect the endocardium, myocardium, or peri-cardium during the early acute phase. It may later affect the heart valves, causing chronic valvular disease. (See *How rheumatic fever affects heart valves*, page 156.)

The extent of damage to the heart depends on where the disorder strikes:

• Myocarditis produces characteristic lesions called Aschoff bodies in the acute stages and cellular swelling and fragmentation of interstitial collagen, leading to formation of progressively fibrotic nodules and interstitial scars.

• Endocarditis causes valve leaflet swelling; erosion along the lines of leaflet closure; and blood, platelet, and fibrin deposits, which form beadlike vegetation. It usually strikes the mitral valve in females and the aortic valve in males. Occasionally, endocarditis affects the tricuspid valve and, rarely, the pulmonic valve.

• Valvular disease may eventually cause chronic valvular stenosis and insufficiency, including mitral stenosis and insufficiency and aortic insufficiency. In children, mitral insufficiency is the major sequela of rheumatic heart disease. Malfunctioning valves can ultimately lead to severe pancarditis and occasionally produce pericardial effusion and fatal heart failure.

With 15 to 20 million new cases reported each year, rheumatic heart disease remains the leading cause of death for young people in many parts of the world, especially in urban slums of the developing world. Children between ages 5 and 15 who experience malnutrition and crowded living conditions are especially at high risk. This disease strikes most often during cool, damp weather in the winter and early spring.

How rheumatic fever affects heart valves

Rheumatic fever causes gross changes in the mitral and aortic valves — edema, erosion of the valve leaflets along the closure line, and formation of beadlike vegetations along the inflamed leaflet edges.

These illustrations show how rheumatic inflammation in a mitral valve may progress to stenosis and regurgitation.

Vegetations form on leaflets
Vegetations form when fibrin and platelets accumulate on the damaged valve surface. Mitral valve leaflets become inflamed, with a thin line of rheumatic vegetations formed along the leaflet edges.

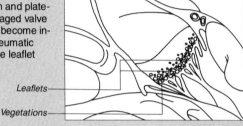

Leaflets

Vegetations

Stenosis reduces movement
In mitral stenosis, the most common valvular defect associated with recurrent rheumatic fever, inflammation causes shrinkage of the chordae tendineae and fusion of adjacent leaflets. This reduces valve movement. The left atrium attempts to force blood through the narrow valve opening into the left ventricle, eventually causing left atrial enlargement, pulmonary congestion, and right ventricular hypertrophy and failure. Symptoms of mitral stenosis don't usually appear until the valve opening narrows by about 50%.

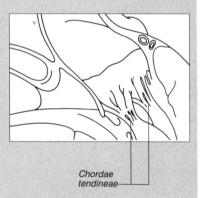

Chordae
tendineae

Mitral insufficiency occurs
Some degree of insufficiency (backflow) of blood into the atrium may coexist with stenosis because the dysfunctional valve can't close tightly.

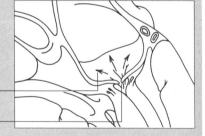

Blood backflow

Narrowed opening

Causes

Rheumatic fever appears to be a hypersensitivity reaction in which antibodies produced to combat streptococci react and create characteristic lesions at specific tissue sites. How and why group A streptococcal infection initiates this process remains unknown. Because fewer than 1% of people infected with *Streptococcus* ever contract rheumatic fever, altered host resistance probably is involved in its development or recurrence.

ASSESSMENT

Your nursing assessment should include a thorough health history, physical examination findings, and diagnostic test results.

Health history

The patient may report migratory joint pain. This pain commonly affects the knees, ankles, elbows, and hips. In two-thirds of all cases, the patient reports having had an infection in the preceding month. He may also report a recent history of a low-grade fever that spikes to at least 100.4° F (38° C) late in the afternoon, unexplained epistaxis, and abdominal pain.

Physical examination

When assessing vital signs, you'll usually discover an elevated temperature.

When inspecting the patient, you may note skin lesions such as *erythema marginatum rheumaticum*, a nonpruritic, macular, transient rash. The lesions are red with blanched centers and well-demarcated borders. They typically appear on the trunk and extremities.

You may notice subcutaneous nodules near tendons or the bony prominences of joints. These nodules commonly appear around the elbows, knuckles, wrists, knees, vertebral spines and, less commonly, on the scalp and backs of the hands. The nodules persist for a few days to several weeks and, like erythema marginatum rheumaticum, frequently accompany carditis, which usually results in scarring of the heart valves. If the patient reports joint pain, look for swelling, redness, and signs of effusion.

Up to 6 months after the original streptococcal infection, you may note transient chorea. Mild chorea may produce hyperirritability, a deterioration in handwriting, or an inability to concentrate. Severe chorea causes purposeless, nonrepetitive, involuntary muscle spasms and speech disturbances; poor muscle coordination; and weakness. Chorea resolves with rest and causes no residual neurologic damage.

Auscultation commonly reveals a murmur. This murmur may occur throughout the patient's life. The most common murmurs include:

• a systolic murmur of mitral insufficiency (high-pitched, blowing, holosystolic, loudest at apex, possibly radiating to the anterior axillary line, usually grade III or more on a scale of I to VI)
• a diastolic murmur of aortic insufficiency (soft, high-pitched, decrescendo, blowing)
• a middiastolic (Carey Coombs) murmur (low-pitched, apical, easily missed).

If the patient has pericarditis, auscultation may also reveal a pericardial friction rub. Palpation may reveal a rapid pulse rate. Palpation of subcutaneous nodules reveal that they are firm, movable, nontender, and about 3 mm to 2 cm in diameter. During your assessment, you may also detect signs of complications, such as heart failure.

Diagnostic test results

No specific laboratory test detecting rheumatic fever exists; however, the following test results support the diagnosis:

• White blood cell count and erythrocyte sedimentation rate may be elevated during the acute phase. Blood studies show slight anemia caused by suppressed erythropoiesis during inflammation. Anemia is a good indicator of severe or chronic presence of rheumatic fever.

- C-reactive protein is positive, especially during the acute phase.
- Cardiac enzyme levels may be increased in severe carditis.
- Antistreptolysin-O (ASO) titer is elevated in 95% of patients within 2 months of onset. Antideoxyribonuclease B (anti-DNase B), along with the ASO titer, is fairly conclusive for diagnosis.
- Throat cultures may continue to show the presence of group A streptococci. Because these organisms usually occur in small numbers, however, isolating them is difficult.

Additional tests

- Electrocardiography (ECG) reveals no diagnostic changes, but 20% of patients show a prolonged PR interval.
- Chest X-rays show a normal heart size, except with myocarditis, heart failure, and pericardial effusion.
- Echocardiography helps evaluate valvular damage, chamber size, ventricular function, and the presence of pericardial effusion.

NURSING DIAGNOSIS

Common nursing diagnoses for a patient with rheumatic heart disease include:
- Decreased cardiac output related to disease process
- Diversional activity deficit related to need for prolonged rest
- Knowledge deficit related to prevention and treatment of rheumatic heart disease
- Pain related to inflammatory joint lesions.

PLANNING

Based on the nursing diagnosis *decreased cardiac output,* develop appro-

priate patient outcomes. For example, your patient will:
- maintain hemodynamic stability as evidenced by vital sign measurements
- show no signs of impaired tissue perfusion, such as a change in mental status or decreased urine output
- not experience chest pain, dizziness, or arrhythmias, as indicated by verbal reports, a physical examination, or diagnostic tests
- maintain warm, dry skin
- not exhibit dyspnea, a dry cough, neck vein distention, or other signs of heart failure.

Based on the nursing diagnosis *diversional activity deficit*, develop appropriate patient outcomes. For example, your patient will:
- express a desire to participate in quiet activities
- select and participate in activities that conform to the prescribed physical restrictions and that are appropriate for his age-group
- report enjoyment in activity and relief from boredom and loneliness.

Based on the nursing diagnosis *knowledge deficit,* develop appropriate patient outcomes. For example, your patient will:
- communicate an understanding of rheumatic heart disease, its causes, and its potential complications
- communicate an understanding of the need for long-term antibiotic therapy and the need for prophylaxis before invasive procedures
- explain the importance of obtaining rest and gradually increasing activities when permitted
- list the warning signs to report to the doctor.

Based on the nursing diagnosis *pain,* develop appropriate patient outcomes. For example, your patient will:
- report an absence of, or decrease in, pain after administration of analgesics
- report increased rest and comfort

Treatments

Medical care of the patient with rheumatic fever and rheumatic heart disease

Treatment focuses on eradicating streptococcal infection, relieving symptoms, and preventing recurrence, thus reducing the chance of permanent cardiac damage.

Drug therapy
During the acute phase, treatment includes penicillin or, if the patient is hypersensitive to penicillin, erythromycin. Salicylates, such as aspirin, relieve fever and minimize joint swelling and pain. Salicylates may be given to children at a daily dose of 15 to 25 mg/kg/24 hours for 1 week, with the dose then decreased by half. If the patient has carditis or if salicylates fail to relieve pain and inflammation, the doctor may prescribe corticosteroids.

After the acute phase subsides, a monthly I.M. injection of penicillin G benzathine or daily doses of oral sulfadiazine or penicillin G may be used to prevent recurrence. If the patient is sensitive to penicillin or sulfadiazine, the doctor may prescribe erythromycin. This regimen usually continues for 5 to 10 years or until age 25.

Supportive measures
The doctor may prescribe strict bed rest for about 5 weeks during the acute phase with active carditis, followed by a progressive increase in physical activity. The degree to which the patient is allowed to increase his activity level depends on clinical and laboratory findings and his response to treatment.

Treatment for heart failure
Heart failure requires continued bed rest and diuretics. If the patient develops persistent heart failure because of severe mitral or aortic valvular dysfunction, he may undergo corrective surgery, such as commissurotomy (separation of the adherent, thickened leaflets of the mitral valve), valvuloplasty (inflation of a balloon within a valve), or valve replacement (with a prosthetic valve). Corrective valvular surgery seldom is necessary before late adolescence.

• experience less pain after the course of treatment, as evidenced by verbal reports or behavior.

IMPLEMENTATION

Focus your nursing care on teaching the patient and family members about rheumatic fever and rheumatic heart disease, encouraging compliance with therapy, providing for the patient's comfort, and helping the patient and family members cope with the effects of illness. You will also participate in implementing medical therapies. (See *Medical care of the patient with rheumatic fever and rheumatic heart disease*.)

Nursing interventions
• Before giving penicillin, ask the patient (or his parents) if he's ever had a hypersensitivity reaction to it. Even if he hasn't, warn him that such a reaction is possible.

• Administer antibiotics on time to maintain consistent drug levels in the blood.

Timesaving tip: To help convince a child to take daily medications, use multicolored stars as a reward. Prepare a medication sheet with the child's name printed across the top in bold letters and the days of the week below. List the prescribed medications down the left side to form a chart.

Each time the child takes his medications, attach a colored adhesive-backed star in the appropriate day's space. Use the medication sheet when teaching the child about drug therapy. Give the medication sheet to the child's parents at discharge.

• Stress the importance of bed rest. Assist with bathing, as necessary.

• Find out the interests of the patient. Help the patient devise activities that are age-appropriate and don't require expending a lot of energy.

⏲ **Timesaving tip:** After the novelty of new coloring books wears off, provide creative suggestions that will help a child occupy his time. For example, if a child loves playing with model cars, help him create a race course with materials at hand. Make a road by taping 8 to 10 paper towels together, use a pillow to represent a mountain, and a food tray to represent a bridge. Encourage the child to add his own twists. By becoming engrossed in projects such as this, the child may learn to cope better with his illness and recovery and you may experience fewer interruptions.

• After the acute phase, encourage the patient's family members and friends to spend as much time as possible with the patient to minimize boredom. Advise the parents to obtain a tutor to help their child keep up with schoolwork.

• Provide analgesics to relieve pain. Monitor their effectiveness.

• Administer oxygen to prevent tissue hypoxia, as needed.

• To reduce anxiety, allow the patient to express concerns. Reassure the patient that the physical restrictions are temporary.

• If the patient is unstable because of chorea, clear the environment of objects that could trip him.

• Help the parents overcome any guilt feelings about their child's illness. Failure to seek treatment for streptococcal infection is common because the illness may seem no worse than a cold.

• Monitor for impending complications, including heart failure, and pericardial effusions.

• Encourage the parents and child to vent their frustrations during the long, tedious recovery. If the child has severe carditis, help them prepare for permanent changes in the child's life-style.

Patient teaching

• Explain the disorder and its causes, symptoms, and complications.

• Discuss all diagnostic tests.

• Stress the importance of rest. Upon recovery, tell the patient to resume activities slowly and to include rest periods in his routine for a while.

• Explain antibiotic therapy. Tell the parents or patient to stop penicillin therapy and call the doctor immediately if the patient develops signs of an allergic reaction.

• Instruct the patient and family members to watch for and report early signs of left ventricular failure, such as dyspnea and a hacking, nonproductive cough.

• Warn the parents to watch for and immediately report signs of recurrent streptococcal infection: a sudden sore throat, diffuse throat redness and oropharyngeal exudate, swollen and tender cervical lymph glands, pain on swallowing, a fever, headache, and nausea. Urge them to keep the child away from people with respiratory tract infections.

• Help the family understand the effects of chorea: nervousness, restlessness, poor coordination, weakness, and inattentiveness. Emphasize that these effects are transient.

• Help the patient and family members understand the need to comply with prolonged antibiotic therapy and follow-up care, as well as the possible need for additional antibiotics before dental work or surgery.

Discharge TimeSaver

Ensuring continued care for the patient with rheumatic fever and rheumatic heart disease

Review the following teaching topics, referrals, and follow-up appointments to ensure that your patient is adequately prepared for discharge.

Teaching topics
Make sure that the following topics have been covered and that your patient's learning has been evaluated:
☐ explanation of rheumatic fever, including its causes, symptoms, and potential complications
☐ activity restrictions
☐ drug therapy, including antibiotics and antipyretics
☐ signs and symptoms to report to the doctor
☐ need for prophylactic antibiotic therapy before invasive procedures
☐ sources of information and support.

Referrals
Make sure the patient has been provided with necessary referrals to:
☐ home health care agency
☐ social services.

Follow-up appointments
Make sure that the necessary follow-up appointments have been scheduled and that the patient has been notified:
☐ doctor
☐ additional diagnostic tests, if necessary.

• Advise the patient about sources of information and support. Arrange for a home health care nurse, if necessary. (See *Ensuring continued care for the patient with rheumatic fever and rheumatic heart disease.*)

EVALUATION

When evaluating a patient's response to your nursing care, gather reassessment data and compare this information with the patient outcomes specified in your plan of care.

Teaching and counseling
Begin by evaluating your patient's response to teaching and counseling. Consider the following questions:
• Does the patient communicate an understanding of rheumatic heart disease, its cause, and its potential complications?
• Does he communicate an understanding of the need for long-term antibiotic therapy and the need for prophylaxis before invasive procedures?
• Can he explain the importance of obtaining rest and gradually increasing activities when permitted?
• Can he list the warning signs to report to the doctor?

Cardiac status
Check the following to assess for hemodynamic stability:
• Note the presence or absence of signs of impaired tissue perfusion, such as a change in mental status or decreased urine output.
• Also note if the patient reports chest pain or dizziness or if his ECG readings indicate the presence of arrhythmias.
• Check whether the patient's skin is warm and dry.
• Finally, note the presence or absence of signs of heart failure, such as dyspnea, a dry cough, or neck vein distention.

Coping with convalescence

Evaluate the patient's ability to cope with the long convalescence associated with rheumatic heart disease and rheumatic fever. Consider the following question:

• Does the patient select and participate in activities that conform to prescribed physical restrictions and that are appropriate for his age-group?

You should also document any patient statements that indicate enjoyment in activity and relief from boredom and loneliness.

Pain relief

Periodically reassess your patient's pain. Consider the following questions:

• After administration of analgesics, does the patient report absent or diminished pain?

• After the course of treatment, does he indicate a decrease in pain?

CHAPTER 7

Caring for patients with valvular disorders

Mitral valve prolapse syndrome

Distressing and poorly understood, mitral valve prolapse syndrome occurs commonly and is often misdiagnosed. In mitral valve prolapse, one or both valve leaflets sink into the left atrium during systole. (See *What happens in mitral valve prolapse.*) When the disorder's cause isn't known, it's called primary mitral valve prolapse. This disorder may be transmitted as an autosomal dominant trait. It may also result from acute rheumatic fever, cardiomyopathies, chest trauma, chronic rheumatic heart disease, myocardial or papillary muscle dysfunction, ischemic heart disease, lupus erythematosus, or complications of mitral valvotomy.

In *mitral valve prolapse syndrome,* the anatomic prolapse is accompanied by a constellation of signs and symptoms unrelated to the valvular abnormality, such as chest pain, palpitations, dyspnea, emotional lability, and others. Researchers speculate that metabolic or neuroendocrine factors (rather than abnormal valve function) cause these signs and symptoms. (See *Key points about mitral valve prolapse syndrome,* page 166.)

ASSESSMENT

A patient with a prolapsed mitral valve may be asymptomatic. In this case, the first diagnostic clues to the disorder may be gathered from the patient's and family histories, a physical examination, and diagnostic test results. Because mitral valve prolapse often has a hereditary component, explore the family history to determine if any close relative has had the disorder. (You may also want to recommend auscultatory screening for all immediate relatives.)

Health history

A patient with mitral valve prolapse syndrome may report chest pain, palpitations, headache, fatigue, exercise intolerance, dyspnea, light-headedness, syncope, mood swings, anxiety, or panic attacks. These signs and symptoms may worsen when the patient is tired or emotionally stressed. In women, they may worsen during menstruation or menopause. In many patients, the symptoms disappear without treatment for months or years before resurfacing.

The patient may mistake the sudden onset of chest pain for a possible myocardial infarction (MI). However, the syndrome is usually benign and doesn't result from coronary artery obstruction or spasm.

Physical examination

When observing the patient, you may note that she's thinner than average, with a height-to-weight ratio greater than average.

Auscultation typically reveals a mobile, midsystolic click, with or without a mid- to late systolic murmur. You'll hear the murmur and click best at the apex.

Timesaving tip: If you're auscultating for a known click and murmur in a supine patient and can't detect it, have her stand up. You may hear the hallmark click and murmur closer to S_1.

Diagnostic test results

Echocardiography helps to confirm the diagnosis. A two-dimensional study reveals prolapse of one or both mitral valve leaflets into the left atrium.

If echocardiography shows thickening and other anatomic abnormalities of the leaflets, the patient has an increased risk for complications, such as infective endocarditis and mitral insufficiency.

What happens in mitral valve prolapse

In this disorder, the mitral valve leaflets protrude into the left atrium. If these leaflets don't close properly, blood flows back into the left atrium.

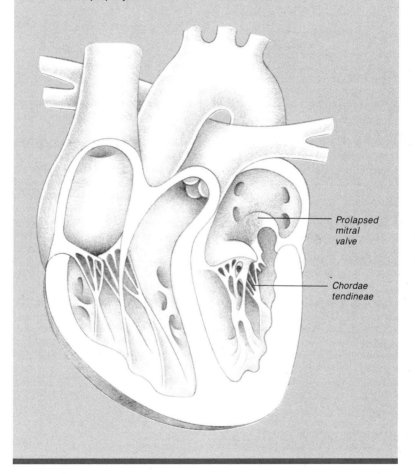

Prolapsed mitral valve

Chordae tendineae

Other test results may indicate the following:

• Color-flow Doppler studies can reveal and evaluate the presence and degree of mitral insufficiency.

• Resting electrocardiography (ECG) may show nonspecific ST-segment changes. It may also disclose biphasic or inverted T waves in leads II, III, or aV_F.

• Radionuclide imaging (thallium 201 or technetium-99m scanning) helps confirm absence of myocardial ischemia.

FactFinder

Key points about mitral valve prolapse syndrome

- *Incidence:* The syndrome most commonly affects young women, but it may occur in both sexes and in all age-groups.
- *Prognosis:* Most patients are only mildly affected and experience no progression of the disorder. If the prolapse is uncomplicated, patients can expect a normal life span. Symptoms directly related to mitral valve dysfunction, if seen, usually occur after age 50 and may require valve surgery.

- *Chief diagnostic methods:* Auscultation and echocardiography.
- *Treatment:* No cure exists. Treatment focuses on alleviating symptoms, if present, and preventing complications.
- *Leading complication:* Severe mitral insufficiency.
- *Other complications:* Although infrequent, other complications may include cardiac arrhythmias, transient ischemic attacks, bacterial endocarditis, and congestive heart failure.

- Exercise ECG testing evaluates chest pain and atrial or ventricular arrhythmias, if present. Be aware that false-positive tests are common.
- Holter monitoring may identify arrhythmias or conduction defects.

NURSING DIAGNOSIS

Common nursing diagnoses for a patient with mitral valve prolapse syndrome include:
- Knowledge deficit related to mitral valve prolapse syndrome, its associated risks, and its management
- Anxiety related to the diagnosis and symptoms
- Activity intolerance related to chest pain, fatigue, or dyspnea.

PLANNING

Because mitral valve prolapse syndrome can't be cured, focus your care on reducing your patient's fears about the disorder and alleviating her symptoms. Also plan to teach her how to avoid complications and recognize warnings signs that warrant medical attention.

Based on the nursing diagnosis *knowledge deficit*, develop appropriate patient outcomes. For example, your patient will:
- communicate an understanding of mitral valve prolapse syndrome, including potential complications and measures to manage symptoms
- express willingness to adhere to follow-up care measures and make necessary life-style changes
- express willingness to take antibiotics before dental work, surgery, or other invasive procedures.

Based on the nursing diagnosis *anxiety,* develop appropriate patient outcomes. For example, your patient will:
- express the understanding that most patients with mitral valve prolapse syndrome lead normal lives
- state at least two measures that will help eliminate or reduce anxiety.

Based on the nursing diagnosis *activity intolerance,* develop appropriate patient outcomes. For example, your patient will:
- agree to begin an exercise program that improves cardiovascular fitness.

Treatments

Medical care of the patient with mitral valve prolapse syndrome

Most patients with mitral valve prolapse syndrome can control their symptoms by carefully managing their diet and life-style. Some patients, however, may require drug therapy especially when their symptoms are severe.

Drug therapy
Generally, drugs are prescribed on a temporary basis. They include:
• beta blockers to treat runs of paroxysmal atrial tachycardia or premature ventricular or atrial contractions and other symptoms, such as migraine headaches.
• antiarrhythmic agents to treat serious arrhythmias, such as ventricular

tachycardia
• calcium channel blockers to control arrhythmias and migraine headaches
• antibiotic agents to provide prophylaxis before dental work, surgery, and other invasive procedures in patients with auscultatory or echocardiographic signs of significant regurgitation and in patients with structurally impaired valve leaflets.

IMPLEMENTATION

Target your nursing interventions to the patient's condition. If she's asymptomatic, focus your care on easing her anxiety and teaching her about measures to prevent complications. (See *Medical care of the patient with mitral valve prolapse syndrome.*)

Nursing interventions
• Obtain baseline assessment data, especially the results of cardiac auscultation and the type and frequency of symptoms, if present.

Patient teaching
• Help alleviate anxiety by allowing the patient to express fears and by providing advice and reassurance. Explain that most patients with mitral valve prolapse syndrome lead normal lives and don't experience serious complications or require heart surgery.
• Explain mitral valve prolapse syndrome and its possible causes and complications.
• Teach the patient about echocardiography and other diagnostic tests, as needed. If the patient has a history of

syncope or symptomatic arrhythmia, explain the Holter monitoring procedure. Also describe the exercise ECG test to evaluate chest pain, as needed.
• Advise the patient on how to prevent or manage symptoms of mitral valve prolapse syndrome. (See *Helping patients cope with mitral valve prolapse syndrome,* page 168.)
• Instruct her to check with her doctor about the need for antibiotics before dental work or invasive procedures.
• Teach about prescribed medications and their possible adverse effects.
• Emphasize the importance of good oral hygiene and regular dental checkups to help reduce the risk of bacterial endocarditis.
• If possible, encourage the patient to join a support group for those with the syndrome.
• Before discharge, explain the importance of keeping follow-up appointments to check for disease progression, even in the absence of symptoms. (See *Ensuring continued care for the patient with mitral valve prolapse syndrome.* page 169.)

Helping patients cope with mitral valve prolapse syndrome

Encourage patients with mitral valve prolapse syndrome to take steps to improve their quality of life and cope better with their condition.

Regular exercise

Encourage your patient to begin carefully planned aerobic exercise. Exercise reduces plasma catecholamines (epinephrine or adrenalin and norepinephrine), lowers resting heart rate, decreases stress, increases cardiac output, and increases blood volume — all beneficial effects that may help relieve symptoms.

Drug precautions

Advise the patient to take over-the-counter (OTC) drugs with caution. Many symptoms of mitral valve prolapse syndrome can be exacerbated by common OTC ingredients, including caffeine, ephedrine, epinephrine, pseudoephedrine hydrochloride, and pseudoephedrine sulfate. Tell the patient to read labels carefully and to seek advice before taking medications to relieve allergies, colds, or pain.

Also tell the patient to avoid caffeine. This nervous system stimulant may bring on or exacerbate symptoms of mitral valve prolapse syndrome, especially chest pain and palpitations.

Dietary habits

Tell the patient not to cut back on salt and fluids (unless specifically ordered to treat a medical condition). Encourage the patient to drink at least eight glasses of fluid a day. This will increase blood volume and may be especially helpful for problems of orthostatic hypotension or syncope.

Warn against crash and fad diets.

Rapidly shedding pounds means losing a lot of essential water and sodium. Using diet pills that contain stimulants may also adversely affect the patient's health. If the patient wants to lose weight, advise her to exercise regularly and practice good eating habits.

Advise the patient to avoid foods with fast-acting carbohydrates, such as candy, cookies, and chocolate. These foods may cause symptoms to become worse.

Symptom management

Advise the patient with mitral valve prolapse syndrome to use the techniques described for managing these symptoms.

Chest pain

Tell the patient to lie flat, raise her legs to a 90-degree angle, and lean them against a wall or couch. The pain will usually subside in 3 to 5 minutes.

Extra heartbeats

Instruct the patient to take a walk or do some other activity that will increase her heart rate. A higher heart rate usually overrides or suppresses extra heartbeats.

Mild dyspnea

Tell the patient to breathe in as much air as possible and then exhale slowly through pursed lips. If she does this three or four times, the dyspnea should disappear.

Discharge TimeSaver

Ensuring continued care for the patient with mitral valve prolapse syndrome

Review the following teaching topics, referrals, and follow-up appointments to ensure that your patient is adequately prepared for discharge.

Teaching topics
Make sure that the following teaching topics have been covered and that your patient's learning has been evaluated:
☐ an explanation of the disorder and its causes, symptoms, and possible complications
☐ need for lifelong follow-up
☐ symptom management, if needed
☐ reportable signs and symptoms
☐ need for antibiotics before dental work or invasive procedures.

Referrals
Make sure that your patient has re-

ceived the following appropriate referrals:
☐ dietitian
☐ smoking cessation program, if necessary
☐ exercise program
☐ support group for people with mitral valve prolapse syndrome, if available.

Follow-up appointments
Make sure that your patient has been provided with the times and dates for these necessary follow-up appointments:
☐ doctor
☐ additional diagnostic tests.

EVALUATION

To evaluate a patient's response to your care, gather reassessment data and compare this information with the patient outcomes specified in your plan of care.

Teaching and counseling
Begin by evaluating the effectiveness of your patient teaching. Listen for statements from the patient indicating:
• an understanding of mitral valve prolapse syndrome and its possible complications
• willingness to adhere to follow-up measures and to seek medical attention if warning symptoms occur
• awareness that most patients with the syndrome lead normal lives
• knowledge of how to prevent or manage symptoms of the syndrome.

Coping with anxiety
Assess your patient's ability to cope with anxiety. Consider the following questions:
• Can your patient describe measures that will help eliminate or reduce anxiety?
• Does she indicate, either through her words or actions, that she'll be able to live with her diagnosis without experiencing severe anxiety?

Coping with activity intolerance
Evaluate your patient's ability to cope with activity intolerance. Consider the following questions:
• Is your patient willing to structure her activities in a way that promotes optimal use of her energy?
• Does she report that episodes of chest pain, fatigue, and shortness of breath are less frequent or absent altogether?

Mitral insufficiency

Mitral insufficiency occurs when an incompetent mitral valve allows blood from the left ventricle to flow back into the left atrium during systole. The condition, also known as mitral regurgitation, may be acute or chronic and tends to be self-perpetuating: as insufficiency progresses, the left atrium enlarges. In patients with chronic mitral insufficiency, the left ventricle dilates to accommodate the increased volume of blood from the left atrium. Left ventricular dilation worsens mitral insufficiency, which further enlarges the left atrium and left ventricle and exacerbates the insufficiency.

As mitral insufficiency progresses, heart failure and pulmonary edema may occur. With acute mitral insufficiency, acute and fulminant heart failure may occur. With chronic mitral insufficiency, atrial fibrillation commonly occurs.

Causes

Mitral insufficiency may result from any of several congenital or acquired conditions. (See *Causes of mitral insufficiency*.)

ASSESSMENT

Your assessment should include a thorough health history, physical examination, and review of diagnostic test results.

Health history

With mild to moderate mitral insufficiency, the patient may be asymptomatic. As the disorder progresses, the patient may report fatigue, orthopnea, exertional dyspnea, weakness and, possibly, atypical chest pain, dysphagia, and palpitations. Be sure to question the patient about the development or worsening of symptoms. Also explore the medical history for a possible causative factor.

Physical examination

Inspection may reveal jugular vein distention with an abnormally prominent v wave. You may also note peripheral edema.

Palpation of the abdomen may reveal hepatomegaly. Palpation of the carotid artery may disclose a pulsation that's sharp on the upstroke. You can probably palpate a systolic thrill at the apex.

Auscultation may reveal a classic sign of mitral insufficiency: a grade III to VI or louder, high-pitched, blowing, holosystolic murmur. (See *Identifying the murmur of mitral insufficiency*, page 172.) You may also hear a soft S_1 and a low-pitched S_3. Usually with severe mitral insufficiency, the systolic murmur starts immediately after the soft S_1 and continues and may obscure A_2. In patients who have a normal sinus rhythm, S_4 may occur in recent, acute mitral insufficiency.

Auscultation of the lungs may reveal crackles if the patient has pulmonary edema.

Diagnostic test results

• Cardiac catheterization may indicate signs of mitral insufficiency, including increased left ventricular end-diastolic volume and pressure, increased atrial and pulmonary artery wedge pressures, and decreased cardiac output.
• Chest X-rays may demonstrate left atrial and ventricular enlargement, pulmonary venous congestion, and calcification of the mitral leaflets.
• Echocardiography may reveal abnormal motion of the valve leaflets, left atrial enlargement, and a hyperdynamic left ventricle.
• Electrocardiography (ECG) may show left atrial and ventricular hypertrophy, sinus tachycardia, or atrial fibrillation.

NURSING DIAGNOSIS

Common nursing diagnoses for a patient with mitral insufficiency include:
• Activity intolerance related to fatigue and dyspnea
• Decreased cardiac output related to mitral insufficiency
• Fatigue related to decreased cardiac output
• Fluid volume excess related to pulmonary edema
• High risk for infection related to invasive procedures or I.V. drug abuse.

PLANNING

Develop a plan of care to help the patient manage his symptoms, especially fatigue and dyspnea. Also plan to implement measures to improve cardiac output and prevent complications.

Based on the nursing diagnosis *activity intolerance,* develop appropriate patient outcomes. For example, your patient will:
• identify and avoid or obtain assistance with activities that worsen fatigue and dyspnea
• demonstrate skill in conserving energy while performing self-care activities to his tolerance level
• maintain vital signs within the prescribed limits during activities.

Based on the nursing diagnosis *decreased cardiac output,* develop appropriate patient outcomes. For example, your patient will:
• maintain hemodynamic stability, as evidenced by vital signs within set limits; warm, dry skin; adequate urine output; and baseline mental status
• report fewer episodes of syncope and dizziness
• report fewer dyspneic episodes
• comply with treatment to enhance cardiac output.

Based on the nursing diagnosis *fatigue,* develop appropriate patient outcomes. For example, your patient will:

FactFinder
Causes of mitral insufficiency

In *chronic* mitral insufficiency, damage to the mitral valve may result from:
• congenital anomalies, such as transposition of the great arteries
• endocarditis
• idiopathic hypertrophic subaortic stenosis
• mitral valve prolapse
• rheumatic heart disease
• dilation of annulus secondary to congestive cardiomyopathies
• ruptured chordae tendineae secondary to trauma.

In *acute* mitral insufficiency, damage to the mitral valve may result from any of the following:
• myocardial infarction
• prosthetic valve malfunction
• trauma
• endocarditis
• ruptured chordae tendineae.

Causes in older patients
In older patients, mitral insufficiency may occur because the mitral annulus has become calcified, a condition that occurs more frequently in females. The cause is unknown, but it may be linked to a degenerative process.

• agree to conserve energy through rest, planning, and setting priorities
• establish a regular sleeping pattern.

Based on the nursing diagnosis *fluid volume excess,* develop appropriate patient outcomes. For example, your patient will:
• demonstrate baseline respiratory rate and pattern
• maintain output greater than intake during initial treatment
• agree to take precautions to prevent or minimize pulmonary edema, such as complying with drug therapy and

Identifying the murmur of mitral insufficiency

If you discover a murmur, try to discern its type through careful auscultation. If you suspect mitral insufficiency, listen for a high-pitched, blowing, holosystolic murmur that may radiate from the mitral area to the left axillary line. Best heard at the apex, this murmur results from turbulent, high-pressure blood flow back through and across the opening of the mitral valve. Notice that when the patient stands suddenly, the murmur sounds softer.

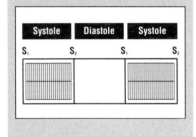

adhering to dietary and activity restrictions

Based on the nursing diagnosis *high risk for infection,* develop appropriate patient outcomes. For example, your patient will:
• comply with prolonged antibiotic treatment
• agree to take antibiotics before dental work, surgery, or other invasive procedures
• express a willingness to initiate measures to help prevent exposure to infection.
• agree to report signs and symptoms of infection or exposure to streptococcal infection to the doctor immediately.

IMPLEMENTATION

Because the nature and severity of symptoms varies among patients, tailor your nursing care to the patient's condition. Expect to provide comprehensive teaching, because all patients must learn how to prevent complications and manage symptoms. Administer medications and prepare the patient for valvular surgery, when necessary. (See *Medical care of the patient with mitral insufficiency.*)

Nursing interventions
• Monitor the patient for signs of heart failure, pulmonary edema, and arrhythmias. Assess vital signs, heart and breath sounds, arterial blood gas levels, intake and output, and daily weight. Monitor blood chemistry studies, chest X-rays, and ECG readings.
• To prevent excessive fatigue, provide periods of rest between activities. Assist the patient, as needed, to minimize fatigue and dyspnea.
• Keep the patient with signs of heart failure on a low-sodium diet. Consult with the dietitian to provide as many favorite foods as possible in light of restrictions.
• Administer diuretics, digitalis glycosides, and other prescribed drugs for heart failure. Monitor drug effectiveness and for possible adverse reactions.
• Before giving penicillin or any other antibiotic, ask the patient if he has ever had a hypersensitivity reaction to the medication. Even if he has never had such a reaction, warn that it's possible. Administer antibiotics on time to maintain consistent drug levels in the blood. Monitor for adverse reactions.
• Provide oxygen to prevent tissue hypoxia, as needed.

Patient teaching
• Teach the patient and family members about the disorder and its causes, symptoms, and complications. Explain

Treatments

Medical care of the patient with mitral insufficiency

Treatment for patients with mitral insufficiency is determined by the nature and severity of associated symptoms and the presence of complications.

Activity restrictions
The patient may need to restrict activities to avoid extreme fatigue and dyspnea.

Treatment for heart failure
A patient who develops heart failure may require digitalis glycosides, diuretics, angiotensin-converting enzyme inhibitors, a sodium-restricted diet and, in acute cases, oxygen. Other measures may include anticoagulant therapy to prevent thrombus formation

around diseased or replaced valves, and prophylactic antibiotics before and after surgery, dental work, or other invasive procedures.

Surgery
If the patient has severe signs and symptoms that can't be managed medically, he may undergo surgery to repair or replace the affected valve. Valve replacement requires open-heart surgery with cardiopulmonary bypass.

---

all diagnostic tests. Provide advice on dietary and activity restrictions, if appropriate. Also teach the patient energy conservation techniques and stress the need for rest.

• Discuss the need for prescribed medications, if appropriate. Review proper administration and possible adverse effects. If the patient requires anticoagulant therapy, discuss foods and medications that may interfere with this therapy.

• Prepare the patient for valve replacement or repair as indicated. Teach about the surgery, preparation, and aftercare.

• Discuss how to minimize exposure to infection. Emphasize the need to promptly report signs of infection or exposure to streptococcal infection.

• Instruct the patient and family members to watch for and report early signs of heart failure, such as dyspnea and a hacking, nonproductive cough.

• Make sure the patient and family members understand the importance of lifelong follow-up. Emphasize the

need to comply with prolonged antibiotic therapy and the need for additional antibiotics before dental work, surgery, and other invasive procedures. (See *Ensuring continued care for the patient with mitral insufficiency,* page 174.)

EVALUATION

When evaluating your patient's response to your care, gather reassessment data and compare this information with the patient outcomes specified in your plan of care.

Teaching and counseling
Begin by determining the effectiveness of teaching and counseling. Listen for statements from the patient indicating:
• an understanding of mitral insufficiency and its symptoms, causes, treatments, and potential complications
• willingness to comply with prescribed therapy and to keep appointments for follow-up care

Discharge TimeSaver

Ensuring continued care for the patient with mitral insufficiency

Review the following teaching topics, referrals, and follow-up appointments to make sure that your patient is adequately prepared for discharge.

Teaching topics
Ensure that the following teaching topics have been covered and that the patient's learning has been evaluated:
□ explanation of mitral insufficiency, including its causes, symptoms, and complications
□ importance of follow-up care
□ activity restrictions, if needed
□ drug therapy
□ sodium-restricted diet, if needed
□ signs and symptoms to report to the doctor
□ need for antibiotics before dental work and invasive procedures
□ surgery, including preoperative and postoperative care, as needed.

Referrals
Make sure that your patient has received the following appropriate referrals:
□ dietitian
□ home health care agency
□ social services
□ cardiac rehabilitation center.

Follow-up appointments
Make sure that your patient has been provided with the times and dates for these necessary follow-up appointments:
□ doctor or clinic
□ surgeon
□ additional diagnostic tests, if needed.

• an intention to take prescribed medications and to report early signs of heart failure
• willingness to make necessary lifestyle changes to reduce excessive fatigue.

Coping with activity intolerance
Evaluate your patient's ability to cope with activity intolerance. Consider the following questions:
• Can the patient identify activities that increase fatigue and dyspnea?
• Does he try to avoid or obtain assistance with such activities?
• Does he demonstrate skill in conserving energy while performing self-care activities?
• Do his vital signs remain within prescribed limits during activity?

Coping with fatigue
Evaluate your patient's ability to cope with fatigue. Consider the following questions:
• Does the patient take steps to conserve energy through rest, planning, and setting priorities?
• Has he established a regular sleeping pattern?

Preventing infection
Evaluate the patient's willingness to take steps to prevent infection. Consider the following questions:
• Does the patient comply with prolonged antibiotic treatment?
• Does he understand the need for antibiotic prophylaxis before dental work, surgery, or other invasive procedures?
• Does he understand the need to avoid exposure to infection and to report signs of infection or exposure to streptococcal infection to the doctor?

Physical condition

Evaluation of the patient's condition should include reassessment of fluid volume and cardiac status.

Fluid volume status

Consider the following questions:
• During initial treatment, has the patient been able to maintain output greater than input?
• Is he willing to take precautions to prevent or minimize pulmonary edema?
• Are his respiratory rate and pattern within established limits?

Cardiac status

Consider the following questions:
• Does the patient demonstrate evidence of hemodynamic stability, including vital signs within set limits; warm, dry skin; adequate urine output; and baseline mental status?
• How often does he experience episodes of syncope and dizziness or dyspnea?

Mitral stenosis

In this disorder, mitral valve leaflets become diffusely thickened by fibrosis and calcification. The mitral commissures fuse, the chordae tendineae fuse and shorten, the valvular cusps become rigid, and the orifice of the valve becomes narrowed, obstructing blood flow from the left atrium to the left ventricle. (See *What happens in mitral stenosis,* page 176.)

Because of progressive narrowing of the mitral valve, left atrial volume and pressure rise and the atrial chamber dilates. The increased resistance to blood flow eventually causes pulmonary hypertension. In time, severe pulmonary hypertension leads to right-sided heart failure and tricuspid insufficiency. These changes can offer a protective effect; the increased precapillary resistance decreases the frequency of symptoms of pulmonary congestion.

In addition, inadequate filling of the left ventricle reduces cardiac output. However, atrial fibrillation and systemic emboli may also occur.

Causes

Two-thirds of all patients with mitral stenosis are female. The disorder most commonly results from rheumatic fever, but it may also be associated with congenital anomalies. Rarely, mitral stenosis is a complication of systemic lupus erythematosus and rheumatoid arthritis.

ASSESSMENT

During your assessment, explore the patient's history to detect possible causes of mitral stenosis.

Health history

In mild mitral stenosis, the patient may have no symptoms. As the disorder progresses, she may report dyspnea on exertion, paroxysmal nocturnal dyspnea, orthopnea, weakness, fatigue, palpitations, and a chronic, nonproductive cough. Hemoptysis and hoarseness may also occur.

Physical examination

Depending on the severity of the disorder, physical findings may vary.

Inspection may reveal a malar rash. In severe mitral stenosis, you may note *mitral facies,* which are pinkish purple patches on the cheeks. You may note jugular vein distention and ascites in the patient with severe mitral stenosis with pulmonary hypertension and right-sided heart failure. The jugular venous pulse usually has a prominent a wave in patients with sinus rhythm.

Abdominal palpation may reveal hepatomegaly, with severe mitral stenosis. Auscultation may reveal a loud S_1 or opening snap and a low-pitched,

What happens in mitral stenosis

In this disorder, the openings of the mitral valve narrow because of progressive fibrosis, scarring, and calcification of the valve leaflets as well as fusion of the commissures and shortening of the chordae tendineae.

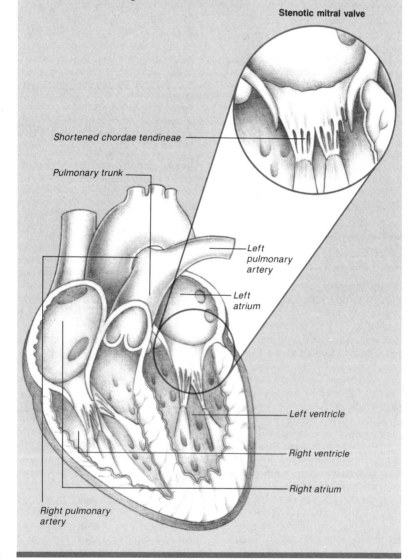

Stenotic mitral valve

Shortened chordae tendineae

Pulmonary trunk

Left pulmonary artery

Left atrium

Left ventricle

Right ventricle

Right atrium

Right pulmonary artery

rumbling, diastolic murmur that's heard best at the apex. The murmur may radiate to the axilla or to the left sternal border. The murmur's duration serves as a guide to the extent of mitral narrowing (a longer duration indicates greater narrowing).

Timesaving tip: For a patient with mitral stenosis, follow these steps to hear the murmur: Place her in a left lateral position. Then, because the murmur is low-pitched, use the bell of the stethoscope, placing it directly on the apical impulse. Listen closely during exhalation because the murmur is best heard then. (See *Identifying the murmur of mitral stenosis.*)

In patients with pulmonary hypertension, S_2 is often accentuated, and its two components are closely split. With further elevation of pulmonary pressure, S_2 becomes a single sound. A pulmonary systolic ejection click may be heard in patients with severe pulmonary hypertension. Crackles may also be heard.

Diagnostic test results

• Cardiac catheterization shows a diastolic pressure gradient across the mitral valve and elevated left atrial and pulmonary artery pressures. It also shows an elevated pulmonary artery wedge pressure (PAWP) that exceeds 15 mm Hg. Catheterization may also reveal elevated right ventricular pressure, decreased cardiac output, and abnormal contraction of the left ventricle. However, this test may not be indicated in patients who have isolated mitral stenosis with mild symptoms.

• Chest X-rays show left atrial and left ventricular enlargement (in severe mitral stenosis), straightening of the left border of the cardiac silhouette, enlarged pulmonary arteries, dilation of the pulmonary veins of the upper lobes of the lungs, and mitral valve calcification.

Identifying the murmur of mitral stenosis

If you discover a murmur, try to determine its type through careful auscultation. If your suspect mitral stenosis, listen for a low-pitched, rumbling, crescendo-decrescendo murmur in the mitral valve area. The murmur results from the turbulent flow of blood across the stiffened and narrowed valvular structure.

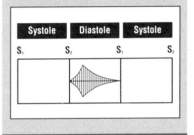

• Echocardiography (one of the most important tests) may disclose thickened mitral valve leaflets and left atrial enlargement.

• Electrocardiography (ECG) may reveal atrial fibrillation, right ventricular hypertrophy, left atrial enlargement (in sinus rhythm), and right axis deviation.

NURSING DIAGNOSIS

Common nursing diagnoses for mitral stenosis include:

• Activity intolerance related to fatigue, dyspnea, or palpitations

• Decreased cardiac output related to the disorder's effects

• High risk for infection related to invasive procedures

• Fatigue related to decreased cardiac output

• Impaired gas exchange related to pulmonary hypertension.

PLANNING

Plan to monitor the patient for signs of complications and teach her about prescribed medications and other measures to alleviate or prevent symptoms.

Based on the nursing diagnosis *activity intolerance,* develop appropriate patient outcomes. For example, your patient will:
• identify and avoid or obtain assistance with activities that increase fatigue, dyspnea, and palpitations
• demonstrate skill in conserving energy while performing self-care activities to her tolerance level
• maintain vital signs within the prescribed limits during activity.

Based on the nursing diagnosis *decreased cardiac output,* develop appropriate patient outcomes. For example, your patient will:
• demonstrate hemodynamic stability, as evidenced by vital signs within set limits; warm, dry skin; adequate urine output; maintenance of baseline mental status; and reduced incidence of syncope and dizziness
• report fewer dyspneic episodes
• agree to comply with treatment to enhance cardiac output
• regain normal cardiac output after valve replacement, commissurotomy, or percutaneous balloon valvuloplasty.

Based on the nursing diagnosis *high risk for infection,* develop appropriate patient outcomes. For example, your patient will:
• express a willingness to comply with prolonged antibiotic treatment, if prescribed, and to take prophylactic antibiotics before dental work, surgery, or other invasive procedures
• initiate measures to help prevent exposure to infection
• agree to report signs of infection or exposure to streptococcal infection to the doctor immediately.

Based on the nursing diagnosis *fatigue,* develop appropriate patient outcomes. For example, your patient will:
• conserve energy through rest, planning, and establishing priorities for activities
• establish a regular sleeping pattern.

Based on the nursing diagnosis *impaired gas exchange,* develop appropriate patient outcomes. For example, your patient will:
• report that she feels comfortable while she's breathing
• maintain a baseline respiratory rate and pattern and adequate breath sounds
• maintain baseline arterial blood gas (ABG) levels
• take precautions to prevent or minimize pulmonary edema, such as adhering to the medication regimen and to dietary and activity restrictions.

IMPLEMENTATION

Provide interventions that are tailored to the nature and severity of the patient's symptoms. For example, if the patient is young and asymptomatic, stress the need for prophylactic antibiotics before invasive procedures. If the patient has symptoms or complications, you may need to administer medications, enforce bed rest and, possibly, prepare her for valvular surgery. (See *Medical care of the patient with mitral stenosis.*)

Nursing interventions

• Monitor the patient for signs of heart failure, pulmonary edema, arrhythmias, and systemic emboli. Assess her vital signs, heart and breath sounds, ABG levels, intake and output, and daily weight. Monitor blood chemistry studies, chest X-rays, and ECG readings.
• Stress the importance of obtaining needed bed rest. Assist the patient with bathing and other activities, as necessary. Provide a bedside commode because

Treatments

Medical care of the patient with mitral stenosis

In mitral stenosis, the nature and severity of associated symptoms and complications determine the type of treatment.

Asymptomatic patient
If the patient is asymptomatic, an appropriate antibiotic is an important prophylactic before dental work, surgery, or other invasive procedures.

Patient with complications
If the patient develops heart failure, she requires bed rest, a digitalis glycoside, diuretics, a sodium-restricted diet and, in acute cases, oxygen. Small doses of beta blockers or calcium channel blockers may also be used to slow the ventricular rate when digitalis glycosides fail to control atrial fibrillation or flutter.

Anticoagulant therapy is indicated for the patient in atrial fibrillation because of the risk of embolization. This therapy is also indicated for a patient who has had an embolic event.

Patient with severe signs and symptoms
If the patient has severe signs and symptoms that can't be managed medically, she may need open-heart surgery with cardiopulmonary bypass for commissurotomy or valve replacement.

Percutaneous balloon valvuloplasty may be used in young patients who have no calcification or subvalvular deformity, in symptomatic pregnant women, and in elderly patients with end-stage disease who can't withstand general anesthesia or who refuse surgery. This procedure is performed in the cardiac catheterization laboratory.

---

using a commode puts less stress on the heart than using a bedpan. Offer an opportunity to participate in physically undemanding activities. Schedule activities to promote sufficient rest periods.
• Place her in an upright position to relieve dyspnea, if needed. Administer oxygen to prevent tissue hypoxia, as needed.
• Keep the patient with signs of heart failure on a low-sodium diet. Consult with the dietitian to plan menus that provide as many favorite foods as possible in light of restrictions.
• Administer diuretics and a digitalis glycoside, as prescribed, for heart failure. Monitor drug effectiveness and for possible adverse reactions.

Patient teaching
• Teach the patient and family members about the disorder, including its causes, symptoms, and potential complications. Also review ordered diagnostic tests and prescribed treatments. Explain dietary or activity restrictions. Teach energy conservation techniques and the need for daily rest periods.
• Provide instructions about the proper use of medications and their possible adverse effects. If the patient is receiving anticoagulants, discuss foods and medications that may interfere with this therapy.
• Advise the patient about how to minimize exposure to infection. Tell her to promptly report signs of infection or exposure to streptococcal infection to the doctor.
• Instruct the asymptomatic patient and her family to watch for and report early

Ensuring continued care for the patient with mitral stenosis

Review the following teaching topics, referrals, and follow-up appointments to ensure that your patient is adequately prepared for discharge.

Teaching topics
Make sure that the following teaching topics have been covered and that the patient's learning has been evaluated:
□ explanation of mitral stenosis, including its causes, symptoms, and possible complications
□ activity restrictions, if needed
□ drug therapy
□ sodium-restricted diet, if needed
□ signs and symptoms to report to the doctor
□ need for antibiotics before dental work and invasive procedures
□ surgery, including preoperative and postoperative care, if appropriate.

Referrals
Make sure that your patient has been provided with the following appropriate referrals:
□ dietitian
□ home health care agency
□ social services
□ cardiac rehabilitation center.

Follow-up appointments
Make sure that your patient has been provided with the times and dates for these necessary follow-up appointments:
□ doctor or clinic
□ surgeon
□ additional diagnostic tests.

signs of heart failure, such as dyspnea and a hacking, nonproductive cough. Stress the importance of reporting hemoptysis.

• If the patient is scheduled for a valve replacement or a percutaneous balloon valvuloplasty, explain the procedure to the patient and family members and tell them what to expect before, during, and after the procedure. Prepare the patient for the procedure, as indicated.

• Before discharge, make sure the patient and her family understand the need to obtain follow-up care and to take antibiotics before and after dental work, surgery, and other invasive procedures. (See *Ensuring continued care for the patient with mitral stenosis.*)

EVALUATION

When evaluating your patient's response to nursing care, gather reassessment data and compare this infor-

mation with the patient outcomes specified in your plan of care.

Teaching and counseling

Begin by determining the effectiveness of teaching and counseling. Listen for statements by the patient indicating:

• willingness to make life-style changes to reduce fatigue, dyspnea, and palpitations

• understanding of mitral stenosis and its causes, symptoms, and complications.

• intention to seek necessary follow-up care and take prophylactic antibiotics, as needed.

• understanding of the purpose of tests and treatments.

Coping with activity intolerance
Assess the patient's ability to cope with activity intolerance. Consider the following questions:

• Is the patient able to identify activities that increase fatigue, dyspnea, and palpitations? If so, does she avoid or obtain assistance with these activities?
• Does she demonstrate skill in conserving energy while performing self-care activities?
• Do her vital signs remain within the prescribed limits during activity?

Coping with fatigue
Assess your patient's ability to cope with fatigue. Consider the following questions:
• Can she conserve energy through rest, planning, and establishing priorities for activities?
• Has she established a regular sleeping pattern?

Preventing infection
Determine whether your patient has taken steps to avoid infection. Consider the following questions:
• Is she willing to comply with prolonged antibiotic treatment?
• Does she initiate measures to help prevent exposure to infection?
• Have signs and symptoms of infection or exposure to streptococcal infection been promptly reported?

Physical condition
Evaluation of the patient's physical condition should include the patient's cardiac and respiratory status.

Cardiac status
Consider the following questions:
• Does the patient demonstrate evidence of hemodynamic stability, including vital signs within set limits; warm, dry skin; adequate urine output; maintenance of baseline mental status; and reduced incidence of syncope and dizziness?
• How frequently does she experience dyspneic episodes?
• If the patient underwent valve replacement, commissurotomy, or percutaneous balloon valvuloplasty, has she regained normal cardiac output?

Respiratory status
Consider the following questions:
• Does the patient indicate that she feels comfortable breathing, either by her words or actions?
• Does she maintain a baseline respiratory rate?
• Are breath sounds adequate?
• Does she maintain ABG levels at established limits?
• Has she taken precautions to prevent or minimize pulmonary edema?

Aortic insufficiency

In this disorder (also called aortic regurgitation), blood flows back into the left ventricle during diastole. This condition may be acute or chronic. In chronic aortic insufficiency, the left ventricle becomes overloaded and dilated and eventually hypertrophies. In advanced stages, the excess fluid volume also overloads the left atrium and, later, the pulmonary system. Aortic insufficiency eventually leads to heart failure. The patient is also at risk for myocardial ischemia because left ventricular dilation and elevated left ventricular systolic pressure alter myocardial oxygen requirements. In acute aortic insufficiency, the normal-sized ventricle can't accommodate the large regurgitant blood volume. Therefore, stroke volume declines and ventricular end pressure rises.

Aortic insufficiency by itself occurs most commonly among males. When associated with mitral valve disease, however, it's more common among females.

Causes
Chronic aortic insufficiency may occur in Marfan syndrome, an inherited dis-

Assessment TimeSaver

Identifying signs of severe chronic aortic insufficiency

Finding	Characteristics
Musset's sign	Heartbeats jar the body and patient's head bobs with each systole.
Water-hammer pulse (Corrigan's pulse)	Pulse rate rises rapidly, then collapses late in systole.
Quincke's sign	Pressure applied to nail tip causes the root to flush and pale.
Pulsus bisferiens	Palpation of peripheral pulse reveals double beating with two systolic peaks.
Pistol-shot sound (Traube's sign)	Auscultation over large arteries reveals loud, intense sound.
Duroziez's murmur	Applying pressure to stethoscope reveals double murmur over femoral artery.

order. It may also result from rheumatic fever, syphilis, endocarditis, ankylosing spondylitis, congenital anomaly, hypertension or aortic aneurysm, or calcification of an aortic valve. In some patients, it may be idiopathic. Acute aortic insufficiency most commonly results from infective endocarditis, aortic dissection, or trauma.

ASSESSMENT

Because signs and symptoms vary with the severity of the disorder, a physical examination and test results are particularly important for establishing the diagnosis. (See *Identifying signs of severe chronic aortic insufficiency*.)

Health history

A patient with mild or moderate aortic insufficiency may remain asymptomatic for years. In severe chronic aortic insufficiency, the patient may report an uncomfortable awareness of his heartbeat, especially when lying down. He may report palpitations along with a pounding headache, especially with emotional stress or exertion.

Dyspnea may occur with exertion, and the patient may experience paroxysmal nocturnal dyspnea with diaphoresis, orthopnea, night sweats, and a cough. He may become fatigued or, rarely, experience syncope. He may also have a history of anginal pain that may or may not be relieved by sublingual nitroglycerin. In acute aortic insufficiency, patients often develop sudden signs of cardiovascular collapse with weakness, severe dyspnea, and hypotension.

The patient's medical history may also reveal a possible cause of aortic insufficiency.

Physical examination

In severe chronic aortic insufficiency, you may note that each heartbeat seems to jar the patient's entire body and that his head bobs with each systole (Musset's sign). Inspection of arterial pulsations shows a rapidly rising pulse rate that collapses suddenly as arterial pressure falls late in systole. This phenomenon, called a water-hammer pulse (or Corrigan's pulse), may especially be noted on inspection of the carotid arteries. It may also be disclosed by palpating the radial artery with the patient's arm elevated.

The patient's nail beds may appear to be pulsating. If you apply pressure at the nail tip, the root will alternately flush and pale (a phenomenon called Quincke's sign). Inspection of the chest may reveal a visible apical impulse. Arterial pulsations in the neck may be visible.

When you palpate the peripheral pulses (especially of the brachial and femoral arteries), you may note a double beating pulse with two systolic peaks (pulsus bisferiens) and collapsing pulses. If the patient has arrhythmias, his pulse rate may be irregular.

When you palpate for the apical impulse, keep in mind that the apex may be displaced laterally and inferiorly. You may be able to palpate a diastolic thrill, usually along the left sternal border, and feel a prominent systolic thrill in the suprasternal notch and over the carotid arteries.

Auscultation may reveal a high-pitched, blowing, decrescendo diastolic murmur, best heard at the left sternal border, at the third or fourth intercostal space. It begins immediately after A₂. (See *Identifying the murmur of aortic insufficiency.*)

Timesaving tip: Use the diaphragm of the stethoscope to hear the murmur in aortic insufficiency. Have the patient sit up, lean forward, and hold his breath in forced expiration.

You may also hear additional heart sounds or murmurs, including:
• an S_1 (in acute aortic insufficiency; may be soft or absent)
• an S_3
• an S_4 (in acute aortic insufficiency)
• a loud P_2 (in acute aortic insufficiency)

Identifying the murmur of aortic insufficiency

If you discover a murmur, try to determine its type. If you suspect aortic insufficiency, listen for a high-pitched, blowing, decrescendo diastolic murmur that radiates from the aortic valve area to the left sternal border.

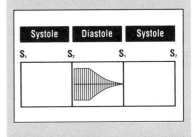

• a loud systolic ejection murmur
• a midsystolic ejection murmur at the base of the heart. This murmur may be grade I to IV and typically is higher pitched, shorter, and less rasping than the murmur heard in aortic stenosis. In acute aortic insufficiency, the murmur is lower pitched and shorter than in chronic aortic insufficiency.
• a soft, low-pitched, rumbling, mid-diastolic murmur (Austin Flint murmur). It may be present briefly in acute aortic insufficiency. This murmur, best heard at the apex of the heart, may be confused with the murmur of mitral stenosis. The absence of a loud S_1 and opening snap distinguishes it.
• a booming pistol-shot sound when the stethoscope is placed lightly over the femoral artery (Traube's sign).
• a to-and-fro or double murmur (Duroziez's murmur) when the stethoscope is placed firmly over the femoral artery.

The patient may develop widened arterial pulse pressure. Therefore, auscultation of blood pressure in chronic aortic insufficiency may reveal greatly increased systolic pressure and muffling of the Korotkoff sounds in phase IV.

Diagnostic test results
The following tests help to confirm the diagnosis and evaluate the severity of the disorder:
• Cardiac catheterization shows reduced arterial diastolic pressure, aortic insufficiency, and valvular abnormalities.
• Echocardiography reveals left ventricular enlargement and changes in left ventricular function. It's helpful in identifying the cause of aortic insufficiency. It may show a dilated aortic root, a flail leaflet, thickening of the cusps, or valve prolapse. Doppler echocardiography readily detects mild degrees of aortic insufficiency that may be inaudible. It also shows a rapid, high-frequency, diastolic fluttering of the anterior mitral leaflet that results from aortic insufficiency.
• Electrocardiography (ECG) may show left ventricular hypertrophy, ST-segment depression, and T-wave inversion.
• Radionuclide angiography is helpful in determining the degree of regurgitant blood flow and assessing left ventricular function.

NURSING DIAGNOSIS

Common nursing diagnoses for aortic insufficiency include:
• Altered cardiopulmonary tissue perfusion related to decreased cardiac output
• High risk for infection related to invasive procedures
• Decreased cardiac output related to the disorder's effects
• Fatigue related to decreased tissue oxygenation with exertion.

PLANNING

Develop a plan of care that incorporates patient teaching and measures to lessen fatigue and prevent infection. Also plan to monitor the patient carefully and prepare him, if necessary, for valvular surgery.

Based on the nursing diagnosis *altered cardiopulmonary tissue perfusion,* develop appropriate patient outcomes. For example, your patient will:
• report decreased frequency of dyspnea
• identify activities that cause dyspnea and avoid or seek assistance with these activities.

Based on the nursing diagnosis *high risk for infection,* develop appropriate patient outcomes. For example, your patient will:
• agree to take antibiotics before dental work, surgery, or other invasive procedures
• initiate measures to help prevent exposure to infection
• agree to report signs of infection or exposure to streptococcal infection to the doctor immediately.

Based on the nursing diagnosis *decreased cardiac output,* develop appropriate patient outcomes. For example, your patient will:
• maintain his pulse rate and blood pressure within established limits
• avoid vigorous sports or exertion
• experience decreased frequency of arrhythmias, as evidenced by ECG readings
• maintain baseline mental status
• maintain adequate urine output
• list signs and symptoms of decreased cardiac output, including dizziness, syncope, clammy skin, fatigue, and dyspnea.
• communicate understanding of the importance of seeking medical attention if signs of decreased cardiac output are present
• show evidence of diminished severity and less frequent episodes of dyspnea

• comply with treatment to enhance his cardiac output.

Based on the nursing diagnosis *fatigue,* develop appropriate patient outcomes. For example, your patient will:
• explain the relationship among his disorder, fatigue, and activity intolerance
• agree to conserve energy during his daily routine through resting, planning, and setting priorities
• agree to establish a regular sleeping pattern.

IMPLEMENTATION

Valve replacement surgery is the treatment of choice for aortic insufficiency but not for patients with chronic aortic insufficiency who are asymptomatic, who have good exercise tolerance, and who have normal left aortic valve function. As needed, prepare the patient for surgery and teach him what to expect before, during, and after the procedure. Ideally, valve replacement is performed before significant left ventricular dysfunction occurs.

If the patient develops left ventricular failure, you'll need to administer prescribed medications, such as digitalis glycosides, diuretics, vasodilators, and angiotensin-converting enzyme inhibitors. Also provide the patient with a low-sodium diet. Stress the importance of taking antibiotics before dental work and invasive procedures. In acute episodes, you may need to administer supplemental oxygen.

Nursing interventions
• Watch for signs of infection, arrhythmias, heart failure, pulmonary edema, and cardiac ischemia. Assess the patient's vital signs, heart and lung sounds, arterial blood gas levels, intake and output, and daily weight. Monitor blood chemistry studies, chest X-rays, and ECG readings.

• Monitor the patient for chest pain, which may indicate myocardial ischemia.
• Observe the patient's level of activity tolerance and his degree of fatigue. Teach energy conservation techniques and stress the need for daily rest periods.
• If the patient needs bed rest, make sure he understands why. Assist with bathing and other activities, as necessary. Provide a bedside commode because using a commode puts less stress on the heart than using a bedpan. Provide an opportunity to participate in physically undemanding activities. Schedule treatments and procedures to promote sufficient rest periods.
• Place the patient in an upright position to relieve dyspnea and administer oxygen to prevent tissue hypoxia, as needed.
• Provide the patient with signs of heart failure with a low-sodium diet; include as many favorite foods as possible in light of restrictions. Provide guidelines about dietary restrictions.
• Administer medications, as prescribed, for heart failure. Monitor drug effectiveness and for possible adverse reactions.
• Teach the patient about the proper use of prescribed medications and possible adverse effects. If anticoagulants are prescribed, discuss foods and medications that may interfere with this therapy.
• Keep the patient's legs elevated while he sits in a chair to improve venous return. Encourage him to use this position whenever he sits.

Patient teaching
• Teach the patient and family members about the disorder, including its causes, symptoms, and potential complications. Be sure to explain all diagnostic tests.
• Provide guidelines to minimize exposure to infection. Urge the patient to

Ensuring continued care for the patient with aortic insufficiency

Review the following teaching topics, referrals, and follow-up appointments to ensure that your patient is adequately prepared for discharge.

Teaching topics
Make sure that the following topics have been covered and that your patient's learning has been evaluated:
□ explanation of aortic insufficiency, including its causes, symptoms, and possible complications
□ activity restrictions as needed
□ drug therapy, including anticoagulant therapy, as needed
□ sodium-restricted diet as needed
□ signs and symptoms to report to the doctor
□ need for antibiotics before dental work or invasive procedures
□ surgery, if needed, including preoperative and postoperative care.

Referrals
Make sure that your patient has been provided with the following appropriate referrals:
□ dietitian
□ home health care agency
□ social services
□ cardiac rehabilitation center.

Follow-up appointments
Make sure that your patient has been provided with the times and dates of these follow-up appointments:
□ doctor or clinic
□ surgeon
□ additional diagnostic tests, if necessary.

promptly report signs of infection or exposure to streptococcal infection.
• Instruct the asymptomatic patient and his family to watch for and report early signs of heart failure, such as dyspnea on exertion and a hacking, nonproductive cough.
• Before discharge, make sure the patient and his family understand the need for follow-up care and for prophylactic antibiotics before and after dental work, surgery, and other invasive procedures. (See *Ensuring continued care for the patient with aortic insufficiency.*)

EVALUATION

When evaluating your patient's response to nursing care, gather reassessment data and compare this information with the patient outcomes specified in your plan of care.

Teaching and counseling
Talk to the patient to determine the effectiveness of teaching and counseling. Consider the following questions:
• Has the patient demonstrated adequate understanding of aortic insufficiency, including its signs and symptoms, potential complications, and treatment?
• Does he know the signs of decreased cardiac output?
• Does he understand the importance of seeking medical attention if he notices signs of decreased cardiac output?
• Has he acknowledged the importance of complying with follow-up care measures, including prophylactic antibiotics?

Evaluating self-care
Evaluate your patient's willingness to comply with treatment and to practice self-care measures to reduce fatigue

and prevent infection. Consider the following questions:
• Does your patient seem to understand the relationship among the disorder, fatigue, and activity tolerance?
• Is he willing to modify his daily routine to reduce fatigue?
• Has he established a regular sleeping pattern?
• Does he take appropriate measures to help prevent exposure to infection?
• Does he intend to promptly report signs of infection or exposure to streptococcal infection?

Cardiopulmonary status
When reassessing your patient's cardiopulmonary status, consider the following questions:
• Does the patient have chest pain?
• Can he identify activities that cause chest pain? Does he avoid or seek assistance with these activities?
• Are his pulse rate and blood pressure within established limits?
• Do his ECG readings indicate an absence of arrhythmias?
• Does reexamination indicate that he has maintained baseline mental status?
• Is his urine output adequate?
• Are episodes of dyspnea less frequent and less severe?

Aortic stenosis

In this disorder, the opening of the aortic valve narrows and the left ventricle exerts increased pressure to drive blood through the opening. The added work load causes the ventricle to hypertrophy. As aortic stenosis worsens, cardiac output declines. The thickened heart muscle, increased systolic pressure, and increased systolic ejection time interfere with coronary artery blood flow, leading to myocardial ischemia and heart failure. (See *Looking at a stenotic aortic valve.*)

Looking at a stenotic aortic valve

The illustrations below point out the effects of aortic stenosis. Normally, the valve leaflets are flexible and move freely. In aortic stenosis, the leaflets become thick and stiffen (with decreased motility), obstructing blood flow across the valve.

Normal aortic valve

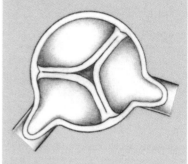

Stenotic valve

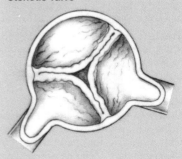

Causes
Aortic stenosis may result from congenital malformations such as a bicuspid valve, or from rheumatic fever or, in elderly patients, degenerative stenosis.

Identifying the murmur of aortic stenosis

If you discover a murmur, try to determine its type through careful auscultation. If you suspect aortic stenosis, listen for a low-pitched, harsh, crescendo-decrescendo murmur that radiates from the aortic valve area to the carotid artery. The murmur results from turbulent, high-pressure blood flow across the stiffened leaflets and through the narrowed opening.

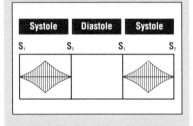

Systole	Diastole	Systole
S₁ S₂		S₁ S₂

ASSESSMENT

Usually, the onset of heart failure is revealed during the patient history. Auscultation of the heart and cardiac studies confirm the diagnosis.

Health history

Even with severe aortic stenosis (narrowing to about one-third of the normal opening), the patient may be asymptomatic. Commonly, the patient develops symptoms when he's in his fifties. He will complain of a cough, dyspnea on exertion, fatigue, exertional syncope, angina, and palpitations. As heart failure progresses, he may complain of orthopnea and paroxysmal nocturnal dyspnea.

Explore the patient's medical history for clues that may reveal the cause of aortic stenosis. Ask the patient if he has a history of rheumatic fever.

Physical examination

While examining your patient, you may note a prominent a wave in the jugular venous pulse. The systolic murmur you hear is low-pitched, harsh, rasping, and crescendo-decrescendo; is loudest at the base of the heart, which is located at the second intercostal space, to the right of the sternal border; and radiates to the neck. In children and adolescents who have a noncalcified aortic valve, you may detect an early systolic ejection sound during auscultation. The sound begins shortly after S_1, has a frequency similar to S_1, and doesn't vary with respiration. It diminishes just before the aortic valve closes.

Timesaving tip: To hear the murmur more easily, place the patient in a sitting position, leaning forward. The murmur will vary in intensity during atrial fibrillation. (See *Identifying the murmur of aortic stenosis.*)

In patients with left ventricular dysfunction, you may detect a paradoxical splitting of S_2. S_2 may be a single sound or it may be inaudible when the valve is rigid. You may also detect an S_4 at the apex, which suggests left ventricular hypertrophy.

When palpating the patient's carotid pulse, you may detect a slowed upstroke and diminished pulse volume. These findings become more marked as the stenosis becomes more severe.

If the patient has left ventricular failure, you may note an exaggerated point of maximal impulse. You may be able to palpate a systolic thrill at the base of the heart, at the suprasternal notch, and along the carotid arteries. The systolic thrill may be palpable only during expiration and when the patient leans forward. In severe aortic stenosis, the pulse pressure and systolic pressure is reduced.

Diagnostic test results

The following tests help to confirm the diagnosis and evaluate the severity of the disorder:

• Cardiac catheterization reveals the pressure gradient across the aortic valve (indicating the severity of obstruction), increased left ventricular end-diastolic pressures (indicating left ventricular dysfunction), and the number of cusps.

• Chest X-rays show valvular calcification, left ventricular enlargement, dilation of the ascending aorta, pulmonary venous congestion and, in later stages, left atrial, pulmonary artery, right atrial, and right ventricular enlargement.

• Echocardiography demonstrates a thickened aortic valve and left ventricular wall and possible coexistent mitral valve stenosis. Doppler echocardiography allows calculation of the aortic pressure gradient.

• Electrocardiography (ECG) reveals left ventricular hypertrophy and ST-segment and T-wave abnormalities. As hypertrophy progresses in severe aortic stenosis, left atrial enlargement is noted. Up to 10% of patients have atrioventricular and intraventricular conduction defects.

NURSING DIAGNOSIS

Common nursing diagnoses for a patient with aortic stenosis include:

• Altered cardiopulmonary tissue perfusion related to decreased coronary artery perfusion and increased demand for oxygen

• Decreased cardiac output related to disease process

• High risk for infection related to threat of bacterial endocarditis associated with invasive procedures

• Fatigue related to decreased tissue oxygenation with exertion.

PLANNING

Focus your plan of care on teaching the patient to comply with treatment and avoid complications. Also plan to monitor him closely for signs of heart failure and to administer medications and prepare him for surgery, as indicated.

Based on the nursing diagnosis *altered cardiopulmonary tissue perfusion,* develop appropriate patient outcomes. For example, your patient will:

• report an absence of chest pain

• identify activities that cause chest pain and avoid or seek assistance with these activities

• maintain his pulse rate and blood pressure within established limits

• show decreased frequency of arrhythmias

• maintain baseline mental status

• maintain adequate urine output.

Based on the nursing diagnosis *decreased cardiac output,* develop appropriate patient outcomes. For example, your patient will:

• list signs and symptoms of decreased cardiac output, including dizziness, syncope, clammy skin, fatigue, and dyspnea

• communicate understanding of the importance of promptly seeking medical attention if any symptoms of aortic stenosis occur

• report a decrease in episodes of dyspnea

• agree to comply with the treatment to enhance cardiac output

• regain normal cardiac output after valve replacement surgery.

Based on the nursing diagnosis *high risk for infection,* develop appropriate patient outcomes. For example, your patient will:

• express willingness to initiate measures to help prevent exposure to infection

Treatments

Medical care of the patient with aortic stenosis

Drug therapy and surgery form the basis for treating aortic stenosis.

Drug therapy
The patient with heart failure may receive digitalis glycosides and diuretics along with nitroglycerin to help relieve angina. Other measures may include a low-sodium diet and, in acute cases, supplemental oxygen.

Surgery
In children who don't have calcified valves, simple commissurotomy under direct visualization is usually effective.

Adults with calcified valves will need valve replacement surgery once they become symptomatic or are at risk for developing left ventricular failure.
Percutaneous balloon aortic valvuloplasty may be performed in children and young adults who have congenital aortic stenosis and in elderly patients with severe calcification. This procedure may improve left ventricular function so that the patient can tolerate valve replacement surgery.

• agree to take antibiotics before dental work, surgery, or other invasive procedures
• agree to report signs of infection or exposure to streptococcal infection to the doctor immediately.

Based on the nursing diagnosis *fatigue,* develop appropriate patient outcomes. For example, your patient will:
• communicate understanding of the relationship between fatigue and the disorder
• agree to conserve energy through rest, planning, and setting priorities
• state his intention to incorporate measures to reduce fatigue during his daily routine
• establish a regular sleeping pattern.

IMPLEMENTATION

Depending on the patient's condition, you may need to administer medications for heart failure or angina or prepare him for surgery. (See *Medical care of the patient with aortic stenosis.)* Provide comprehensive patient teaching, and include family members whenever possible.

Nursing interventions
• Observe the patient for signs of infection, arrhythmias, heart failure, pulmonary edema, and myocardial ischemia. Also monitor him for chest pain, which may indicate myocardial ischemia.
• Assess the patient's vital signs, heart and lung sounds, arterial blood gas levels, intake and output, and daily weight. Monitor his blood chemistry studies, chest X-rays, and ECG readings.
• Observe his activity tolerance and degree of fatigue. Teach him about activity restrictions, if appropriate. Review energy conservation techniques and the need for daily rest periods.
• If the patient needs bed rest, explain why. Assist with bathing and other activities, as necessary. Provide a bedside commode because using a commode puts less stress on the heart than using a bedpan. Provide opportunities to participate in physically undemanding activities. Schedule activities to promote sufficient rest periods.
• Place him in an upright position to relieve dyspnea, and administer oxygen to prevent tissue hypoxia, as needed.

• Tell him to elevate his legs when sitting to improve venous return to the heart.

• If the patient has signs of heart failure, keep him on a low-sodium diet; provide as many favorite foods as possible in light of restrictions. Give him written instructions about following a low-sodium diet.

• Administer prescribed medications for heart failure. Monitor drug effectiveness and for possible adverse reactions.

• Administer other prescribed medications. Teach the patient and family members about possible adverse effects. If the patient requires anticoagulants, review the foods and medications that may cause harmful interactions.

• Allow the patient to express concerns about the disorder and its impact on his life. Discuss any fears he harbors about impending surgery. Reassure him as needed.

• Prepare the patient for valve replacement surgery or percutaneous balloon aortic valvuloplasty, if indicated. Explain the procedure to the patient and his family and tell them what to expect before, during, and after the procedure.

Patient teaching

• Teach the patient and family members about aortic stenosis and its causes, symptoms, and complications. Explain all diagnostic tests.

• Warn the patient and family members that even though he's symptom-free, he'll need follow-up care and continuing assessment to detect further disease progression. Explain that it's important to report any symptoms related to aortic stenosis, such as angina, dyspnea, or syncope.

• Make sure that the patient and family members understand the need for antibiotics before and after undergoing dental work, surgery, and other invasive procedures.

• Advise the patient about ways to minimize exposure to infection. Discuss the need to promptly report signs of infection or exposure to streptococcal infection. (See *Ensuring continued care for the patient with aortic stenosis*, page 192.)

EVALUATION

When evaluating your patient's response to nursing care, gather reassessment data and compare this information with the patient outcomes specified in your plan of care.

Teaching and counseling

Next, evaluate the patient's response to your teaching. Consider the following questions:

• Do the patient's statements demonstrate an understanding of aortic stenosis and its signs and symptoms, possible complications, and treatments?

• Does he intend to comply with treatment and obtain regular follow-up care?

• Does he understand the relationship of fatigue to his disorder?

• Is he willing to modify activities to reduce fatigue?

• Does he understand the need to establish a regular sleep pattern?

• Does he know the signs of decreased cardiac output?

• Does he understand the need to report signs and symptoms that require medical attention?

• Can he identify activities that cause chest pain, and will he avoid or seek assistance with these activities?

Preventing infection

Evaluate the patient's risk for infection. Consider the following questions:

• Does the patient appear willing to initiate measures to help prevent exposure to infection?

Ensuring continued care for the patient with aortic stenosis

Review the following teaching topics, referrals, and follow-up appointments to ensure that your patient is adequately prepared for discharge.

Teaching topics
Make sure that the following topics have been covered and that your patient's learning has been evaluated:
☐ explanation of aortic stenosis, including its causes, symptoms, and complications
☐ activity restrictions as needed
☐ medications, including anticoagulant therapy, if prescribed
☐ sodium-restricted diet as needed
☐ signs and symptoms to report to the doctor
☐ need for antibiotics before dental work and invasive procedures
☐ surgery, preoperative and postoperative care, as indicated.

Referrals
Make sure that your patient has received the following appropriate referrals:
☐ dietitian
☐ home health care agency
☐ social services
☐ cardiac rehabilitation center.

Follow-up appointments
Make sure that your patient has been provided with the times and dates for these follow-up appointments:
☐ doctor or clinic
☐ surgeon
☐ additional diagnostic tests, if necessary.

• Does he understand the need to take antibiotics before dental work, surgery, or other invasive procedures?
• If the patient developed signs of infection or was exposed to streptococcal infection, were these events reported promptly to the doctor?

Physical condition
When evaluating the patient's physical condition, consider the following questions:
• Has his cardiac output improved?
• Does he report less dyspnea?
• Does he report absence of chest pain?
• Are his pulse rate and blood pressure within established limits?
• Do ECGs show no arrhythmias?
• Is the patient able to maintain baseline mental status and adequate urine output?
• If the patient has undergone valve replacement surgery, is his cardiac output adequate?

Tricuspid insufficiency

In tricuspid insufficiency, also known as tricuspid regurgitation, an incompetent tricuspid valve allows blood to flow from the right ventricle back into the right atrium during systole. This backflow elevates right atrial pressure, which leads to systemic venous congestion and pulmonary hypertension. Tricuspid insufficiency also reduces blood flow to the lungs and left side of the heart, decreasing cardiac output. Right-sided heart failure is a common complication of tricuspid insufficiency. Mitral valve disease may also be present.

Causes
Tricuspid insufficiency results from marked dilation of the right ventricle and tricuspid valve ring (annulus). Its

etiology varies. (See *Causes of tricuspid insufficiency*.)

ASSESSMENT

Your assessment of the patient should include a health history, physical examination, and consideration of diagnostic test findings.

Health history
The patient with tricuspid insufficiency may report symptoms of reduced cardiac output, including dyspnea, fatigue, weakness, and syncope. He may feel uncomfortable because of peripheral edema and ascites. The patient also may report anorexia.

Physical examination
You may observe jugular vein distention with prominent v waves. In the patient with severe tricuspid insufficiency, extensive peripheral edema and ascites may be present.

During auscultation, you may hear a high-pitched, blowing, holosystolic murmur at the fourth intercostal space, at the left sternal border. The murmur increases with inspiration (Carvallo sign) and decreases with expiration and Valsalva's maneuver. A right ventricular S_3 is common and increases on inspiration. (See *Identifying the murmur of tricuspid insufficiency,* page 194.)

In patients with right-sided heart failure, you may palpate systolic pulsations of the liver, a positive hepatojugular reflux, and hepatomegaly. You also may feel a prominent right ventricular pulsation along the left parasternal region. If the patient exhibits signs of hepatomegaly, inspect for jaundice and palpate his spleen for splenomegaly.

Inspect the patient for peripheral cyanosis, a sign of slow perfusion resulting from reduced cardiac output.

FactFinder
Causes of tricuspid insufficiency

Tricuspid insufficiency commonly occurs as a complication of right-sided heart failure. The causes of heart failure may include ischemic heart disease, cardiomyopathy, right ventricular infarction, and rheumatic or congenital heart disease with severe pulmonary hypertension.

Other possible causes include:
• carcinoid heart disease
• congenital deformity of the tricuspid valves
• congenital defects in the atrioventricular canal
• Ebstein's anomaly of the tricuspid valve
• endomyocardial fibrosis
• infective endocarditis
• right atrial myxoma
• trauma
• tricuspid valve prolapse.

Diagnostic test results
The following tests help to establish a diagnosis of tricuspid insufficiency:
• Cardiac catheterization shows markedly decreased cardiac output. The mean right atrial and right ventricular end-diastolic pressures often are elevated.
• Chest X-ray reveals right atrial and ventricular enlargement.
• Echocardiography shows right ventricular dilation and paradoxical septal motion. It may show prolapsing or flailing of the tricuspid valve leaflets. Estimates of pulmonary artery and right ventricular systolic pressure are obtained by Doppler echocardiography.
• Electrocardiography (ECG) shows right atrial hypertrophy and right or left ventricular hypertrophy. ECG also may reveal atrial fibrillation or incomplete right bundle-branch block.

Identifying the murmur of tricuspid insufficiency

If you discover a murmur, try to determine its type through careful auscultation. If you suspect tricuspid insufficiency, listen for a high-pitched, blowing, holosystolic murmur in the tricuspid area that increases with inspiration. This sound is caused by blood flowing backward, through the tricuspid valve.

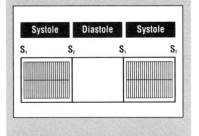

NURSING DIAGNOSIS

Common nursing diagnoses for a patient with tricuspid insufficiency include:
• High risk for infection related to invasive procedures
• Fatigue related to decreased cardiac output
• Fluid volume excess related to elevated right atrial pressure, systemic venous congestion, and hepatic congestion
• Decreased cardiac output related to tricuspid stenosis and possible mitral valve disease.

PLANNING

Goals of nursing care for the patient with tricuspid insufficiency include relieving the patient's symptoms, preventing complications, and teaching the patient about the disorder and its treatment.

Based on the nursing diagnosis *high risk for infection,* develop appropriate patient outcomes. For example, your patient will:
• agree to comply with the prescribed antibiotic treatment
• state his intention to take antibiotics before dental work, surgery, or other invasive procedures
• express a willingness to take measures to help prevent exposure to infection
• agree to report signs of infection or exposure to streptococcal infection to the doctor immediately.

Based on the nursing diagnosis *fatigue,* develop appropriate patient outcomes. For example, your patient will:
• explain the relationship of fatigue to the disease process
• demonstrate willingness to conserve energy by resting and by planning and setting priorities for activities
• agree to make life-style changes to reduce fatigue
• establish a regular sleeping pattern.

Based on the nursing diagnosis *fluid volume excess,* develop appropriate patient outcomes. For example, your patient will:
• maintain his intake and output, daily weight, and blood pressure within established limits.
• maintain his blood urea nitrogen (BUN), serum creatinine, serum electrolyte, hemoglobin, and hematocrit levels within established limits
• express willingness to comply with a sodium-restricted diet and the prescribed medications
• maintain hemodynamic stability as evidenced by warm, dry skin; adequate urine output; baseline mental status; and absence of syncope and dizziness.

Based on the nursing diagnosis *decreased cardiac output,* develop appropriate patient outcomes. For example, your patient will:

• experience fewer dyspneic episodes, as evidenced by verbal reports or behavior

• agree to comply with the treatment regimen to enhance cardiac output

• show evidence of enhanced cardiac output after tricuspid or mitral valve surgical procedures.

IMPLEMENTATION

Treatment of tricuspid insufficiency is based on the patient's symptoms. Expect to provide measures to reduce the patient's fatigue, dyspnea, and other symptoms.

If the patient has heart failure, provide a sodium-restricted diet and administer digoxin and diuretics, as prescribed. Stress the importance of antibiotic prophylaxis for endocarditis and rheumatic fever.

If your patient requires surgery, prepare him for tricuspid annuloplasty or tricuspid valve replacement, as indicated. Surgery for associated mitral valve disease also may be necessary.

Nursing interventions

• Monitor the patient for signs of heart failure and arrhythmias. Assess his vital signs, heart and breath sounds, arterial blood gas levels, intake and output, daily weight, blood chemistry studies, chest X-rays, and ECG.

• Allow the patient to express his fears and concerns about the disorder and about any impending surgery. Encourage discussions about the impact he feels the disorder or surgery will have on his life. Reassure him as needed.

• If the patient needs bed rest, stress its importance. Assist with bathing and other activities, as necessary. Provide a bedside commode, which places less stress on the heart than use of a bedpan.

• Provide the patient with opportunities to participate in physically unde-

manding activities. Schedule activities to promote sufficient rest periods.

• Place the patient in an upright position to relieve dyspnea, if needed. Administer oxygen to prevent tissue hypoxia, as needed.

• Keep the patient who shows signs of heart failure on a low-sodium diet.

• Administer prescribed medications for heart failure. Monitor drug effectiveness and for possible adverse reactions.

Patient teaching

• Teach the patient and family members about the disorder and its causes, symptoms, and complications. Explain all diagnostic tests.

• If the patient is scheduled for valvular surgery, explain the procedure to him and family members. Tell them what to expect before, during, and after the procedure.

• Teach the patient about dietary and activity restrictions.

• Teach energy conservation techniques and the need for daily rest periods. Help the patient learn to adjust to life-style changes.

• Review the prescribed medications, their proper administration, and their possible adverse effects.

• If the patient requires anticoagulant therapy, review with him and family members which foods and medications may interact adversely with this therapy.

• Advise the patient on how to minimize exposure to infection. Explain the need to promptly report signs of infection or exposure to streptococcal infection.

• Instruct him to elevate his legs whenever he's sitting.

• Inform the patient about the warning signs of progressive valvular dysfunction and reportable complications.

• Teach the patient how to measure his intake and output and how to obtain his daily weight, as needed. Instruct

Discharge Timesaver

Ensuring continued care for the patient with tricuspid insufficiency

Review the following teaching topics, referrals, and follow-up appointments to ensure that your patient is adequately prepared for discharge.

Teaching topics
Make sure that the following topics have been covered and that your patient's learning has been evaluated:
☐ nature of the disorder and its causes, symptoms, and possible complications
☐ activity restrictions as needed
☐ medications, including anticoagulant therapy, if indicated
☐ sodium-restricted diet as needed
☐ signs and symptoms to report to the doctor
☐ need for antibiotics before dental work or invasive procedures
☐ surgery, including preoperative and postoperative care, as needed.

Referrals
Be sure that your patient has been provided with the following appropriate referrals:
☐ dietitian
☐ home health care agency
☐ social services
☐ cardiac rehabilitation center.

Follow-up appointments
Be sure that your patient has been provided with the times and dates of these necesssary follow-up appointments:
☐ doctor or clinic
☐ surgeon
☐ additional diagnostic tests, if necessary.

him to report results that exceed established limits.

• Before the patient leaves the hospital, make sure he and family members understand the need to comply with follow-up care. Confirm their understanding of the patient's need for antibiotics before and after dental work, surgery, and other invasive procedures. (See *Ensuring continued care for the patient with tricuspid insufficiency*.)

EVALUATION

To evaluate the patient's response to your nursing care, gather reassessment data and compare this information with the patient outcomes specified in your plan of care.

Teaching and counseling

To evaluate the effectiveness of teaching and counseling, consider the following questions:
• Is the patient complying with the prescribed antibiotic treatment?
• Does he intend to take antibiotics before undergoing dental work, surgery, or other invasive procedures?
• Is he willing to take measures that will help reduce his exposure to infection?
• Does he intend to immediately report signs of infection or exposure to streptococcal infection?
• Does he understand the relationship between fatigue and his disorder?
• Is he willing to conserve energy by resting and by planning and setting priorities for activities?
• Has he acknowledged the need to adopt life-style changes that reduce fatigue?

• Does he intend to establish a regular sleeping pattern?

• Is he complying with a sodium-restricted diet and medication prescriptions?

Physical condition

Continue your evaluation by reassessing the patient's physical condition. Consider the following questions:

• Does the patient's skin show signs of infection?

• Is he maintaining sufficient intake and output?

• Is his weight stable?

• Are his blood pressure and BUN, serum creatinine, serum electrolyte, hemoglobin, and hematocrit levels within established limits?

• Does he demonstrate evidence of hemodynamic stability, including warm, dry skin; adequate urine output; maintenance of baseline mental status; and absence of syncope and dizziness?

• How often does he experience dyspnea?

• If the patient has undergone tricuspid or mitral valve surgery, is his cardiac output improved?

Tricuspid stenosis

A relatively uncommon disorder, tricuspid stenosis obstructs blood flow from the right atrium to the right ventricle, which causes the right atrium to dilate and hypertrophy. Eventually, this leads to heart failure and increased pressure in the vena cava. Tricuspid stenosis rarely occurs alone and most often is associated with mitral stenosis. It's most common in women.

Causes

Tricuspid stenosis almost always results from rheumatic fever. Other causes are infrequent and include tricuspid atresia and atrial myxomas (if the myxoma obstructs the valvular orifice). Tricuspid stenosis also may occur as a sequela to cancer if fibrous plaques develop on the tricuspid valve or its components.

ASSESSMENT

During your assessment, keep in mind that mitral stenosis is often associated with tricuspid stenosis. If your patient has both disorders, signs and symptoms of mitral stenosis may overshadow those of tricuspid stenosis.

Health history

The patient with tricuspid stenosis may complain of dyspnea, fatigue, weakness, and syncope resulting from low cardiac output. Some patients report neck pulsations, which result from distended jugular veins.

When exploring the possible cause of tricuspid stenosis, be sure to question the patient about a history of rheumatic fever.

Physical examination

During inspection, you may observe jugular vein distention with giant a waves in the patient with a normal sinus rhythm. In the patient with severe tricuspid stenosis, you may note increased peripheral edema and ascites. The patient may also appear malnourished and jaundiced.

During palpation, you may detect signs of hepatomegaly in patients with right-sided heart failure and subsequent venous congestion.

During auscultation, you may hear a diastolic murmur at the fourth intercostal space at the lower left sternal border and over the xiphoid process. The murmur is most prominent during presystole in sinus rhythm. The murmur increases with inspiration and decreases with expiration and during Valsalva's maneuver. An opening snap may be heard. (See *Identifying the murmur of tricuspid stenosis*, page 198.)

Identifying the murmur of tricuspid stenosis

If you discover a murmur, try to determine its type through careful auscultation. If you suspect tricuspid stenosis, listen for a low, rumbling, crescendo-decrescendo murmur in the tricuspid area. The murmur results from turbulent blood flow across the stiffened and narrowed valvular leaflets.

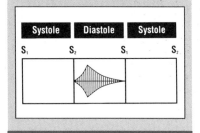

Systole	Diastole	Systole	
S_1	S_2	S_1	S_2

Diagnostic test results
The following tests help to establish the diagnosis and evaluate the severity of the disorder:
• Cardiac catheterization shows increased right atrial pressure and decreased cardiac output. This test may also show an increased pressure gradient across the tricuspid valve, but the gradient is usually small (4 to 8 mm Hg).
• Chest X-ray shows right atrial and superior vena cava enlargement.
• Echocardiography shows a thick tricuspid valve with reduced mobility and right atrial enlargement.
• Electrocardiography (ECG) shows right atrial hypertrophy and right ventricular hypertrophy. Atrial fibrillation may be present. Tall, peaked P waves are seen in lead II and prominent, upright P waves are seen in lead V_1, indicating right atrial enlargement.

NURSING DIAGNOSIS

Common nursing diagnoses for a patient with tricuspid stenosis include:
• High risk for infection related to the threat of bacterial endocarditis from invasive procedures
• Fatigue related to decreased cardiac output
• Fluid volume excess related to elevated right atrial pressure, systemic venous congestion, and hepatic congestion
• Decreased cardiac output related to the disorder's effects.

PLANNING

Develop a plan of care that focuses on preventing complications and providing the patient with symptomatic relief. Incorporate patient teaching into your plan, especially about valvular surgery, if indicated.

Based on the nursing diagnosis *high risk for infection,* develop appropriate patient outcomes. For example, your patient will:
• express understanding of the need for antibiotic treatment
• agree to receive prophylactic antibiotics for dental work, surgery, or other invasive procedures
• express willingness to initiate measures to help prevent exposure to infection
• agree to report signs of infection or exposure to streptococcal infection to the doctor immediately.

Based on the nursing diagnosis *fatigue,* develop appropriate patient outcomes. For example, your patient will:
• communicate understanding of the relationship of fatigue to the disorder
• demonstrate willingness to conserve energy through rest, planning, and setting priorities
• agree to incorporate measures to reduce fatigue into her daily life-style
• establish a regular sleeping pattern.

Based on the nursing diagnosis *fluid volume excess,* develop appropriate patient outcomes. For example, your patient will:

• maintain her intake, output, and weight within established limits

• maintain intact, infection-free skin

• demónstrate compliance with a sodium-restricted diet and prescribed drugs.

Based on the nursing diagnosis *decreased cardiac output,* develop appropriate patient outcomes. For example, your patient will:

• maintain her blood pressure and blood urea nitrogen (BUN), serum creatinine, serum electrolyte, hemoglobin, and hematocrit levels within established limits

• maintain hemodynamic stability, as evidenced by vital signs within established limits; warm, dry skin; no decrease in urine output; no deterioration in mental status; and absence of syncope and dizziness

• experience fewer dyspneic episodes, as evidenced by her reports or behavior

• comply with treatment to enhance her cardiac output

• exhibit improved cardiac output after tricuspid and possible mitral valve surgery.

IMPLEMENTATION

Because treatment aims to relieve symptoms, focus your interventions on reducing the patient's fatigue and dyspnea. Also implement measures to prevent complications, such as heart failure and hepatic congestion.

For patients with moderate to severe stenosis, tricuspid valve repair or replacement is usually indicated. Some patients also require mitral valve replacement. If valvular surgery is planned, provide a sodium-restricted diet and administer diuretics before the procedure, as prescribed, to reduce hepatic congestion.

Nursing interventions

• Monitor the patient for signs of heart failure and arrhythmias. Assess her vital signs, heart and breath sounds, arterial blood gas levels, intake and output, and daily weight. Also review her blood chemistry studies, chest X-rays, and ECG readings.

• If the patient needs bed rest, explain why. Assist with bathing and other activities, as necessary. Provide a bedside commode because using a commode puts less stress on the heart than using a bedpan. Schedule activities to promote sufficient rest periods.

• Explain the need for activity restrictions. Teach energy conservation techniques and the need for daily rest periods. Help the patient adjust to life-style changes. Provide opportunities for her to participate in physically undemanding activities.

• Place the patient in an upright position to relieve dyspnea, and administer oxygen to prevent tissue hypoxia, as needed.

• Keep the patient with signs of heart failure on a low-sodium diet; provide as many favorite foods as possible in light of dietary restrictions. Teach the patient about her diet.

• Administer prescribed medications for heart failure. Monitor drug effectiveness and for possible adverse reactions.

• Allow the patient to express her concerns about the disorder and its potential impact on her life-style. Discuss any fears she expresses about impending surgery. Reassure her as needed.

• Prepare the patient for valvular surgery, as indicated. Before surgery, explain the procedure to her and her family. Tell them what to expect before, during, and after the procedure.

Patient teaching

• Teach the patient and family members about the disorder, including its causes, symptoms, and potential com-

Discharge TimeSaver

Ensuring continued care for the patient with tricuspid stenosis

Review the following teaching topics, referrals, and follow-up appointments to make sure that your patient is adequately prepared for discharge.

Teaching topics
Make sure that the following topics have been covered and that your patient's learning has been evaluated:
□ explanation of tricuspid stenosis, including its causes, symptoms, and potential complications
□ activity restrictions as needed
□ medications, including anticoagulant therapy, if indicated
□ sodium-restricted diet as needed
□ signs and symptoms to report to the doctor
□ need for antibiotics before dental work or invasive procedures
□ surgery, if needed, including preoperative and postoperative care.

Referrals
Make sure that your patient has been provided with the following appropriate referrals:
□ dietitian
□ home health care agency
□ social services
□ cardiac rehabilitation center.

Follow-up appointments
Make sure that your patient has been provided with the times and dates for these necessary follow-up appointments:
□ doctor or clinic
□ surgeon
□ additional diagnostic tests, if necessary.

plications. Also, explain all diagnostic tests.

• Instruct her to take prescribed medications correctly and to report any adverse reactions. If she requires anticoagulants, review foods and medications that may interfere with this therapy.

• Tell her how to minimize exposure to infection. Instruct her to report signs of infection or exposure to streptococcal infection immediately.

• Inform her about warning signs of progressive valvular dysfunction and reportable complications.

• Teach her how to measure intake and output and how to obtain daily weight, as needed. Instruct her to report results that exceed established limits.

• Tell her to elevate her legs when she sits.

• Before discharge, make sure the patient and her family understand the need to comply with follow-up care and to take antibiotics before and after dental work, surgery, and other invasive procedures. (See *Ensuring continued care for the patient with tricuspid stenosis.*)

EVALUATION

When evaluating your patient's response to nursing care, gather reassessment data and compare this information with the patient outcomes specified in your plan of care.

Teaching and counseling
Begin by determining the effectiveness of teaching and counseling. Take note of statements from the patient indicating:

• understanding of tricuspid stenosis and its causes, symptoms, treatments, and possible complications
• understanding of the need for antibiotic therapy to prevent or treat infection
• understanding of the relationship of fatigue to the disorder
• willingness to make life-style changes to reduce fatigue and minimize exposure to infection
• intention to comply with treatment, adhere to a schedule for follow-up care, and report signs of complications
• willingness to take prophylactic antibiotics for dental work or invasive procedures
• understanding of the need for a sodium-restricted diet
• understanding of the purpose for prescribed medications and their potential adverse effects.

Evaluating self-care
Additional questions to consider during your evaluation include the following:
• If the patient noticed signs of infection or was exposed to streptococcal infection, did she promptly report the information to the doctor?
• Has she taken steps to conserve her energy by resting, planning, and setting priorities?
• Has she established a regular sleeping pattern?
• Has she maintained her intake, output, and weight within established limits?
• Is her skin intact and free of infection?

Cardiac status
When evaluating the patient's cardiac status, consider the following questions:
• Are blood pressure and BUN, serum creatinine, serum electrolyte, hemoglobin, and hematocrit levels within established limits?

• Does the patient demonstrate evidence of hemodynamic stability, including vital signs within established limits; warm, dry skin; no decrease in urine output; no deterioration in mental status; and an absence of syncope and dizziness?
• Have dyspneic episodes increased or decreased in frequency?

Pulmonic insufficiency

In pulmonic insufficiency, blood ejected into the pulmonary artery during systole flows back into the right ventricle during diastole, causing fluid overload in the ventricle, ventricular hypertrophy and, eventually, right-sided heart failure.

Causes
Pulmonic insufficiency may be congenital or may result from pulmonary hypertension. The most common acquired cause is dilation of the pulmonic valve ring resulting from severe pulmonary hypertension. Repair of pulmonic stenosis may also cause pulmonic insufficiency.

Other causes include infective endocarditis, tumors, and syphilitic aneurysm of the main pulmonary artery. Rarely, pulmonic insufficiency may result from rheumatic fever or prolonged use of a pulmonary artery catheter.

ASSESSMENT

Most patients are asymptomatic. Rarely, the patient may complain of dyspnea on exertion, fatigue, chest pain, and syncope.

Physical examination
Inspection doesn't usually reveal characteristic signs. However, if pulmonic insufficiency causes right-sided heart failure, you may notice severe periph-

Identifying the murmur of pulmonic insufficiency

In patients with pulmonic insufficiency, you may auscultate a characteristic blowing, diastolic, decrescendo murmur at Erb's point (the mid–left sternal border). If the patient has elevated pulmonary pressures, the murmur is high-pitched. If the patient doesn't have elevated pulmonary pressures, the murmur is low-pitched.

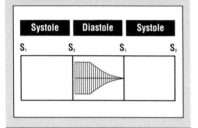

Systole	Diastole	Systole	
S_1	S_2	S_1	S_2

eral edema, jugular vein distention, and ascites.

Palpation may reveal hepatomegaly when right-sided heart failure is present. If the patient has elevated pulmonary pressures, auscultation may reveal a high-pitched, decrescendo, diastolic blowing murmur along the mid–left sternal border. Known as Graham Steell's murmur, it may be difficult to differentiate from the murmur of aortic insufficiency, but is accompanied by an accentuated P_2.

If the patient doesn't have elevated pulmonary pressures, auscultation may disclose a medium-pitched, decrescendo, diastolic murmur with inspiration. (See *Identifying the murmur of pulmonic insufficiency.*)

Diagnostic test results

The following tests help to confirm the diagnosis and evaluate the disorder's severity:

• Cardiac catheterization shows pulmonic insufficiency, increased right ventricular pressure, and associated cardiac defects.
• X-ray shows enlargement of the right ventricle and pulmonary artery.
• Echocardiography visualizes the pulmonary valve's abnormality.
• Electrocardiography (ECG) may be normal in mild cases or show right ventricular or right atrial hypertrophy.

NURSING DIAGNOSIS

Common nursing diagnoses for pulmonic insufficiency include:
• High risk for infection related to the threat of bacterial endocarditis from invasive procedures
• Fatigue related to decreased cardiac output
• Fluid volume excess related to systemic venous hypertension and congestion because of right-sided heart failure
• Decreased cardiac output related to right ventricular failure.

PLANNING

Design your plan of care to address the severity of the patient's condition. The patient with mild pulmonic insufficiency may require only instruction; the patient with severe insufficiency may also require preparation for surgery and treatment for heart failure.

Based on the nursing diagnosis *high risk for infection*, develop appropriate patient outcomes. For example, your patient will:
• agree to take antibiotics before dental work, surgery, or other invasive procedures
• state his intention to initiate measures that help prevent infection
• express his willingness to report signs of infection or exposure to streptococcal infection to the doctor immediately.

Based on the nursing diagnosis *fatigue,* develop appropriate patient outcomes. For example, your patient will:
• express an understanding of the relationship between fatigue and pulmonic insufficiency
• demonstrate willingness to conserve energy through rest, planning, and setting priorities
• agree to incorporate measures to reduce fatigue into his daily life
• establish a regular sleeping pattern.

Based on the nursing diagnosis *fluid volume excess,* develop appropriate patient outcomes. For example, your patient will:
• maintain his intake, output, and daily weight within established limits
• maintain intact, infection-free skin
• agree to comply with a sodium-restricted diet and the prescribed medication regimen.

Based on the nursing diagnosis *decreased cardiac output,* develop appropriate patient outcomes. For example, your patient will:
• maintain his blood pressure and blood urea nitrogen (BUN), serum creatinine, serum electrolyte, hemoglobin, and hematocrit levels within established limits
• maintain hemodynamic stability, as evidenced by vital signs within set limits; warm, dry skin; no decrease in urine output; no deterioration in mental status; and absence of syncope and dizziness
• experience fewer dyspneic episodes
• agree to comply with treatment to enhance cardiac output
• demonstrate enhanced cardiac output after valvular surgery.

IMPLEMENTATION

Direct your care toward relieving the patient's symptoms, if present. If he's asymptomatic, no special treatment is warranted.

If the patient has severe pulmonic insufficiency, prepare him for valve repair or replacement, as needed. Before surgery, provide a sodium-restricted diet and diuretics, as prescribed.

Nursing interventions
• Monitor the patient for signs of heart failure. Assess his vital signs, heart and breath sounds and, as needed, arterial blood gas levels, intake and output, daily weight, blood chemistry studies, chest X-rays, and ECG.
• Provide sufficient rest if he experiences fatigue. Assist with activities of daily living, if needed. Help him to identify measures to relieve fatigue and to incorporate them into his lifestyle, as needed.
• Place the patient in an upright position to relieve dyspnea, if needed. Administer oxygen to prevent tissue hypoxia, as needed.
• Keep the patient with signs of heart failure on a low-sodium diet; provide as many favorite foods as possible in light of restrictions. Administer prescribed drugs, monitor their effectiveness, and be alert for adverse reactions.

Patient teaching
• Teach the patient and family members about the disorder and its causes, symptoms, and complications. Explain all diagnostic tests.
• Prepare him for valve repair or replacement surgery, as indicated. Explain the procedure to the patient and family members and tell them what to expect before, during, and after the procedure.
• Allow him to express his fears and concerns about the disorder, its perceived impact on his lifestyle, and impending surgery. Reassure him as needed.
• Teach the asymptomatic, stable patient or his family members about the importance of follow-up care to detect

possible complications or progression of the valvular disorder.
• If needed, teach the patient about dietary and activity restrictions and medications. Teach energy conservation techniques and the need for daily rest periods. Help the patient adjust to lifestyle changes.
• Tell him how to minimize exposure to infection and of the need to promptly report signs of infection or exposure to streptococcal infection.
• If appropriate, teach the patient to elevate his legs whenever he's sitting.
• Educate the patient and family members about anticoagulants, if indicated. Review the foods and medications that may interfere with this therapy.
• Inform him about warning signs of progressive valvular dysfunction or reportable complications.
• For a patient with edema and ascites, explain how to measure his intake and

output and how to obtain his daily weights, as needed. Instruct him to report results that exceed established limits.
• Before discharge, make sure the patient and family members understand the need for antibiotics before and after dental work, surgery, and other invasive procedures. (See *Ensuring continued care for the patient with pulmonic insufficiency.*)

EVALUATION

To evaluate the patient's response to your care, gather reassessment data and compare this information with the patient outcomes specified in your plan of care.

Teaching and counseling
Talk to the patient to determine the effectiveness of teaching and counseling.

Document statements by the patient indicating:

• understanding of the disorder and its symptoms, possible complications, and any prescribed treatments

• intention to initiate measures to help prevent exposure to infection

• willingness to comply with antibiotic therapy before invasive procedures, as needed

• intention to immediately report signs of infection or exposure to streptococcal infection

• understanding of the relationship of fatigue to the disorder

• willingness to conserve energy by resting, planning, and setting priorities

• willingness to comply with the treatment regimen to enhance cardiac output

• willingness to adopt measures to reduce fatigue in daily life

• willingness to adopt a regular sleeping pattern

• compliance with the prescribed medication therapy and dietary restrictions, if appropriate.

Physical condition

Next, gather reassessment data by reviewing diagnostic tests and examining the patient. Consider the following questions:

• Are the patient's vital signs within established limits?

• Is his skin warm and dry?

• Is his skin intact and free of infection?

• Has he shown no decrease in urine output or a deterioration in mental status?

• Are syncope and dizziness absent?

• Are intake, output, and daily weight within established limits?

• Have dyspneic episodes decreased?

• Are appropriate laboratory values (BUN, serum creatinine, serum electrolyte, hemoglobin, and hematocrit) within established limits?

• If the patient has undergone valvular surgery, does he exhibit evidence of enhanced cardiac output?

Pulmonic stenosis

In pulmonic stenosis, a narrowing of the pulmonic valve obstructs right ventricular outflow and eventually leads to right ventricular hypertrophy. Heart failure may ultimately result, although patients with mild to moderate pulmonic stenosis usually are stable and tolerate the disorder well. Pulmonic stenosis is rare in elderly patients. (See *Looking at a stenotic pulmonic valve,* page 206.)

Causes

Pulmonic stenosis usually results from congenital stenosis of the valve cusp. It's often associated with other congenital heart defects, such as tetralogy of Fallot.

Rheumatic fever occasionally causes fibrous thickening, contractures, or fusion of the valve cusps, leading to pulmonic stenosis.

Cancer also may cause the disorder if fibrous plaques form on the valve surfaces, right ventricular endocardium, and intima of the pulmonary artery.

ASSESSMENT

Your assessment should include the patient's health history, the presence of risk factors, physical examination findings, and a review of diagnostic test results. Because this disorder may be familial, check for its presence among family members.

Health history

A patient with mild pulmonic stenosis may be asymptomatic if the obstruction isn't severe. A patient with moderate to severe stenosis may report dys-

Looking at a stenotic pulmonic valve

The illustrations below point out the effects of pulmonic stenosis. Narrowing of the pulmonic valve interferes with the outflow of blood from the right ventricle, leading to right ventricular hypertrophy.

Normal pulmonic valve

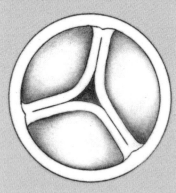

Stenotic pulmonic valve

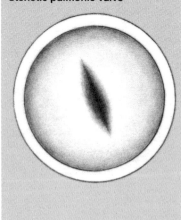

pnea on exertion, fatigue, chest pain, and syncope.

Physical examination

Your examination of the patient with pulmonic stenosis may reveal a prominent a wave in the jugular venous pulse. During auscultation, you may hear a harsh systolic crescendo-decrescendo ejection murmur. Auscultate the murmur at the second intercostal space at the left sternal border. If stenosis is congenital, the murmur will be present at an early age. (See *Identifying the murmur of pulmonic stenosis.*)

S_2, if present, is widely split. S_3 and S_4 are frequently heard and sound louder with inspiration. You may palpate a thrill at the upper left sternal border.

In patients with severe stenosis that has progressed to right-sided heart failure, you may observe severe peripheral edema, ascites, and jugular vein distention. During palpation, you may detect hepatomegaly, presystolic pulsations of the liver, and a right parasternal lift. Right-sided heart failure is rarely seen in infants and children with pulmonic stenosis, and many adults exhibit no signs other than a murmur.

Diagnostic test results

The following tests help establish a diagnosis of pulmonic stenosis and detect and evaluate complications:
• Cardiac catheterization reveals increased right ventricular pressure, decreased pulmonary artery pressure, and an abnormal valve orifice.
• Chest X-ray usually reveals a normal heart size and normal lung vascularity, although the pulmonary arteries may be evident. With severe obstruction and right-sided heart failure, right atrial and ventricular enlargement usually are seen.
• Echocardiography often reveals the pulmonic valve's abnormality.

• Electrocardiography (ECG) results may be normal in mild cases, or they may indicate right axis deviation and right ventricular hypertrophy. High-amplitude P waves in leads II, III, aV_F, and V_1 indicate right atrial enlargement.

NURSING DIAGNOSIS

Common nursing diagnoses for a patient with pulmonic stenosis include:
• High risk for infection related to invasive procedures
• Fatigue related to decreased cardiac output
• Fluid volume excess related to systemic venous congestion caused by right-sided heart failure
• Decreased cardiac output related to right-sided heart failure.

PLANNING

Your plan of care for the patient with pulmonic stenosis should reflect the severity of his condition. A patient with mild stenosis may require only instruction. For a patient with severe stenosis, you also may need to prepare him for surgery and treatment for heart failure.

Based on the nursing diagnosis *high risk for infection,* develop appropriate patient outcomes. For example, your patient will:
• agree to comply with prescribed antibiotic treatment
• state his intention to take prophylactic antibiotics before dental work, surgery, or other invasive procedures
• express willingness to take measures that help prevent infection
• agree to report signs of infection or possible exposure to streptococcal infection to the doctor immediately.

Based on the nursing diagnosis *fatigue,* develop patient outcomes. For example, your patient will:
• explain the relationship between fatigue and the disorder

Identifying the murmur of pulmonic stenosis

During auscultation of a patient with suspected pulmonic stenosis, carefully listen for a medium-pitched, systolic, harsh crescendo-decrescendo murmur in the area of the pulmonary valve. This characteristic murmur is caused by turbulent blood flow across the stiffened, narrow valve.

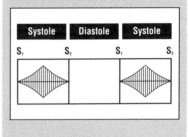

Systole	Diastole	Systole	
S_1	S_2	S_1	S_2

• express willingness to conserve energy by resting and by planning and setting priorities for activities
• state his intention to take measures to reduce fatigue in his daily life
• agree to establish a regular sleeping pattern.

Based on the nursing diagnosis *fluid volume excess,* develop appropriate patient outcomes. For example, your patient will:
• express understanding of the need to maintain appropriate fluid intake and output and daily weight.
• agree to comply with a sodium-restricted diet and the prescribed medications
• maintain his blood pressure and blood urea nitrogen (BUN), serum creatinine, serum electrolyte, hemoglobin, and hematocrit levels within established limits
• maintain hemodynamic stability, as evidenced by warm, dry skin; adequate

urine output; baseline mental status; and absence of syncope and dizziness.

Based on the nursing diagnosis *decreased cardiac output,* develop appropriate patient outcomes. For example, your patient will:
• demonstrate fewer dyspneic episodes, as evidenced by reports or behavior
• demonstrate compliance with treatment to enhance cardiac output
• exhibit evidence that cardiac output is enhanced or maintained after valvuloplasty.

IMPLEMENTATION

A patient with mild pulmonic stenosis usually is asymptomatic. In this case, treatment primarily consists of teaching the patient how to prevent complications and recognize warning signs of disease progression. Special treatments usually aren't prescribed, although prophylaxis for infective endocarditis may be indicated.

If your patient has severe pulmonic stenosis, prepare him for surgery, as indicated. Percutaneous balloon valvuloplasty (also called cardiac catheter balloon valvuloplasty) is usually effective, even for patients with moderate to severe obstruction. Before surgery, provide a sodium-restricted diet and diuretics, if prescribed, to treat signs of heart failure.

Nursing interventions
• Monitor the patient for signs of heart failure. Assess his vital signs, heart and breath sounds, arterial blood gas levels, intake and output, and daily weight. Monitor blood chemistry studies, chest X-rays, and ECG readings.
• Provide sufficient rest for the patient experiencing fatigue and assist him with activities, if necessary. Help him identify and incorporate measures to reduce fatigue in his life.
• Place him in an upright position to relieve dyspnea, and administer oxygen to prevent tissue hypoxia, as needed.
• Keep the patient with signs of heart failure on a low-sodium diet.
• Administer medications, as prescribed, for heart failure and other complications. Monitor drug effectiveness and for possible adverse reactions.
• Allow the patient to express his fears and concerns about the disorder and any impending surgery. Encourage discussion about the impact the disorder or surgery will have on his life. Reassure him as needed.

Patient teaching
• Teach the patient and family members about pulmonic stenosis and its causes, symptoms, and complications. Explain all diagnostic tests.
• Review with the patient and family members the proper use of medications and their possible adverse reactions. If he requires anticoagulants, discuss the foods and medications that may interfere with treatment.
• If the patient is scheduled for percutaneous balloon valvuloplasty, explain the procedure to him and family members. Tell them what to expect before, during, and after the procedure.
• Instruct the asymptomatic, stable patient and his family members about the importance of follow-up care. Describe how to detect warning signs of progressive valvular dysfunction or reportable complications.
• Teach the patient about dietary and activity restrictions, as needed. Explain the importance of energy conservation techniques and the need for daily rest periods. Help him adjust to lifestyle changes.
• When appropriate, advise the patient to elevate his legs while he's sitting.
• For the patient with edema and ascites, explain how to measure his intake and output and how to obtain his daily weight, as needed. Instruct him to re-

Discharge TimeSaver
Ensuring continued care for the patient with pulmonic stenosis

Review the following teaching topics, referrals, and follow-up appointments to ensure that your patient is adequately prepared for discharge.

Teaching topics
Make sure that the following topics have been covered and that your patient's learning has been evaluated:
☐ a review of pulmonic stenosis and its causes, symptoms, and possible complications
☐ activity restrictions as needed
☐ administration of medications, including anticoagulant therapy, if indicated
☐ details of a sodium-restricted diet
☐ signs and symptoms to report to the doctor
☐ need for lifelong follow-up care
☐ need for antibiotics before dental work and invasive procedures.

Referrals
Make sure that the patient has been provided with the following appropriate referrals:
☐ dietitian
☐ home health care agency
☐ social services
☐ cardiac rehabilitation center.

Follow-up appointments
Be sure that your patient is aware of the times and dates for these necessary follow-up appointments:
☐ doctor or clinic
☐ additional diagnostic tests.

port results that exceed the established limits.

• Tell him how to minimize exposure to infection, and explain the importance of promptly reporting signs of infection or exposure to streptococcal infection.

• Before discharge, make sure he and his family understand the need for antibiotics before and after undergoing dental work, surgery, and other invasive procedures. (See *Ensuring continued care for the patient with pulmonic stenosis.*)

EVALUATION

When evaluating a patient's response to your nursing care, gather reassessment data and compare this information with the patient outcomes specified in your plan of care.

Teaching and counseling

Begin by evaluating the effectiveness of your teaching. Document statements by the patient indicating:

• understanding of the disorder and its symptoms, possible complications, and treatments

• willingness to comply with antibiotic therapy and follow-up care

• intention to take antibiotics before dental work and invasive procedures

• intention to take measures to help prevent infection and to report signs of infection or exposure to streptococcal infection to the doctor immediately

• understanding of how fatigue affects the disorder

• willingness to reduce fatigue, conserve energy, and set priorities for activities

• intention to establish a regular sleeping pattern

• understanding of the need to maintain appropriate intake, output, and daily weight

• adherence to a sodium-restricted diet and compliance with related medication therapy.

Physical condition
Gather reassessment data from ongoing examination and testing of the patient. Obtain current blood pressure and BUN, serum creatinine, serum electrolyte, hemoglobin, and hematocrit levels and compare this information with target levels specified in your plan of care. To evaluate cardiac status, consider the following questions:

• Does the patient demonstrate evidence of hemodynamic stability, including warm, dry skin; adequate urine output; baseline mental status; and an absence of syncope and dizziness?

• Does he experience fewer dyspneic episodes, as evidenced by reports or behavior?

• Does he comply with treatment to enhance cardiac output?

• Following valvuloplasty, does the patient exhibit evidence that cardiac output is enhanced or maintained?

Caring for patients with arrhythmias

Arrhythmias

Arrhythmias result from disturbances in impulse generation (ectopic tachyarrhythmias), impulse conduction (reentrant arrhythmias), or both. They occur when abnormal electrical impulses alter the heart's rate and rhythm.

A patient with a normal heart may experience an arrhythmia without developing symptoms. However, persistently rapid rates or highly irregular rhythms may impair cardiac output. The threat to hemodynamic stability increases if the patient has a cardiac disorder, particularly left ventricular dysfunction.

Arrhythmias are classified by their site of origin and by the heart rate produced. Mild, asymptomatic arrhythmias don't require treatment. Other arrhythmias, such as ventricular fibrillation, require immediate treatment.

Causes

Arrhythmias may be congenital or may result from myocardial ischemia, myocardial infarction (MI), organic heart disease, drug toxicity, or degeneration of myocardial conductive tissue. In addition, arrhythmias may be precipitated by hypokalemia, hyperkalemia, hypocalcemia, hypercalcemia, hypoxia, fever, acidosis, alkalosis, exercise, or an increase in catecholamine levels.

ASSESSMENT

During an arrhythmia, your patient may be symptomatic or asymptomatic. Complaints of syncope, dizziness, dyspnea, chest pain, or altered mental status may indicate inadequate cerebral or myocardial perfusion resulting from a life-threatening arrhythmia. Also, complaints of palpitations, diaphoresis, mild weakness, fear, anxiety, or panic may be associated with the rhythm disturbance.

If you suspect an arrhythmia and the patient has a pulse, immediately determine the patient's tolerance for the abnormal rhythm. If possible, document the rhythm. If he complains of dyspnea or chest pain, has a urine output of less than 30 ml/hour, or exhibits a decreased level of consciousness (LOC), consider his condition serious, especially if he has a systolic blood pressure below 90 mm Hg or a coexisting complication, such as shock, heart failure, pulmonary congestion, or MI. Your patient may have an life-threatening arrhythmia, such as unstable ventricular tachycardia (VT), advanced atrioventricular (AV) block, or paroxysmal supraventricular tachycardia (SVT).

If the patient is stable, listen to his complaints and focus on the most serious ones first. Then, carefully review his health history, physical examination findings, and diagnostic test results.

Health history

During the health history, discuss the patient's use of medications. Ask him if he has been taking digoxin (arrhythmias commonly result from digoxin toxicity). Also ask whether he uses cocaine or other illicit drugs. Discuss factors that may precipitate an arrhythmia, including caffeine intake, stress, or vagal stimulation. In addition, find out if any family members have a history of cardiac disorders.

Review the patient's medical history for preexisting arrhythmias or heart disease or other causative factors.

Timesaving tip: If the patient has had a previous electrocardiogram (ECG), obtain his rhythm strips for comparison. If the strips are on file at another hospital, they can be faxed to you.

Physical examination

During inspection, you may note signs of hypoperfusion, including pale, dusky, or grayish skin; altered LOC; and decreased urine output. You may observe signs of anxiety, such as facial tension, restlessness, or trembling.

During palpation of the patient's pulse, you may note an abnormal rate or rhythm, or both. Document the rate and rhythm and the intensity of the apical and peripheral pulses. You may also note cool, clammy skin, a sign of peripheral hypoperfusion.

When auscultating breath sounds, you may detect crackles, a sign of progressive heart failure. When auscultating heart sounds, you may detect murmurs, a possible sign of underlying valvular disorders. In a patient with heart failure, you may hear an S_3 gallop.

Measuring the patient's blood pressure may reveal hypotension, a result of altered tissue perfusion.

Diagnostic test results

An ECG allows detection and identification of an arrhythmia. If the patient is asymptomatic, the doctor may prescribe 24-hour ambulatory (Holter) monitoring. (See *Interpreting ECGs,* pages 214 to 232.)

Electrolyte studies and toxicology screening may help pinpoint the cause of the arrhythmia. If not, the doctor may order more sophisticated tests, such as esophageal ECG or echocardiography.

NURSING DIAGNOSIS

Common nursing diagnoses for the patient with an arrhythmia include:
• Altered tissue perfusion (renal, cerebral, cardiopulmonary, or peripheral) related to decreased cardiac output from shortened left ventricular filling time
• Anxiety related to the potential for life-threatening complications

• Knowledge deficit related to the treatment and prevention of arrhythmias.

PLANNING

Based on the nursing diagnosis *altered tissue perfusion (renal, cerebral, cardiopulmonary, or peripheral),* develop appropriate patient outcomes. For example, your patient will:
• achieve a systolic blood pressure above 90 mm Hg and a mean arterial pressure (MAP) above 80 mm Hg
• exhibit a normal sinus rhythm or an arrhythmia that doesn't compromise hemodynamic status
• avoid developing complications of altered cerebral tissue perfusion, such as stroke or seizure
• state that he experiences fewer episodes of dyspnea, chest pain, or syncope
• maintain baseline mental status
• exhibit warm, dry skin
• maintain urine output of at least 30 ml/hour.

Based on the nursing diagnosis *anxiety,* develop appropriate patient outcomes. For example, your patient will:
• express his feelings of anxiety
• demonstrate effective coping techniques
• express a willingness to use outside sources of support
• experience less anxiety, as evidenced by the absence of trembling, restlessness, and facial tension.

Based on the nursing diagnosis *knowledge deficit, develop appropriate patient outcomes. For example, your patient will:*
• communicate an understanding of therapies used to treat and prevent arrhythmias
• participate in making decisions related to his care.

(Text continues on page 233.)

Interpreting ECGs

Each cardiac arrhythmia has a distinct appearance and defining characteristics on an electrocardiogram (ECG). Becoming familiar with these ECG characteristics will help you interpret your patient's arrhythmia.

Most arrhythmias are classified by their point of origin: sinus, atrial, junctional, or ventricular arrhythmias. Ventricular arrhythmias are perhaps the most life-threatening type because of their immediate effect on cardiac output. The most common supraventricular arrhythmias, which originate above the ventricles, are supraventricular tachycardias.

In contrast, atrioventricular (AV) blocks are classified by severity, not location. AV blocks, which may be total or partial, result from an interruption or delay in conduction between the atria and ventricles.

Sinus bradycardia

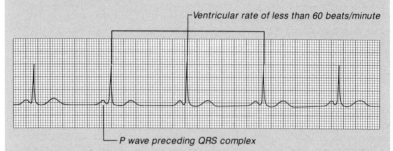

Ventricular rate of less than 60 beats/minute

P wave preceding QRS complex

ECG characteristics
- *Atrial rhythm:* regular
- *Ventricular rhythm:* regular
- *Atrial rate:* less than 60 beats/minute
- *Ventricular rate:* less than 60 beats/minute
- *P wave:* precedes each QRS complex
- *PR interval:* normal, remaining constant at 0.12 to 0.20 second
- *QRS complex:* duration and configuration usually normal

Causes
- May occur normally in athletes
- Increased intracranial pressure
- Increased vagal tone from myocardial infarction (MI) or from straining at defecation, vomiting, intubation, or mechanical ventilation
- Carotid massage
- Sick sinus syndrome
- Hypothyroidism
- Drugs such as anticholinesterases, beta blockers, digoxin, and morphine

Interpreting ECGs *(continued)*

Sinus tachycardia

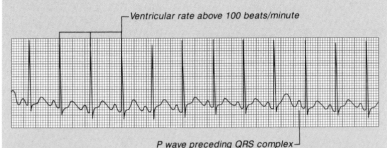

Ventricular rate above 100 beats/minute

P wave preceding QRS complex

ECG characteristics
- *Atrial rhythm:* regular
- *Ventricular rhythm:* regular
- *Atrial rate:* greater than 100 beats/minute (usually 100 to 160 beats/minute)
- *Ventricular rate:* greater than 100 beats/minute (usually 100 to 160 beats/minute)
- *P wave:* precedes each QRS complex
- *PR interval:* normal, remaining constant at 0.12 to 0.20 second
- *QRS complex:* duration and configuration usually normal

Causes
- Exercise
- Fever
- Hypoxia
- Pain
- Stress
- Volume depletion
- Ingestion of alcohol or caffeine
- Cigarette smoking
- Shock
- Left ventricular failure
- Cardiac tamponade
- Anemia
- Hyperthyroidism
- Pulmonary embolus

(continued)

Interpreting ECGs *(continued)*

Premature atrial contractions

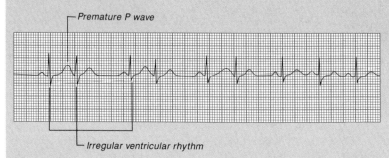

Premature P wave

Irregular ventricular rhythm

ECG characteristics
- *Atrial rhythm:* irregular, due to the premature beat; underlying rhythm may be regular
- *Ventricular rhythm:* irregular, due to the premature beat; underlying rhythm may be regular
- *Atrial rate:* varies according to the underlying rhythm
- *Ventricular rate:* varies according to the underlying rhythm
- *P wave:* premature and abnormally shaped, possibly lost in previous T wave
- *PR interval:* usually within normal limits (0.12 to 0.20 second)
- *QRS complex:* duration and configuration usually normal
- *T wave:* usually of normal duration and configuration

Note: Premature atrial beats depolarize the sinoatrial (SA) node early, disrupting the normal cycle; therefore, the next sinus beat occurs sooner than it normally would. This results in an incomplete compensatory pause. By contrast, a premature ventricular contraction is usually followed by a full compensatory pause.

Causes
- Stress
- Cigarette smoking
- Alcohol, caffeine, or cocaine use
- Congestive heart failure (CHF)
- Ischemic heart disease
- Mitral or tricuspid valvular insufficiency
- Acute respiratory failure
- Chronic obstructive pulmonary disease (COPD)
- Hyperthyroidism
- Hypokalemia
- Digitalis toxicity

Interpreting ECGs *(continued)*

Paroxysmal atrial tachycardia

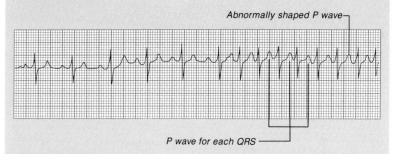

Abnormally shaped P wave

P wave for each QRS

ECG characteristics
- *Atrial rhythm:* regular
- *Ventricular rhythm:* regular
- *Atrial rate:* 160 to 250 beats/minute
- *Ventricular rate:* 160 to 250 beats/minute
- *P wave:* abnormal configuration
- *QRS complex:* duration and configuration usually normal
- *Other:* one P wave for each QRS complex

Causes
- Digitalis toxicity
- Cardiomyopathy
- Congenital heart disease
- MI
- Valvular disease
- Wolff-Parkinson-White syndrome
- Cor pulmonale
- Hyperthyroidism
- Systemic hypertension
- Excessive ingestion of caffeine or alcohol
- Use of marijuana or cocaine
- Cigarette smoking
- Stress

(continued)

Interpreting ECGs *(continued)*

Atrial tachycardia with AV block

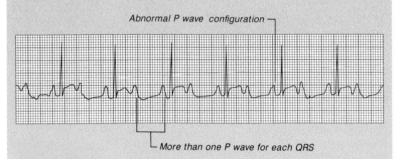

Abnormal P wave configuration ⌐

More than one P wave for each QRS

ECG characteristics
- *Atrial rhythm:* regular
- *Ventricular rhythm:* regular if block is constant; irregular if block is variable
- *Atrial rate:* 160 to 250 beats/minute; will be a multiple of ventricular rate
- *Ventricular rate:* varies
- *P wave:* slightly abnormal configuration
- *QRS complex:* duration and configuration usually normal
- *Other:* more than one P wave for each QRS complex

Causes
- Digitalis toxicity
- Hypokalemia
- Cardiomyopathy
- Congenital heart disease
- MI
- Valvular disease
- Wolff-Parkinson-White syndrome
- Cor pulmonale
- Hyperthyroidism
- Systemic hypertension

Interpreting ECGs *(continued)*

Multifocal atrial tachycardia or chaotic atrial tachycardia

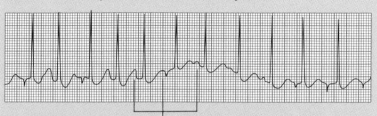

Varying P wave configuration⌐

ECG characteristics
- *Atrial rhythm:* irregular
- *Ventricular rhythm:* irregular
- *Atrial rate:* 100 to 250 beats/minute
- *Ventricular rate:* 100 to 250 beats/minute
- *P wave:* configuration varies
- *PR interval:* varies
- *QRS complex:* duration and configuration usually normal

Causes
- CHF, valvular disease, COPD, electrolyte disturbances, septicemia
- Theophylline toxicity
- May occur postoperatively due to hypoxia secondary to general anesthesia
- May occur in healthy individuals

Atrial flutter

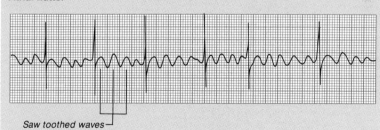

Saw toothed waves⌐

ECG characteristics
- *Atrial rhythm:* regular
- *Atrial rate:* 250 to 350 beats/minute
- *Flutter or F waves:* saw-toothed appearance
- *QRS complex:* duration and configuration usually normal

Causes
- Acute or chronic heart disease, cor pulmonale, inferior-wall MI, intracardiac infection, or mitral or tricuspid valve disease
- Excessive ingestion of caffeine or alcohol

(continued)

Interpreting ECGs *(continued)*

Atrial fibrillation

Coarse

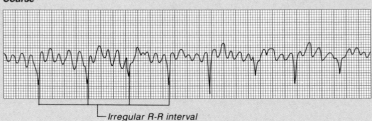

└─*Irregular R-R interval*

Fine

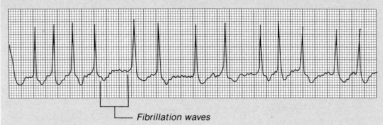

└─ *Fibrillation waves*

ECG characteristics
- *Atrial rhythm:* grossly irregular
- *Ventricular rhythm:* grossly irregular
- *Atrial rate:* almost indiscernible; usually greater than 400 beats/minute
- *Ventricular rate:* 60 to 150 beats/minute
- *P wave:* absent; instead, erratic baseline f waves (fibrillary waves) appear; coarse atrial fibrillation has pronounced f waves; fine atrial fibrillation has less pronounced f waves
- *QRS complex:* duration and configuration usually normal

Causes
- Rheumatic heart disease, constrictive pericarditis
- Valvular disorders (particularly mitral stenosis)
- CHF, cardiomyopathy
- Ischemic heart disease, coronary artery disease (CAD)
- Thyrotoxicosis
- COPD
- Hypertension
- Excessive ingestion of alcohol or caffeine

Interpreting ECGs *(continued)*

Junctional rhythm

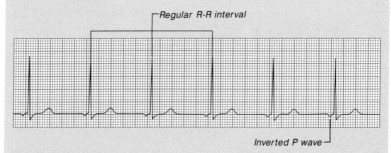

┌Regular R-R interval

Inverted P wave┘

ECG characteristics
- *Atrial rhythm:* regular
- *Ventricular rhythm:* regular
- *Atrial rate:* 40 to 60 beats/minute
- *Ventricular rate:* 40 to 60 beats/minute
- *P wave:* usually inverted, may be upright; may precede, follow, or be hidden in the QRS complex; may be absent
- *PR interval:* if P wave precedes QRS complex, PR interval is shortened (less than 0.12 second); otherwise, not measurable.
- *QRS complex:* duration and configuration usually normal
- *T wave:* usually of normal configuration

Causes
- Digitalis toxicity
- Inferior-wall MI
- Myocardial ischemia
- Increased vagal tone
- Rheumatic heart disease
- Valvular disease
- Organic disease of the SA node, such as sick sinus syndrome or SA node ischemia
- Verapamil toxicity
- Anticholinesterase toxicity
- May occur immediately after cardiac surgery

(continued)

Interpreting ECGs *(continued)*

Junctional tachycardia

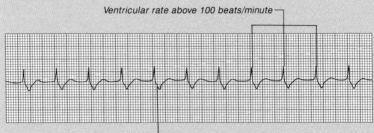

Ventricular rate above 100 beats/minute ⌐

P wave hidden in QRS complex ⌐

ECG characteristics
• *Atrial rate:* if P wave is present, exceeds 100 beats/minute (usually between 100 and 180 beats/minute); rate may be impossible to determine if P wave is absent or hidden in QRS complex or preceding T wave
• *Ventricular rate:* exceeds 100 beats/minute (usually between 100 and 180 beats/minute)
• *P wave:* usually inverted, may be upright or absent; may precede, follow, or be hidden in the QRS complex
• *PR interval:* if P wave precedes QRS complex, PR interval is shortened (less than 0.12 second); otherwise, not measurable
• *QRS complex:* duration and configuration usually normal

Causes
• Digitalis toxicity
• Hypoxia
• Vagal stimulation
• Myocardial ischemia
• MI
• Myocarditis
• Cardiomyopathy
• Valve replacement surgery
• Acute rheumatic fever
• Enhanced automaticity
• May occur immediately after cardiac surgery

Interpreting ECGs *(continued)*

Premature junctional contractions

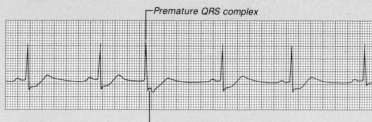

Premature QRS complex

P wave hidden in QRS complex

ECG characteristics
- *P wave:* usually inverted, but may be upright; may precede, follow, or be hidden in the QRS complex; may be absent
- *PR interval:* if P wave precedes QRS complex, PR interval is shortened (less than 0.12 second); otherwise, not measurable
- *QRS complex:* duration and configuration usually normal
- *Other:* commonly accompanied by a noncompensatory pause

Causes
- Digitalis toxicity, MI, myocardial ischemia, ingestion of caffeine or amphetamines

Wolff-Parkinson-White syndrome

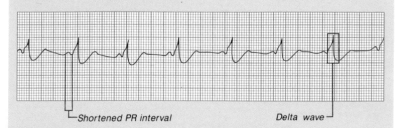

Shortened PR interval

Delta wave

ECG characteristics
- *PR interval:* less than 0.12 second
- *QRS complex:* duration greater than 0.12 second; beginning of complex may be slurred, producing a delta wave. In Type A Wolff-Parkinson-White (WPW) syndrome, the delta wave and QRS complex are upright in the anterior precordial leads. In Type B WPW syndrome, the delta wave and QRS complex are inverted in V_1 and V_2 and upright in V_5 and V_6.
- *ST segment:* changes, generally in a direction opposite the delta wave
- *T wave:* changes, generally in a direction opposite the delta wave

Causes
- Congenital origin

(continued)

Interpreting ECGs *(continued)*

Premature ventricular contractions

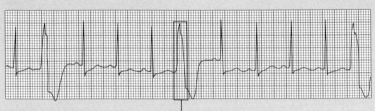

Wide QRS complex with bizarre shape⏎

ECG characteristics
• *P wave:* absent
• *PR interval:* not measurable
• *QRS complex:* occurs earlier than expected; duration exceeds 0.12 second;
bizarre configuration
• *T wave:* occurs in direction opposite QRS complex
• *Other:* a compensatory pause may follow the T wave. (The underlying rhythm doesn't
reset itself, and the next normal beat doesn't occur when expected. The interval between
the normal beat preceding the premature ventricular contraction [PVC] and the normal
beat following the PVC is equal to twice the normal sinus [P-P] interval.)

Causes
• Digitalis toxicity
• Sympathomimetic drugs, such as epinephrine or isoproterenol
• Hypokalemia
• Hypocalcemia
• Exercise
• Excessive ingestion of caffeine or alcohol
• Cigarette smoking
• Hypoxia
• MI
• Myocardial irritation from pacemaker electrodes during insertion
• Hypercapnia associated with COPD

Interpreting ECGs *(continued)*

Ventricular tachycardia

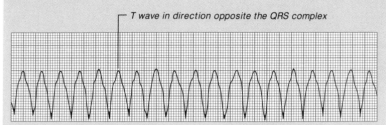

T wave in direction opposite the QRS complex

ECG characteristics
- *Atrial rhythm:* can't be determined
- *Ventricular rhythm:* usually regular but may be slightly irregular
- *Atrial rate:* can't be determined
- *Ventricular rate:* usually rapid (100 to 200 beats/minute)
- *P wave:* usually absent but may be obscured by the QRS complex; retrograde
P waves may be present
- *PR interval:* not measurable
- *QRS complex:* duration exceeds 0.12 second; bizarre appearance, usually with increased amplitude
- *T wave:* direction is opposite that of QRS complex
- *Other:* fusion beats, capture beats

Causes
- Acute MI
- CAD
- Rheumatic heart disease
- Mitral valve prolapse
- CHF
- Cardiomyopathy
- Pulmonary embolism
- Electrolyte imbalance, such as hypokalemia or hypomagnesemia
- Drug toxicity, for example, from quinidine, disopyramide, or procainamide
- Digitalis toxicity
- Hypertensive heart disease
- Cardiac tumors
- Ventricular aneurysm

(continued)

Interpreting ECGs *(continued)*

Ventricular flutter

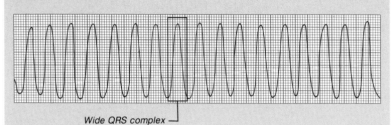

Wide QRS complex ⏐

ECG characteristics
- *Atrial rhythm:* can't be determined
- *Ventricular rhythm:* regular or irregular
- *Atrial rate:* can't be determined
- *Ventricular rate:* 150 to 300 beats/minute
- *P wave:* absent
- *QRS complex:* wide and continuous with zigzag pattern; can't be distinguished from ST segment and T wave

Causes
- Acute MI
- Untreated ventricular tachycardia
- CAD
- Mitral valve failure
- Heart failure
- Cardiomyopathy
- R-on-T phenomenon
- Hypokalemia
- Hyperkalemia
- Hypercalcemia
- Acid-base imbalance
- Epinephrine toxicity
- Quinidine toxicity
- Electric shock
- Hypothermia

Interpreting ECGs *(continued)*

Torsades de pointes

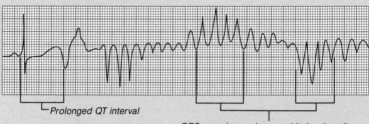

Prolonged QT interval

QRS complexes above and below baseline

ECG characteristics
- *Atrial rhythm:* can't be determined
- *Ventricular rhythm:* regular or irregular
- *Atrial rate:* can't be determined
- *Ventricular rate:* 150 to 250 beats/minute
- *P wave:* hidden in QRS complex; can't be identified
- *QRS complex:* usually wide with phasic variation, complexes deflect downward for several beats and then upward for several beats
- *QT interval:* prolonged preceding arrhythmia
- *Other:* arrhythmia may start and stop suddenly

Causes
- Acute MI
- CAD
- Rheumatic heart disease
- Mitral valve prolapse
- Heart failure
- Cardiomyopathy
- Pulmonary embolism
- Electrolyte imbalance, such as hypokalemia or hypomagnesemia
- Drug toxicity, for example, from quinidine, disopyramide, or procainamide
- Central nervous system disorders, such as intracranial lesions
- QT prolongation syndrome
- Myocarditis
- Liquid protein diets

(continued)

Interpreting ECGs *(continued)*

Ventricular fibrillation

Coarse

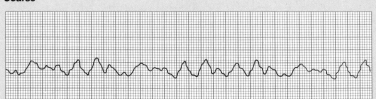

Fine

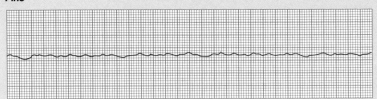

ECG characteristics
- *Atrial rhythm:* can't be determined
- *Ventricular rhythm:* no pattern or regularity
- *Atrial rate:* can't be determined
- *Ventricular rate:* can't be determined
- *P wave:* indiscernible
- *QRS complex:* duration indiscernible
- *Other:* waveform is a wavy line; when waves are large, the rhythm is coarse fibrillation; when waves are small, the rhythm is fine fibrillation

Causes
- Acute MI, CAD
- Untreated ventricular tachycardia, R-on-T phenomenon
- CHF
- Cardiomyopathy
- Blunt or penetrating cardiac trauma
- Electrolyte imbalance, such as hypokalemia, hyperkalemia, or hypercalcemia
- Acid-base imbalance
- Epinephrine or quinidine toxicity
- Digitalis toxicity
- Procainamide toxicity
- Electric shock
- Hypothermia

Interpreting ECGs *(continued)*

Asystole

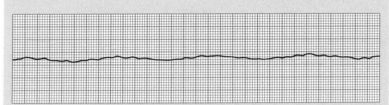

ECG characteristics
- *Atrial rhythm:* usually indiscernible
- *Ventricular rhythm:* none
- *Atrial rate:* usually indiscernible
- *Ventricular rate:* none
- *P wave:* may be present in ventricular asystole; may be absent in atrial asystole
- *QRS complex:* absent; occasionally a wide QRS complex (agonal rhythm) is present
- *T wave:* absent
- *Other:* waveform is a nearly flat line when asystole affects atrium and ventricles

Causes
- Any condition that prevents an adequate flow of blood, such as pulmonary embolism, air embolism, or hemorrhage
- Heart failure
- Cardiac tamponade
- CAD
- Cardiomyopathy
- Rheumatic heart disease
- Blunt or penetrating heart trauma
- Heart rupture
- Ventricular arrhythmias
- AV block
- Pulseless electrical activity
- Hypoxemia
- Electrolyte imbalance such as hypokalemia or hyperkalemia
- Severe acidosis
- Digitalis toxicity
- Electric shock
- Cocaine overdose

(continued)

Interpreting ECGs *(continued)*

First-degree AV block

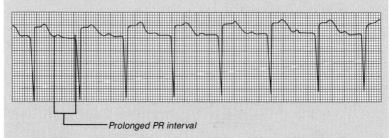

Prolonged PR interval

ECG characteristics
- *Atrial rhythm:* regular
- *Ventricular rhythm:* regular
- *Atrial rate:* usually normal (60 to 100 beats/minute)
- *Ventricular rate:* usually normal (60 to 100 beats/minute)
- *P wave:* present; configuration uniform
- *PR interval:* constant; more than 0.20 second
- *QRS complex:* duration and configuration usually normal
- *Other:* each P wave is followed by a QRS complex; there are no nonconducted beats

Causes
- Digitalis toxicity
- Acute inferior-wall MI
- Degeneration of the conduction system
- Hyperkalemia
- Rheumatic fever
- Acute myocarditis
- Calcium channel blocker use
- May occur in well-trained athletes
- Common in elderly patients without evidence of heart disease
- Quinidine toxicity

Interpreting ECGs *(continued)*

Second-degree AV block, Mobitz Type I (Wenckebach phenomenon)

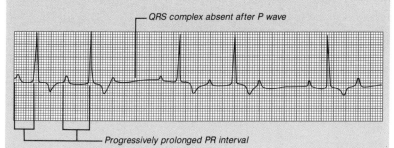

QRS complex absent after P wave

Progressively prolonged PR interval

ECG characteristics
- *Atrial rhythm:* regular
- *Ventricular rhythm:* irregular; R-R interval shortens progressively until P wave appears without QRS complex; cycle then repeats
- *Atrial rate:* exceeds ventricular rate
- *P wave:* present; configuration usually uniform
- *PR interval:* progressively longer, but often only slightly longer with each cycle until P wave appears without QRS complex; PR interval after the nonconducted beat is shorter than the preceding interval
- *QRS complex:* duration and configuration usually normal; complex is periodically absent

Causes
- Inferior-wall MI
- Heart surgery
- Acute infection, such as acute rheumatic fever
- Vagal stimulation
- Digitalis toxicity
- Propranolol use
- Quinidine use
- Procainamide use
- Verapamil use
- Bacterial, viral, or fungal infection
- Electrolyte imbalance
- Uremia
- May occur in well-trained athletes

Interpreting ECGs *(continued)*

Second-degree AV block, Mobitz Type II

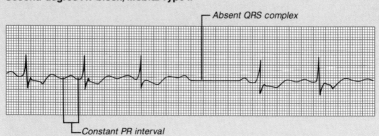

Absent QRS complex

Constant PR interval

ECG characteristics

- *Atrial rhythm:* regular
- *Ventricular rhythm:* regular or irregular; pauses correspond to nonconducted beat
- *P wave:* normal size and configuration
- *PR interval:* remains constant until a QRS complex is absent
- *QRS complex:* duration and configuration usually normal; complex is periodically absent

Causes

- Organic heart disease, such as anterior-wall MI, severe CAD, or acute myocarditis

Third-degree AV block

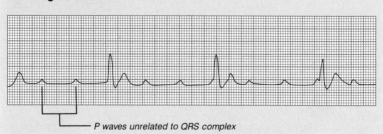

P waves unrelated to QRS complex

ECG characteristics

- *Atrial rhythm:* regular; no relationship between atrial and ventricular rhythm
- *Ventricular rhythm:* regular
- *Atrial rate:* usually exceeds ventricular rate
- *Ventricular rate:* usually less than 40 beats/minute
- *PR interval:* varies; no relationship between P wave and QRS complex
- *QRS complex:* configuration varies

Causes

- Severe digitalis toxicity or anterior-wall or inferior-wall MI (acute blocks)
- Cardiac catheterization or angioplasty (transient blocks)
- Bilateral bundle-branch block, congenital abnormality, rheumatic fever, hypoxia, or mitral valve replacement surgery (chronic blocks)

IMPLEMENTATION

Treatment for arrhythmia focuses on returning pacemaker function to the sinoatrial node, reestablishing a normal ventricular rate and AV synchrony, and maintaining normal sinus rhythm. (See *Medical care of the patient with arrhythmia.*)

• For a symptomatic patient, start cardiac monitoring and insert an I.V. line with a large-bore catheter for emergency drug access.

• Quickly obtain a 12-lead ECG to evaluate the patient's arrhythmia. Have resuscitative equipment available.

• Determine whether the arrhythmia is a life-threatening bradyarrhythmia or tachyarrhythmia. If the patient doesn't have a pulse and you detect ventricular fibrillation (VF), VT, or asystole or if the ECG indicates pulseless electrical activity, immediately implement your hospital's established protocols for the arrhythmia and call a code. (See "Cardiac arrest," page 241.)

• If your patient has a pulse, continue to monitor his condition to determine whether he's stable or unstable. Never rely on the patient's heart rate alone to determine his hemodynamic stability. Instead, interpret his pulse and ECG findings in light of his appearance.

• If the patient is unstable and has serious signs and symptoms, administer drugs or carry out defibrillation or cardioversion according to your hospital's protocol. Perform advanced procedures only if you're qualified and you've taken necessary precautions. Monitor the patient for adverse reactions: antiarrhythmics can cause severe GI, dermatologic, and hematologic effects and may cause proarrhythmias (arrhythmias that occur when another is already present).

• If the patient's arrhythmia isn't life-threatening and he's stable, you have more time to investigate the cause.

Treatments
Medical care of the patient with arrhythmia

Treatment for an arrhythmia focuses on returning pacing function to the sinoatrial node, increasing or decreasing ventricular rate to normal, reestablishing atrioventricular synchrony, and maintaining normal sinus rhythm. The treatment regimen may include any or all of the following interventions:
• Antiarrhythmic therapy
• Electrical conversion with precordial shock (defibrillation and cardioversion)
• Physical maneuvers, such as carotid sinus massage or Valsalva's maneuver
• Temporary or permanent placement of a pacemaker to maintain heart rate
• Surgical removal or cryotherapy of an irritable ectopic focus to prevent recurring arrhythmias.

Ongoing treatment
Treating the underlying disorder, such as hypoxia or electrolyte imbalance, may help control or eliminate arrhythmias. Arrhythmias associated with heart disease, however, may require ongoing and complex treatment. If the patient has recurrent, life-threatening arrhythmias that aren't responsive to drug therapy, the doctor may implant an automatic implantable cardioverter defibrillator.

Bradycardia with a pulse
Treat symptomatic bradycardia according to your hospital's protocol. (See *Treating symptomatic bradycardia*, page 234.)

• If prompt intervention is necessary, administer atropine by rapid I.V. push. If the patient is intubated and the I.V. line has yet to be established (or has infiltrated), give atropine through the en-

Treating symptomatic bradycardia

The following algorithm shows the steps for treating bradycardia in a patient who is not in cardiac arrest.

Perform assessment and early interventions:
- Assess airway, breathing, and circulation.
- Secure airway.
- Administer oxygen.
- Start I.V. line.
- Attach monitor, pulse oximeter, and automatic sphygmomanometer.
- Assess vital signs.
- Review patient history.
- Perform physical examination.
- Order 12-lead electrocardiogram.
- Order portable chest X-ray.

↓

If assessment indicates bradycardia, monitor for serious signs or symptoms or complications. These may include chest pain, shortness of breath, decreased level of consciousness, low back pain, shock, pulmonary congestion, congestive heart failure, or acute myocardial infarction.

Serious signs, symptoms, or complications absent.

Serious signs, symptoms, or complications present.

Assess for Type II second-degree atrioventricular heart block or third-degree atrioventricular heart block.

Administer atropine, 0.5 to 1 mg. Repeat doses every 3 to 5 minutes to total of 0.04 mg/kg. Consider shorter dosing intervals in acute clinical conditions.

Absent   *Present*

Perform transcutaneous pacing, if available. Don't delay transcutaneous pacing while awaiting I.V. access or for atropine to take effect.

Continue to observe the patient.

Prepare the patient for transvenous pacing.

Administer dopamine, 5 to 20 µg/kg/minute.

Administer epinephrine, 2 to 10 µg/minute.

Use transcutaneous pacing as bridge to transvenous pacing. Verify patient tolerance and mechanical capture. Use analgesics and sedatives as needed.

Administer isoproterenol. Keep in mind that this drug can be harmful at higher doses and must be administered with extreme caution.

dotracheal tube at a dosage of 2 to 2½ times the recommended I.V. dose. If atropine fails to boost the heart rate sufficiently or if severe symptoms persist, anticipate temporary pacing.

• Administer isoproterenol cautiously if prescribed. Be aware that some clinicians believe this potent inotropic drug shouldn't be given to patients with coronary artery disease (CAD), diabetes mellitus, hyperthyroidism, left ventricular pathology, or sensitivity to sympathomimetic amines.

• If your patient has symptomatic second-degree (Mobitz Type I or Type II) or third-degree AV block, place him in the supine position to reduce hypotension.

• Stable symptomatic patients may require temporary pacing. If no correctable underlying cause is discovered, further studies or a permanent pacemaker may be ordered. Provide appropriate patient teaching.

Tachycardia
Treat tachycardia according to your hospital's protocol. (See *Treating tachycardia*, pages 236 and 237.) Differentiation among sinus tachycardia, VT, paroxysmal SVT, and nonparoxysmal SVT may be difficult; however, it's critical.

• If your patient is unstable, has serious signs and symptoms, and has a ventricular rate above 150 beats/minute, prepare for immediate cardioversion. A trial of emergency medications may be administered, if they're immediately available.

• When you're unable to determine whether wide QRS-complex tachycardia originates in the ventricle or above the ventricle, give procainamide, not verapamil. Administering verapamil (the standard drug for SVT) to a patient with VT can increase his heart rate, lower his blood pressure, and cause death.

When time permits, vagal maneuvers or adenosine may be used to dis-

tinguish SVT from VT. Vagal stimulation will terminate some SVTs, but it rarely affects VT.

• If the patient is unstable, be prepared for imminent cardiac arrest and initiation of a code.

• If you're assisting with cardioversion, make sure that the patient receives oxygen and is connected to a cardiac monitor, an oxygen saturation monitor, and a noninvasive sphygmomanometer. Keep resuscitation equipment on hand.

• If time permits and the patient is hemodynamically stable, administer the prescribed sedative before cardioversion. Cardioversion causes pain and anxiety for a conscious patient.

• If your patient is taking digoxin or any long-term medication, be extremely careful during cardioversion because toxic drug levels may precipitate severe arrhythmias.

• If the patient is stable, expect to administer drugs before cardioversion. If the patient is unstable, expect to perform cardioversion first and then administer drugs to maintain normal sinus rhythm.

Ventricular tachycardia
• Treat the patient with VT according to your hospital's protocol.

• If the patient is clinically stable, expect to administer lidocaine, the drug of choice.

• Monitor his serum electrolyte levels, especially potassium; abnormal levels can worsen the VT or interfere with treatment.

• If VT is converted to a stable rhythm, continue to monitor the patient for recurrence of the arrhythmia. Assess femoral and carotid pulses to detect pulseless electrical activity. Continue to infuse the medication that converted the VT at the recommended dosage.

• Help identify and manage or eliminate the cause of VT. Possible causes

(Text continues on page 238.)

Treating tachycardia

The following algorithm is based on the most recent American Heart Association guidelines for intervening in tachycardia.

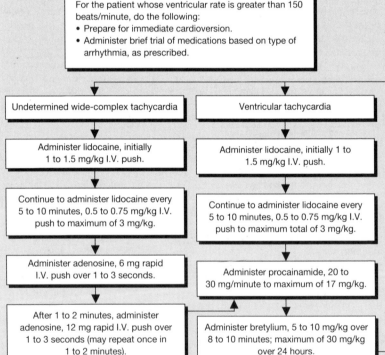

Perform assessment and early interventions:
- Assess airway, breathing, and circulation.
- Secure airway.
- Administer oxygen.
- Start I.V. line.
- Attach monitor, pulse oximeter, and automatic sphygmomanometer.
- Assess vital signs.
- Review health history.
- Perform physical examination.
- Order 12-lead electrocardiogram.
- Order portable chest X-ray.

Unstable with serious signs and symptoms
For the patient whose ventricular rate is greater than 150 beats/minute, do the following:
- Prepare for immediate cardioversion.
- Administer brief trial of medications based on type of arrhythmia, as prescribed.

Undetermined wide-complex tachycardia

Ventricular tachycardia

Administer lidocaine, initially 1 to 1.5 mg/kg I.V. push.

Administer lidocaine, initially 1 to 1.5 mg/kg I.V. push.

Continue to administer lidocaine every 5 to 10 minutes, 0.5 to 0.75 mg/kg I.V. push to maximum of 3 mg/kg.

Continue to administer lidocaine every 5 to 10 minutes, 0.5 to 0.75 mg/kg I.V. push to maximum total of 3 mg/kg.

Administer adenosine, 6 mg rapid I.V. push over 1 to 3 seconds.

Administer procainamide, 20 to 30 mg/minute to maximum of 17 mg/kg.

After 1 to 2 minutes, administer adenosine, 12 mg rapid I.V. push over 1 to 3 seconds (may repeat once in 1 to 2 minutes).

Administer bretylium, 5 to 10 mg/kg over 8 to 10 minutes; maximum of 30 mg/kg over 24 hours.

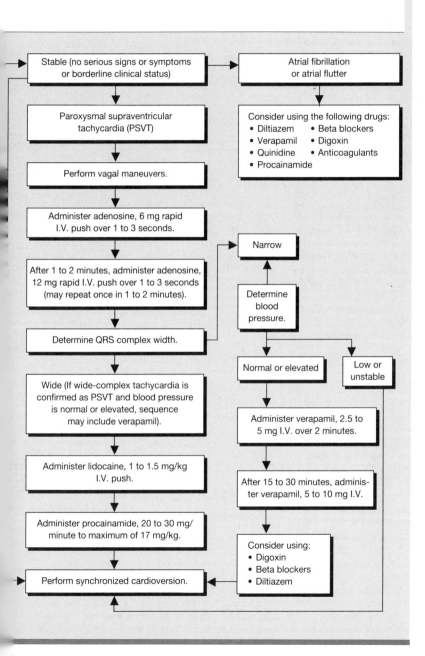

include drug toxicity, electrolyte imbalances, or recent MI.

• If VT proves refractory to first-line drugs, anticipate the use of other drugs, such as amiodarone. Monitor the patient carefully. Adverse effects of amiodarone include proarrhythmia, hepatotoxicity, thyrotoxicity, and pulmonary fibrosis. Also, sotalol shows great promise for terminating VT.

• If your patient has symptomatic, life-threatening, recurrent VT (or VF) that fails to respond to drug therapy, he may receive an implantable cardioverter defibrillator. If so, provide preoperative and postoperative care and patient teaching.

Torsades de pointes

A form of VT associated with prolonged QT interval, torsades de pointes is usually drug induced and may be treated differently than conventional VT. When the patient's symptoms warrant intervention, expect to administer I.V. magnesium sulfate, lidocaine, or isoproterenol or assist with overdrive electrical pacing.

Paroxysmal supraventricular tachycardia

• Treat the patient with paroxysmal SVT according to your hospital's protocol.

• If the patient is stable, use vagal maneuvers, such as carotid sinus massage or Valsalva's maneuver, before drug therapy. These maneuvers produce vagal stimulation, which slows conduction through the AV node. The goal is to trigger atrial standstill, which allows the SA node to reestablish itself as the main pacemaker.

• If vagal maneuvers aren't successful in terminating the arrhythmia, you may need to administer antiarrhythmics.

• If the patient's condition isn't life-threatening, you may have time to investigate the cause before administering drugs. Ask him about the use of al-

cohol, caffeine, or any illicit drugs, particularly cocaine.

• When antiarrhythmics are required, therapy usually begins with adenosine. This drug is considered safer than verapamil, which may cause severe hypotension and bradycardia or precipitate heart failure. Administer adenosine rapidly and warn the patient that he may experience momentary chest pain, flushing, and shortness of breath.

• If verapamil is prescribed, monitor the patient closely to detect adverse reactions quickly.

• For refractory paroxysmal SVTs, administer prescribed medications, such as digoxin or beta blockers.

• If drug therapy fails to control paroxysmal SVT or causes intolerable effects, anticipate cardioversion, atrial overdrive pacing, or catheter ablation of the reentry pathway. Assist with care and provide appropriate patient teaching.

Atrial fibrillation or flutter

• Treat the patient with atrial fibrillation or flutter according to your hospital's protocol.

• If your patient is unstable, help determine the cause of the arrhythmia and monitor the ventricular rate. If this rate becomes rapid (even if the patient is hemodynamically stable), notify the doctor. Even a small elevation can adversely affect ventricular filling time and coronary perfusion. Keep in mind that the patient with atrial flutter is usually less stable than the patient with atrial fibrillation.

• When drug therapy is warranted, administer the prescribed antiarrhythmic. However, if an antiarrhythmic, such as digoxin, caused atrial fibrillation or flutter, don't use it for treatment.

• If your patient is stable but has chronic atrial fibrillation or flutter, or if the arrhythmia has persisted for several days, expect to administer anticoagulants. Such therapy helps prevent pulmonary, cerebral, or peripheral emboli resulting from loosening of mural atrial thrombi. If cardioversion is performed, anticoagulants are especially important because atrial contraction may force a thrombus into the circulation.

Premature ventricular contractions

• Assess the frequency of premature ventricular contractions (PVCs). Six or more PVCs per minute require treatment. Also, if the patient's ECG shows a dangerous pattern, such as multiform PVCs (PVCs that look different from one another), bigeminy (PVCs that occur with every other beat), the R-on-T phenomenon (PVC falls on the T wave of the preceding beat), or three or more PVCs in a row (considered a run of ventricular tachycardia), anticipate treatment.

Frequent PVCs aren't usually treated unless the patient is symptomatic (dizziness, syncope). If ventricular escape beats are present instead of PVCs, they shouldn't be suppressed.

• Help determine the cause of symptomatic or dangerous PVCs, such as an acid-base or electrolyte imbalance or a drug such as digoxin. PVCs may terminate when the underlying cause is corrected. If PVCs result from bradycardia, expect to administer atropine.

• If antiarrhythmic therapy is warranted (such as when three or more PVCs occur in an MI or CAD patient whose ejection fraction is below 30%), administer prescribed I.V. drugs. These include lidocaine, procainamide, or bretylium (unless contraindicated) to suppress ventricular irritability. Expect to continue the drug by I.V. drip for up to 24 hours or until the patient is stable.

Premature atrial contractions

Infrequent premature atrial contractions (PACs) generally don't require treatment. However, if your patient has frequent PACs in conjunction with ischemic heart disease, the arrhythmia may lead to decreased cardiac output and congestive heart failure (CHF).

• When treatment is needed, identify and eliminate the cause — for example, excessive caffeine or alcohol intake.

• If antiarrhythmics are prescribed, administer drugs such as digoxin to suppress atrial irritability.

• Monitor serum digoxin and potassium levels.

• If PACs persist or become more frequent, anticipate increasingly severe atrial arrhythmias.

• If your patient has ischemic heart disease, monitor for signs and symptoms of angina or CHF.

Follow-up care for all arrhythmias

After treating your patient's arrhythmia, take the following steps to ensure his safety.

• Document the arrhythmia. Continue to monitor the patient carefully. Notify the doctor if there's a significant change in the patient's condition.

• Recognize that the patient may be extremely anxious. Encourage him to express his feelings.

• Provide the patient and family members with emotional support. If necessary, explain stress reduction techniques.

Patient teaching

• Teach your patient about his specific arrhythmia, and explain the importance of complying with treatment to prevent serious complications.

• Explain all interventions. When possible, encourage him to participate in care decisions.

• Prepare him for all ordered diagnostic tests, such as ECG, ambulatory ECG (Holter) monitoring, and blood studies.

• Teach the patient or a family member how to take a pulse and how to recognize an irregular rhythm. Explain that any deviation from the established baseline must be reported to the doctor.

• Teach about all prescribed medications, including their dosage and possible adverse effects. Explain the importance of taking all prescribed medications at the proper time intervals, even if symptoms disappear. Advise the patient to call his doctor if he experiences adverse reactions.

• Warn the patient to avoid excessive ingestion of alcohol or caffeine and, if applicable, to stop using tobacco.

• When appropriate, teach your patient how to perform procedures for managing specific arrhythmias, such as carotid sinus massage or Valsalva's maneuver. If the patient will receive a temporary pacemaker or cardioversion while in the hospital, describe how these procedures manage the arrhythmia.

• If surgery is required, teach the patient about the appropriate procedure, for example, open-heart surgery to correct structural defects, insertion of a permanent pacemaker, or insertion of an implantable cardioverter defibrillator. Explain preoperative, postoperative, and home care measures, including care of the incision.

• If your patient receives a permanent pacemaker or an implantable cardioverter defibrillator, provide detailed guidelines for its use and maintenance. Explain precautions, such as the need to carry special identification and the need to avoid strong magnetic fields.

• Stress the importance of scheduling and keeping appointments for regular checkups. For the patient with a pacemaker, stress the importance of monitoring battery function and explain how he can check his pacemaker by telephone.

• Suggest that a family member learn CPR.

• Tell the patient to report dangerous signs and symptoms to his doctor — for example, light-headedness or syncope, altered mental status, dyspnea, chest pain, reduced urine output, increased palpitations, change in pulse, or increasing fatigue.

• Provide the patient and family members with sources of information and support, such as the local chapters of the American Heart Association, Coronary Club, or Heart Disease Research Foundation. (See *Ensuring continued care for the patient with an arrhythmia*.)

EVALUATION

When evaluating the patient's response to your nursing care, gather reassessment data and compare this information to the patient outcomes specified in your plan of care.

Teaching and counseling
Talk to the patient and family members to determine the effectiveness of teaching and counseling. Consider the following questions:

• Can the patient communicate an understanding of the arrhythmia, its treatment, and all medications and devices used in treatment?

• Is he using effective coping mechanisms and support systems to alleviate feelings of anxiety?

Physical condition
If interventions are successful, your evaluation should indicate the following:

• systolic blood pressure above 90 mm Hg

• MAP above 80 mm Hg

• urine output of 30 ml/hour or more

• the presence of a normal sinus rhythm or an arrhythmia that doesn't compromise hemodynamic status (as evidenced by ECG readings)

• absence of complications, such as cerebrovascular accident or seizure

Discharge TimeSaver

Ensuring continued care for the patient with an arrhythmia

Review the following teaching topics, referrals, and follow-up appointments to ensure that your patient is adequately prepared for discharge.

Teaching topics
Make sure that the following topics have been covered and that your patient's learning has been evaluated:
☐ explanation of specific arrhythmia
☐ dietary modifications, including limits for alcohol and caffeine consumption and the need for increased dietary potassium, if prescribed
☐ antiarrhythmic therapy, including possible adverse reactions
☐ methods to correct the arrhythmia, such as Valsalva's maneuver, if appropriate
☐ proper method for measuring pulse rate
☐ symptoms indicating complications and the need to notify the doctor
☐ cardiopulmonary resuscitation (for family members)

☐ the importance of scheduling and attending follow-up appointments.

Referrals
Make sure the patient has been provided with all of these necessary referrals:
☐ social services
☐ sources for information and support, such as the American Heart Association, Coronary Club, or Heart Disease Research Foundation.

Follow-up appointments
Make sure the patient has been provided with the times and dates for these follow-up appointments:
☐ cardiologist
☐ surgeon
☐ additional diagnostic tests.

• absence of dyspnea, chest pain, or syncope (as evidenced by verbal reports or behavior)
• maintenance of baseline mental status
• warm, dry skin.

Failure to achieve outcomes
If the patient outcomes haven't been achieved, investigate further to determine the reason. Consult with the patient, his family members, and the health care team to determine the nature and extent of the problem. Consider the following questions:
• Does the patient understand the treatment regimen?
• Has he participated in decisions about his care?
• Is he taking prescribed medications?

• Does he understand that medications are necessary even when symptoms aren't present?
• Is he avoiding caffeine or alcoholic beverages?
• Are there additional stressors, such as family or financial problems, that are preventing the patient from obtaining relief from anxiety?

Cardiac arrest

Cardiac arrest is the abrupt and complete cessation of the heart's pumping action. Without prompt, aggressive intervention, it leads to circulatory failure, unconsciousness, respiratory arrest, and death. Overall, men have four

Understanding pulseless electrical activity

Pulseless electrical activity is the absence of a detectable pulse and the presence of some type of electrical activity other than ventricular tachycardia or ventricular fibrillation.

The term pulseless electrical activity incorporates electromechanical dissociation, pseudo–electromechanical dissociation, idioventricular rhythms, ventricular escape rhythms, and bradyasystolic rhythms.

Pulseless electrical activity is *nonarrhythmic* cardiac arrest and can't be assessed solely by cardiac monitoring; the cardiac monitor may show organized, normal electrical activity. A physical examination, however, reveals that audible heart sounds, pulse, and blood pressure are absent.

Causes
Causes of pulseless electrical activity include profound hypovolemia, cardiac tamponade, myocardial rupture, massive myocardial infarction, tension pneumothorax, pulmonary embolism, acidosis, and hypoxemia. If you suspect pulseless electrical activity, begin cardiopulmonary resuscitation while the cause is being investigated.

cardial blood flow, such as coronary artery spasm, hypertensive heart disease, cardiac tamponade, or prolonged QT interval syndrome. In addition, cardiac arrest may be caused by pulmonary embolism, air embolism, hemorrhage, hypoxemia, hypokalemia, hypotension, anaphylaxis, severe acidosis, electric shock, and cocaine overdose.

ASSESSMENT

Because cardiac arrest is a medical emergency, limit your initial assessment to verifying that your patient is in arrest. Symptoms include a loss of consciousness; the absence of a pulse, respiration, and blood pressure; and the presence of lethal arrhythmias.

If your patient suddenly loses consciousness, shake his shoulder and ask him if he's all right. If he fails to respond, immediately assess his airway, breathing, and circulation (ABCs).

Diagnostic test results
Cardiac monitoring or an electrocardiogram (ECG) provides information about the patient's cardiac rhythm during an arrest. This information can help guide treatment. (For guidelines on assessing the patient's cardiac rhythm, see *Interpreting ECGs*, pages 214 to 232, and *Understanding pulseless electrical activity*.)

NURSING DIAGNOSIS

Common nursing diagnoses for the patient in cardiac arrest include:
• Altered tissue perfusion (renal, cerebral, cardiopulmonary, or gastrointestinal) related to cessation of the heart's pumping function
• Impaired gas exchange related to cessation of the heart's pumping function

times the risk of cardiac arrest than women, and the risk for both men and women increases greatly with age.

Cardiac arrest has a better prognosis when it results from ventricular fibrillation than from asystole or pulseless electrical activity. Prognosis is poor if it's associated with a noncardiac condition.

Causes
Cardiac arrest may result from any condition that causes inadequate myo-

• Ineffective breathing pattern related to cessation of the heart's pumping function
• Inability to sustain spontaneous ventilation related to cessation of the heart's pumping function
• High risk for injury related to basic life support (BLS) or advanced cardiac life support (ACLS) procedures.

PLANNING

Because cardiac arrest is an emergency, you won't have time to write a plan of care. However, you should be familiar with your hospital's protocol or other prepared plan for a patient in arrest. After the medical emergency, you may need to amend the plan of care to reflect your patient's individual needs.

Based on the nursing diagnosis altered tissue perfusion (renal, cerebral, cardiopulmonary, or gastrointestinal), develop appropriate patient outcomes. For example, your patient will:
• regain normal sinus rhythm or a controlled arrhythmia as evidenced by systolic blood pressure above 90 mm Hg and pulse rate at baseline
• demonstrate palpable carotid and femoral pulses, with pulse rate within established limits
• return to his baseline level of consciousness (LOC)
• exhibit warm, dry skin
• maintain urine output of 30 ml/hour or more
• exhibit constriction of the pupils in response to light.

Based on the nursing diagnosis *impaired gas exchange,* develop appropriate patient outcomes. For example, your patient will:
• achieve adequate ventilation as indicated by arterial blood gas (ABG) levels within established ranges: pH, 7.35 to 7.45; partial pressure of oxygen in arterial blood, 75 to 100 mm Hg; partial pressure of carbon dioxide in arterial blood ($PaCO_2$), 35 to 45 mm Hg;

and arterial oxygen saturation, 94% to 100%
• demonstrate clear bilateral breath sounds.

Based on the nursing diagnosis *ineffective breathing pattern,* develop appropriate patient outcomes. For example, your patient will:
• demonstrate baseline respiratory rate and depth
• not experience dyspnea.

Based on the nursing diagnosis *inability to sustain spontaneous ventilation,* develop appropriate patient outcomes. For example, your patient will:
• demonstrate the ability to maintain respirations without experiencing muscle fatigue
• demonstrate baseline respiratory rate and depth.

Based on the nursing diagnosis *high risk for injury,* develop appropriate patient outcomes. For example, your patient will:
• not sustain fractured ribs, liver laceration, lung puncture, or gastric distention during cardiopulmonary resuscitation (CPR)
• not sustain complications of electric shock, such as burns, during defibrillation or cardioversion.
• not sustain esophageal or tracheal laceration or subcutaneous emphysema during emergency intubation.

IMPLEMENTATION

Because cardiac arrest occurs suddenly and often without warning, successful intervention depends on thorough preparation. (See *Effective code management,* page 244.) Before cardiac arrest, make sure that you know:
• BLS and ACLS procedures
• your hospital's code policy and procedures
• the names of the members of the code team, their departments, and their duties during a code

Effective code management

To be properly prepared for a code, you must be familiar with basic life support (BLS) and advanced cardiac life support (ACLS) procedures, know your hospital's code policy, know who to call when a code occurs, and be familiar with the contents of the crash cart.

BLS and ACLS interventions

BLS interventions focus on maintaining organ perfusion until the patient recovers or until ACLS is initiated. Measures include recognizing cardiac arrest, clearing an obstructed airway, and performing cardiopulmonary rescuscitation.

ACLS interventions are more aggressive efforts to achieve adequate ventilation, control arrhythmias, stabilize the patient's hemodynamic status, and restore organ perfusion. Measures include using a cardiac monitor to detect an abnormal heart rate and rhythm, insertion of peripheral and central I.V. lines, drug therapy, cardiac defibrillation, and the insertion of an artificial pacemaker.

The code team

Most hospitals have code teams that respond to respiratory and cardiac emergencies, and specific standard procedures for code management. Members of the code team represent many different departments, including anesthesia, respiratory therapy, electrocardiography, critical care, and I.V. therapy. Each member has a specific role during a code; some members, including nurses with specialized training, may have standing orders to initiate specific ACLS procedures, such as defibrillation or drug administration.

Know your role and be prepared to vary the sequence of your duties depending on the patient's needs and the setting. For example, besides giving emergency care, you may have to move the patient's roommate, call for staff members to help, get additional equipment, call a member of the clergy to sit with the patient's family members, or direct others to perform these tasks.

Crash carts

Crash carts include all equipment and drugs necessary for ACLS. However, the cart should be checked periodically to make sure that everything is in place; otherwise, valuable time can be lost during a code while a team member searches for missing equipment. If you're responsible for maintaining the crash cart in your hospital, periodically check the cart to be sure it contains all equipment and that the expiration dates for the drugs haven't passed. A typical crash cart contains:

• a manual resuscitation bag
• a cardiac monitor
• a defibrillator
• conductive jelly or paste, saline gel pads, or gauze sponges and 0.9% sodium chloride solution
• emergency medications
• I.V. therapy equipment, including central line catheters and equipment
• needles and syringes
• emergency airway equipment and oxygen supplies
• a cardiac arrest board
• endotracheal tubes
• tonsil-tipped and straight suction catheters
• a laryngoscope
• stylets
• a nasogastric tube and water-soluble lubricant, and a catheter-tip syringe
• adhesive tape
• suction equipment
• arterial blood gas syringes and vascular cutdown tray
• transvenous or transthoracic pacemaker equipment (optional).

• the method for notifying members of the code team of an emergency
• the location of the crash cart and the equipment it contains.

Each time you're assigned a cardiac patient, assess him for critical conditions that, if unrecognized and untreated, could lead to cardiac arrest. Such conditions include shock, acute pulmonary edema, acute myocardial infarction, or arrhythmias that threaten hemodynamic stability. Be familiar with the patient's advance directives.

Essential steps during cardiac arrest

If your patient is unresponsive, assess his airway, breathing, and circulation and call for help. Have a colleague call a code and get the crash cart.
• Assess the patient's breathing by first opening the airway, and then looking, listening, and feeling for signs of respiration.
• If he isn't breathing, begin resuscitation with two slow breaths. Then, palpate for a carotid pulse. If you fail to discern a pulse, place a hard surface, such as the headboard from the bed, under the patient and begin CPR. (A hard surface makes chest compression more effective.) When the crash cart arrives, replace the headboard with the cardiac arrest board.
• If you witness the arrest and a defibrillator isn't immediately available, use the hypothenar aspect of your fist to deliver a single precordial thump to the center of the patient's sternum from a height of 12″ or less. This may convert the abnormal rhythm even before your patient is attached to a cardiac monitor. (Don't administer a precordial thump to a patient with ventricular tachycardia who exhibits a pulse unless a defibrillator is available. The precordial thump may induce ventricular fibrillation.)
• Attach the manual resuscitation bag from the cart to a supplemental oxygen

source. Use the bag to ventilate the patient while your colleague continues chest compressions. Insert the airway, being careful not to displace the tongue into the hypopharynx.
• As members of the code team arrive, relinquish ventilation to the appropriate team member. When documenting the code, record the course of events and the participants. As the nurse assigned to this patient, you should stay in the room during the code to provide information about the patient's medical history and to describe the events that preceded the arrest.

Additional steps

You and members of the code team will continue to perform emergency procedures. These procedures will vary from code to code, depending on the number of staff available and the cause of the cardiac arrest.
• Turn on the cardiac monitor. Apply one electrode in the hollow below each clavicle and another at the fourth intercostal space on the left sternal border. Placement of the remaining electrodes will vary, depending on the type of cardiac monitor.
• Assess the patient's cardiac rhythm to help select the correct treatment. Perform ACLS procedures appropriate for the arrhythmia that appears on the monitor.
• If a diagnosis of asystole is established, defibrillation isn't needed. Continue CPR. Be cautious: Asystole should always be confirmed in two leads (for example, leads I and III) to avoid confusing asystole with fine ventricular fibrillation. If the diagnosis is uncertain, treat the patient for ventricular fibrillation. (*See Treating asystole*, page 246.)
• If a diagnosis of ventricular fibrillation or pulseless ventricular tachycardia is established, expect to defibrillate immediately. Speed in implementing defibrillation greatly improves the chance of successful resuscitation. When possi-

Treating asystole

The algorithm below, for treating asystole, is based on the most recent guidelines from the American Heart Association.

Perform initial assessment and early interventions:
- Assess airway, breathing, and circulation (ABCs).
- Perform cardiopulmonary resuscitation.
- Intubate patient at once.
- Establish an I.V. line.
- Confirm diagnosis of asystole in more than one lead.

⬇

Consider possible causes of asystole:
- Hypoxia
- Hyperkalemia
- Hypokalemia
- Preexisting acidosis
- Drug overdose
- Hypothermia.

⬇

Consider performing transcutaneous pacing immediately.

⬇

Administer epinephrine, 1 mg I.V. push; repeat every 3 to 5 minutes.

⬇

Administer atropine, 1 mg I.V.; repeat every 3 to 5 minutes up to 0.04 mg/kg.

⬇

Consider terminating resuscitation efforts.

ble, defibrillate before inserting an endotracheal tube and establishing an I.V. line. Continue CPR while the defibrillator is being charged. (See *Treating ventricular fibrillation or pulseless ventricular tachycardia,* pages 248 and 249.)
• Assist with endotracheal intubation, if performed. After intubation, check bilateral breath sounds for evidence of adequate ventilation in both lungs. Then, use the highest possible oxygen concentration (100% is preferred).
• Establish an I.V. line to administer fluids and emergency drugs. If a vein hasn't been cannulated before cardiac arrest, initiate therapy in a peripheral vein. Don't interrupt CPR to start a central I.V. line. Choose a large blood vessel, such as the brachial vein; smaller peripheral vessels tend to collapse quickly during cardiac arrest. Use a large-gauge needle that won't dislodge or injure the vein and cause extravasation and vessel collapse.
• Start an infusion of 0.9% sodium chloride solution. Later, other fluids, such as dextrose 5% in water, may be used to keep the vein open for emergency drug administration and to help prevent circulatory collapse from hypovolemia.
• Prepare and administer emergency medications as prescribed or according to standing orders. Drugs that may be given include epinephrine, lidocaine, procainamide, bretylium tosylate, epinephrine, atropine, isoproterenol, sodium bicarbonate, calcium chloride, magnesium sulfate, verapamil, dopamine, dobutamine, and norepinephrine. When using a peripheral I.V. line, administer I.V. medications rapidly by bolus injection, followed by a 20-ml bolus of I.V. fluid to flush the line of medication. If possible, elevate the extremity.
• Administer most drugs I.V., although lidocaine, atropine, and epinephrine may be given endotracheally if an I.V. line isn't yet in place or if it has been

infiltrated. When administering medications endotracheally, increase the dose to 2 to 2½ times the recommended I.V. dose and dilute the drug in 10 ml of 0.9% sodium chloride solution or distilled water.
• Set up portable or wall suction equipment and suction the patient's endotracheal and oral secretions as necessary to maintain an open airway.
• Take the patient's central pulses (carotid or femoral) frequently during ACLS, especially after drug administration or defibrillation. Remember that the cardiac monitor only shows the heart's electrical activity; it doesn't show the effectiveness of cardiac compressions.
• During the code, insert a nasogastric (NG) tube to relieve gastric distention, if needed. Otherwise, insert an NG tube after the patient is stabilized.

Essential steps after resuscitation

• Monitor the patient carefully. Intervene as necessary to maintain cardiac output and hemodynamic stability.
• When the patient's condition has stabilized, obtain a chest X-ray to detect any complications stemming from chest compressions. The X-ray will also indicate whether or not the endotracheal and NG tubes are properly placed.
• Provide the patient and family members with emotional support. Be prepared to discuss the patient's sudden death experience. Refer them for counseling, if needed.

Documenting the code

After the patient is stabilized, review your documentation to be sure you have a complete record of the code. Your documentation should indicate:
• the time the patient was found, the name of the person who found him, whether he experienced cardiac or respiratory arrest, and the names of staff members who responded to the code

Treating ventricular fibrillation or pulseless ventricular tachycardia

In the hospital, cardiac arrest most often results from ventricular fibrillation (VF) or pulseless ventricular tachycardia (VT). The following algorithm, based on the most recent information from the American Heart Association, shows the critical steps to take during cardiac arrest caused by VF or pulseless VT.

Perform assessment and early interventions:
- Assess airway, breathing, and circulation.
- Perform cardiopulmonary resuscitation (CPR) until defibrillator is attached.
- Administer a precordial thump *if you witnessed the arrest and the patient* *has no pulse and if a defibrillator isn't immediately available.*
- Confirm VF or pulseless VT on the defibrillator and confirm absence of a pulse.

Defibrillate up to three times (200 joules, 200 to 300 joules, 360 joules) as needed for persistent VF or pulseless VT.

Determine heart rhythm.

Pulseless electrical activity, including:
- Electromechanical dissociation (EMD)
- Pseudo-EMD
- Idioventricular rhythms
- Ventricular escape rhythms
- Bradyasystolic rhythms
- Postdefibrillation idioventricular rhythms

Return of spontaneous circulation
- Assess vital signs.
- Support airway.
- Support breathing.
- Provide medications appropriate for blood pressure, heart rate, and rhythm.

- Continue CPR.
- Intubate at once.
- Establish an I.V. line.
- Assess blood flow using Doppler ultrasound.

Consider possible causes and anticipate treatment. Causes include:
- Hypovolemia
- Hypoxia
- Cardiac tamponade
- Tension pneumothorax
- Hypothermia
- Massive pulmonary embolism
- Overdose of drugs, for example, tricyclic antidepressants, digoxin, beta blockers, or calcium channel blockers
- Hyperkalemia
- Acidosis
- Massive acute myocardial infarction

Asystole
Refer to algorithm on page 246.

Persistent or recurring VF
or pulseless VT
- Continue CPR.
- Intubate at once.
- Establish an I.V. line.
- Administer epinephrine, 1 mg I.V.
  push; repeat every 3 to 5 minutes.

Defibrillate with 360 joules
within 30 to 60 seconds.

Administer prescribed medications,
which may include one or more of
the following:
- Lidocaine, 1.5 mg/kg I.V. push;
  repeat every 3 to 5 minutes to
  a maximum of 3 mg/kg.
- Bretylium, 5 mg/kg I.V. push;
  if VF persists, repeat every 5 minutes
  with 10 mg/kg to a maximum of
  30 to 35 mg/kg.
- Magnesium sulfate, 1 to 2 g I.V.
- Procainamide, 30 mg/minute to
  a maximum of 17 mg/kg.

Administer epinephrine, 1 mg I.V. push;
repeat every 3 to 5 minutes.

For absolute bradycardia (below
60 beats/minute) or relative bradycardia,
administer atropine, 1 mg I.V.;
repeat every 3 to 5 minutes
to a maximum of 0.04 mg/kg.

Defibrillate with 360 joules 30 to 60 seconds after each dose of medication (pattern should be *drug, shock, drug, shock*).

• the site of the I.V. line, the time of insertion, the size of the needle used, and the fluids and drugs administered
• the patient's ECG before defibrillation (if administered), the number of joules used, and his ECG after defibrillation
• medications, doses, and the routes by which they were given
• whether a manual resuscitation bag was used
• the name of the person who performed endotracheal intubation (if done), the size of the tube used, and whether you heard bilateral breath sounds afterward
• any special procedures performed
• the patient's vital signs and responses to all interventions
• the patient's ABG levels and other laboratory test results
• recommended follow-up therapy and, if the patient is to be transferred, the transfer location and the patient's condition before transfer
• any complications and the interventions taken to correct them.

blood pressure above 90 mm Hg and pulse rate at baseline
• achieves adequate ventilation, as demonstrated by ABG measurements
• demonstrates adequate respiratory rate and depth
• demonstrates clear bilateral breath sounds
• maintains carotid or femoral pulses within established limits
• maintains baseline LOC
• maintains urine output of at least 30 ml/hour
• demonstrates adequate pupillary constriction upon exposure to light
• maintains warm, dry skin.

Also note the presence or absence of complications resulting from CPR (sustained fractured ribs, liver laceration, lung puncture, or gastric distention), defibrillation or cardioversion (electric shock, burns), or emergency intubation (esophageal or tracheal laceration or subcutaneous emphysema).

EVALUATION

Every code team performs a critique after the code. During this evaluation, keep in mind that even the most diligent and aggressive ACLS efforts can't successfully resuscitate all patients.

When resuscitation is successful, evaluate the patient's response to your nursing care. Gather reassessment data and compare this information to the patient outcomes specified in your plan of care.

Physical condition

Successful resuscitation is, by itself, evidence of effective intervention. A physical examination and diagnostic tests should further indicate whether the patient:
• regains normal sinus rhythm or a controlled arrhythmia with a systolic

Caring for patients with peripheral vascular disorders

Thoracic aortic aneurysm

A potentially life-threatening disorder, thoracic aortic aneurysm is characterized by abnormal weakening and widening of the ascending, descending, or transverse part of the aorta. This aneurysm may be *saccular* or *fusiform*. A saccular aneurysm is an outpouching of one portion of the arterial wall. In contrast, a fusiform aneurysm is a spindle-shaped enlargement that completely surrounds the aorta. (See *Key points about thoracic aortic aneurysm.*)

Complications include *aortic wall dissection*, a circumferential or transverse tear in the aortic wall intima, usually in the medial layer. Dissection requires emergency treatment; a dissecting hematoma may compromise major arteries originating from the aorta and coronary arteries. If a hematoma extends into the pericardium, cardiac tamponade may result.

Rupture of the aorta results in extravasation of blood through the walls of the aneurysm. Quick recognition of this surgical emergency can head off primary problems, such as hypovolemic shock, and secondary problems, such as myocardial ischemia or pulmonary edema.

Neurologic complications may include syncope, cerebrovascular accident, and paraplegia. (See *Classifying aortic dissection,* page 254.)

Causes

Ascending thoracic aortic aneurysm commonly results from weakening of the aortic wall and gradual distention of the lumen secondary to atherosclerosis. Descending thoracic aortic aneurysm usually results from blunt chest trauma that transversely shears the aorta or from penetrating chest injury such as a knife wound. It also may be a complication of hypertension. Trans-

verse thoracic aortic aneurysm commonly occurs with Marfan's syndrome.

Other causes of thoracic aortic aneurysm include infection or inflammation of the aorta resulting from bacterial aortitis, mycotic aneurysm, syphilitic aortitis, and ankylosing spondylitis.

In pregnant patients and in those with hypertension or Marfan's syndrome, the aneurysm may follow cystic medial necrosis caused by degeneration of collagen and elastic fibers in the medial layer of the aortic wall. Cystic medial necrosis also may occur without an underlying condition.

In rare cases, congenital disorders such as coarctation of the aorta may cause thoracic aortic aneurysm.

ASSESSMENT

Your assessment should include the patient's health history and physical examination findings and a review of diagnostic test results.

Health history

A patient with thoracic aortic aneurysm usually is asymptomatic until the aneurysm expands or begins to dissect. Dissection may lead to sudden pain and possible syncope. The patient may report back pain, caused by the retroperitoneal position of the aorta. Compression of the surrounding structures or dissection of the aneurysm may lead to pain in the neck, arms, legs, or epigastrium. If a transverse aneurysm compresses surrounding structures, the patient may report hoarseness, dyspnea, throat pain, dysphagia, or a dry cough.

A patient with a *dissecting ascending aneurysm* may report boring, tearing, or ripping pain in the thorax or right anterior chest. Pain may extend to the neck, shoulders, lower back, and abdomen, but rarely radiates to the jaw or arms. Pain is most intense at its onset

FactFinder

Key points about thoracic aortic aneurysm

• *Prognosis:* If dissecting thoracic aortic aneurysm isn't treated within 24 hours, death occurs in 30% to 50% of patients. If it's untreated for 1 to 2 weeks, mortality rises to 50% to 75%. If it's untreated for 1 to 3 months, mortality climbs to 90%.
• *Risk factors:* Hypertension, hypercholesterolemia, hyperlipidemia, and smoking
• *Sites:* Aneurysm in the ascending thoracic aorta is most common, especially in hypertensive men over age 60. Descending thoracic aortic aneurysm is most common in younger patients with a history of chest trauma. Transverse thoracic aortic aneurysm is the least common and is associated with Marfan's syndrome.
• *Complications:* The patient with an aortic aneurysm is at risk for rupture of the aorta and for aortic wall dissection, both of which are potentially life-threatening. Acute dissection of the thoracic aorta occurs more often than aneurysm rupture.

and frequently is misdiagnosed as a transmural myocardial infarction (MI).

The patient with a *dissecting descending aneurysm* may report sharp, tearing pain between the shoulder blades, often radiating to the chest. The patient with a *dissecting transverse aneurysm* may report sharp, boring, tearing pain radiating to the shoulders.

Physical examination

In your initial examination of a patient with dissecting thoracic aortic aneurysm, you may see skin pallor or cyanosis, diaphoresis, trunk mottling, dyspnea, leg weakness, or transient paralysis. Physical examination findings may help you distinguish between dissecting descending and ascending aneurysms.

Dissecting descending aneurysm

• During palpation, you may note that carotid and radial pulses are equal bilaterally.
• During percussion of the chest, you may detect an increasing area of flatness over the heart, suggesting cardiac tamponade and hemopericardium.

• During auscultation, you may hear bilateral crackles and rhonchi, suggesting pulmonary edema.
• Blood pressure measurements may reveal that systolic blood pressure is equal bilaterally.

Dissecting ascending aneurysm

• When palpating the peripheral pulses, you may note abrupt loss of radial and femoral pulses and right and left carotid pulses.
• During auscultation, you may hear a diastolic murmur of aortic insufficiency and if hemopericardium is present, a pericardial friction rub.
• Blood pressure readings may be at baseline or significantly elevated, with a difference in blood pressure, especially systolic, between the right and left arms.

Diagnostic test results

In an asymptomatic patient, diagnosis of thoracic aortic aneurysm commonly occurs accidentally, through routine posteroanterior and oblique chest X-rays. X-rays may show widening of the aorta. The aortic silhouette may be widened wherever the dissection ex-

Classifying aortic dissection

These drawings illustrate the DeBakey classification of aortic dissections. For each type of dissection, the shaded area represents its possible location along the aorta. Dissections can also be classified by their location in relation to the aortic valve. Type I and Type II are proximal. Type IIIa and Type IIIb are distal.

Type I
This is the most common and lethal type of dissection. Intimal tearing occurs in the ascending aorta, and dissection extends into the descending aorta.

Type II
This type of dissection is limited to the ascending or transverse aorta. It occurs most commonly in patients with Marfan's syndrome.

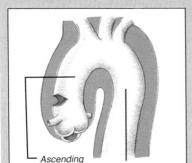

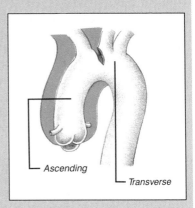

Type III
This type of dissection has two variations:
• The intimal tear in Type IIIa is in the descending aorta with distal propagation of the dissection.

• The intimal tear in Type IIIb also originates in the descending aorta, but may extend to the aortic bifurcation.

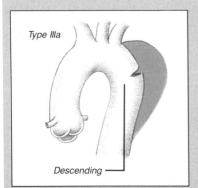

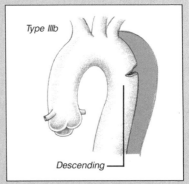

tends. Widening of the mediastinum with left pleural effusion may indicate aortic dissection.

The following additional tests help establish a diagnosis of thoracic aortic aneurysm:

• Aortography, a definitive test, shows the lumen of the aneurysm, its size, location, and possible dissection.

• Echocardiography and transesophageal echocardiography help delineate the aneurysm.

• Electrocardiography (ECG) helps rule out MI.

• Magnetic resonance imaging or computed tomography helps locate and confirm aortic dissection.

• Analysis of cardiac enzyme levels may help rule out MI.

• Decreased hemoglobin levels may indicate blood loss or a leaking aneurysm.

• Blood urea nitrogen and serum creatinine levels may determine renal artery involvement.

• Renal testing helps to determine baseline electrolyte levels.

• Pulse oximetry assesses oxygen delivery to tissues.

NURSING DIAGNOSIS

Common nursing diagnoses for a patient with thoracic aortic aneurysm include:

• Altered tissue perfusion (cerebral, cardiopulmonary, peripheral) related to rupture or dissection

• Fluid volume deficit related to impaired renal function caused by rupture

• Pain related to aortic dissection, rupture, or pressure on surrounding structures

• Anxiety related to the medical diagnosis

• Knowledge deficit related to thoracic aortic aneurysm and associated cardiovascular risk factors.

PLANNING

Goals of nursing care include relieving the patient's pain, teaching him about the disorder and its treatment, and preparing him for surgery, if indicated.

Based on the nursing diagnosis *altered tissue perfusion,* develop appropriate patient outcomes. For example, your patient will:

• maintain baseline level of consciousness (LOC)

• continue to have warm, dry skin

• maintain systolic blood pressure within established limits (usually between 90 and 140 mm Hg)

• maintain mean arterial pressure (MAP) within established limits (usually between 80 and 100 mm Hg)

• keep central venous pressure (CVP), pulmonary artery pressure (PAP), and pulmonary artery wedge pressure (PAWP) at established levels

• maintain heart rate at less than 100 beats/minute, with a regular rhythm

• regularly demonstrate peripheral pulses that are palpable, strong, and equal

• maintain respiratory rhythm and depth at baseline, and respiratory rate within 5 breaths of baseline

• maintain baseline breath sounds.

Based on the nursing diagnosis *fluid volume deficit,* develop appropriate patient outcomes. For example, your patient will:

• maintain urine output greater than 30 ml/hour or 0.5 ml/kg/hour, depending on the patient's body size and physical condition.

Based on the nursing diagnosis *pain,* develop appropriate patient outcomes. For example, your patient will:

• describe characteristics of his pain

• express feelings of comfort or reduced pain

• demonstrate adequate motor function, as evidenced by absence of paresthesia or neurologic deficits.

Based on the nursing diagnosis *anxiety,* develop appropriate patient outcomes. For example, your patient will:
• express characteristics of anxiety
• demonstrate that anxiety is reduced, either verbally or through behavior
• express willingness to use support systems to assist in coping with illness.

Based on the nursing diagnosis *knowledge deficit,* develop appropriate patient outcomes. For example, your patient will:
• express an understanding of surgical procedures, preoperative and postoperative care measures, and home care
• express the need for reducing risk factors for cardiovascular disease.

IMPLEMENTATION

Treatment for the patient with thoracic aortic aneurysm depends on whether he is acutely ill. (See *Medical care of the patient with thoracic aortic aneurysm.*)

Acute care
If the patient is acutely ill, perform these interventions:
• Monitor the patient's vital signs upon admission to the intensive care unit. Check his blood pressure, PAWP, PAP, and CVP. Assess his LOC, pain, breathing, urine output, and heart rate and rhythm. Also assess his carotid, radial, and femoral pulses. Monitor for neurologic disturbances.
• Administer analgesics, as prescribed, and watch for adverse reactions.
• Ensure that laboratory tests are performed, including complete blood count with differential, electrolyte measurements, typing and crossmatching for whole blood, arterial blood gas analysis, and urinalysis.
• Insert an indwelling urinary catheter and monitor hourly output.
• Administer dextrose 5% in water or lactated Ringer's solution and antibiotics, as prescribed.

• Carefully infuse nitroprusside using a separate I.V. line to reduce systolic blood pressure. Nitroglycerin may be added to protect the myocardium. Adjust the dosage by gradually increasing the infusion rate.
• Check blood pressure every 5 minutes until the desired systolic level is achieved. If bleeding from an aneurysm is suspected, give whole blood transfusions as prescribed.
• Administer I.V. propranolol or labetalol as prescribed.
• Monitor the patient's heart rhythm.
• Prepare the patient for emergency surgery, if necessary.

Preoperative care
Before surgery, expect to perform the following interventions:
• Weigh the patient.
• Insert an indwelling urinary catheter.
• Establish an I.V. line.
• Assist with insertion of the arterial line and pulmonary artery catheter to monitor hemodynamic balance.
• Insert a nasogastric tube for intestinal decompression. Irrigate the tube frequently to ensure patency.
• Administer prophylactic antibiotics as ordered.

Postoperative care
After emergency or elective surgery, perform the following interventions.
• Monitor the patient's LOC and compare to baseline.
• Monitor vital signs, PAP, CVP, PAWP, pulse rate and rhythm, urine output, and pain.
• Check respiratory function.
• Carefully observe and record type and amount of chest tube drainage, and frequently assess heart and breath sounds.
• Monitor pulse oximeter to assess arterial oxygen saturation.
• Monitor I.V. therapy and intake and output to assess renal function.

Treatments

Medical care of the patient with thoracic aortic aneurysm

The patient with thoracic aortic aneurysm may require emergency or elective surgery and long-term interventions.

Emergency care
With dissecting ascending aortic aneurysm, an emergency surgical resection of the aneurysm, using Dacron or Teflon graft replacement, can restore normal blood flow. Surgery is the treatment of choice for aneurysms measuring 2¾″ (7 cm) or more, or for smaller aneurysms if they produce symptoms. Surgery may be performed on an emergency basis for dissection or electively in a nonemergency situation.

Postoperative measures
Postoperative interventions may include careful monitoring in the intensive care unit and continuous assessment, antibiotic therapy, insertion of endotracheal and chest tubes, electrocardiogram monitoring and, frequently,

pulmonary artery catheterization and arterial monitoring.

Other emergency measures
Other treatments may include administering antihypertensives (such as nitroprusside), beta blockers (such as labetalol), oxygen (to treat respiratory distress), narcotic analgesics, I.V. fluids, or tranfusions of whole blood.

Long-term measures
For undissected thoracic aortic aneurysm, treatment may include administering beta-adrenergic blockers and other drugs to control hypertension and cardiac output. For aortic dissection after surgery, long-term medical treatment consists of maintaining systolic blood pressure below established parameters (usually 130 mm Hg).

• Administer analgesics, as prescribed, especially before the patient performs breathing exercises or is moved. If the patient is eligible to use a patient-controlled analgesia (PCA) system, set up a PCA system, as ordered, and demonstrate how it works. Alternatively, assist with inserting an epidural catheter for administering analgesics, as prescribed.
• After the patient's vital signs stabilize, encourage and assist him to turn, cough, and breathe deeply using incentive spirometry. Help the patient walk as soon as he is able.
• Watch for signs of infection, including fever and drainage.
• Monitor for signs of dissecting aneurysm, which may indicate a tear at the graft site.

• Assist with range-of-motion exercises for the legs to prevent thromboemboli from venostasis during prolonged bed rest. Also, provide antiembolism stockings to prevent deep vein thrombophlebitis.

Patient teaching
If the patient isn't acutely ill, focus on providing teaching and on alleviating his anxiety.
• Allow the patient to express fears and concerns about the diagnosis, diagnostic tests and procedures, and any impending surgery. Provide reassurance as needed.
• Offer the patient and family psychological support. Answer all their questions directly and honestly.

Discharge TimeSaver
Ensuring continued care for the patient with thoracic aortic aneurysm

Review the following topics and referrals to ensure that your patient is adequately prepared for discharge.

Teaching topics
Make sure that the following topics have been covered and that your patient's learning has been evaluated:
☐ explanation of the disorder, its risk factors, and its complications
☐ importance of eliminating cardiovascular risk factors or minimizing their effects
☐ activity guidelines
☐ prescribed medications
☐ procedure for measuring blood pressure
☐ warning signs to report to the doctor, including signs of rupture or hypertension
☐ sources of additional information and support
☐ home care measures, including the importance of obtaining follow-up care.

Referrals
Make sure your patient has been given appropriate referrals to :
☐ social services
☐ home health care agency
☐ smoking cessation program, if appropriate
☐ cardiac rehabilitation center
☐ dietitian.

Follow-up appointments
Make sure that the necessary follow-up appointments are scheduled and that the patient is notified:
☐ doctor or cardiologist
☐ follow-up diagnostic tests, if necessary, including chest X-ray, magnetic resonance imaging, and echocardiogram
☐ surgeon, if necessary.

• Direct the patient to call the doctor immediately to report any sharp pain in the chest or back of the neck.

• Explain the purposes and procedures for all diagnostic tests.

• If the patient is to be discharged without surgery, explain the importance of follow-up care. Emphasize the importance of adhering to specified activity guidelines.

• Suggest ways the patient can incorporate life-style changes to reduce cardiovascular disease risk factors.

• Instruct the patient to follow prescribed guidelines for antihypertensive drugs and describe any expected adverse effects.

• Teach the patient and family how to monitor blood pressure.

• If indicated, instruct the patient to avoid over-the-counter products containing aspirin or foods containing caffeine. Explain how aspirin hinders blood clot formation, which increases bleeding if the aneurysm ruptures. Mention that caffeine is a stimulant that can raise blood pressure.

• Encourage the patient and family to contact agencies that provide further support and assistance. (See *Ensuring continued care for the patient with thoracic aortic aneurysm.*)

• If elective surgery is scheduled, describe the procedure and any necessary preoperative care and testing. Describe equipment that will be used, such as I.V. and arterial lines, endotracheal and drainage tubes, cardiac monitoring and ventilation equipment, dressings, and indwelling urinary catheters.

EVALUATION

To evaluate the patient's response to your nursing care, gather reassessment data and compare this information with the patient outcomes specified in your plan of care.

Teaching and counseling

Begin by evaluating the effectiveness of patient teaching and counseling. Document statements made by the patient indicating:
• reduced anxiety
• willingness to use support systems to help with coping
• understanding of surgery and preoperative, postoperative, and home care
• intention to implement measures to reduce cardiovascular risk factors.

Also, talk to the patient and family members. Consider the following questions:
• Do they understand the need for follow-up care and prescribed activity and dietary guidelines?
• Can they correctly measure blood pressure?
• Are they familiar with all guidelines for administering prescribed medications?
• Do they know the signs and symptoms that should be reported to the doctor immediately?

Physical condition

Conclude your evaluation by reassessing the patient's physical condition. Consider the following questions:
• Does the patient's LOC remain at baseline?
• Is his skin warm and dry?
• Are his peripheral pulses palpable, strong, and equal?
• In answer to your questions, does the patient report feeling more comfortable or experiencing less pain?

Determine if the following target levels are being maintained:

• urine output greater than 30 ml/hour or 0.5 ml/kg/hour, depending on the patient's body size and physical condition
• systolic blood pressure within established limits (usually between 90 and 140 mm Hg)
• MAP within established limits (usually between 80 and 100 mm Hg)
• CVP, PAP, and PAWP within established limits
• heart rate less than 100 beats/minute with a regular rhythm
• respiratory rate within 5 breaths of baseline with adequate rhythm and depth.

Abdominal aortic aneurysm

Abdominal aortic aneurysm refers to an abnormal dilation in an arterial wall, which generally occurs in the aorta between the renal arteries and the aortic bifurcation. This type of aneurysm develops slowly and may be spindle-shaped (fusiform) or pouchlike (saccular).

An aneurysm occurs when degenerative changes in the aorta cause focal weakness in the vessel's muscular layer (tunica media). This allows the inner layer (tunica intima) and the outer layer (tunica adventitia) of the aorta to stretch outward. Blood pressure in the aorta progressively weakens the vessel wall and enlarges the aneurysm.

The patient with an abdominal aortic aneurysm risks experiencing a rupture, which results in extravasation of blood from the affected vessel. The risk of rupture is directly related to aneurysm size. Rupture of an abdominal aortic aneurysm is a surgical emergency; hemorrhagic shock may ensue rapidly. It also may entail secondary problems, such as myocardial ischemia, pulmonary edema, and renal failure.

Mortality for abdominal aortic aneurysms, with or without rupture, is high. (See *Key points about abdominal aortic aneurysm*.)

Causes

About 95% of abdominal aortic aneurysms result from arteriosclerosis or atherosclerosis. Other causes include cystic medial necrosis, trauma, syphilis, and other infections.

ASSESSMENT

Most patients with abdominal aortic aneurysms are asymptomatic until the aneurysm enlarges enough to put pressure on lumbar nerves, the inferior vena cava, or the duodenum. In many cases, the aneurysm is discovered during a routine physical examination or through X-rays taken for another purpose. In nonemergencies, take an extensive patient health history focusing on associated cardiovascular disease and risk factors.

Health history

The patient with an advanced aneurysm may report dull, generalized, steady abdominal pain or low back pain that is unaffected by movement. He also may report a sensation of gastric or abdominal fullness, caused by pressure on GI structures.

The patient may report sudden onset of severe abdominal pain or lumbar pain radiating to the flank and groin, indicating that the aneurysm has ruptured into the peritoneal cavity. If the aneurysm ruptures into the duodenum, the patient experiences GI bleeding with massive hematemesis and melena. Symptoms associated with hemorrhagic shock appear quickly. These include hypotension, diaphoresis, dysuria, arrhythmias, syncope, weakness, nausea, vomiting, and decreased level of consciousness (LOC).

Physical examination

Inspection of a patient with an intact abdominal aortic aneurysm usually does not provide significant findings. However, if the patient has low body fat, you may detect a pulsating mass in the periumbilical area.

During auscultation of the abdomen, you may detect a systolic bruit over the aorta. The sound you hear is caused by turbulent blood flow in the widened arterial segment. You also may detect bruits by auscultating over femoral arteries.

During palpation of the abdomen you may detect a pulsatile mass. You also may notice some tenderness over the affected area. Severe tenderness suggests an imminent rupture. Aneurysms should *always* be palpated cautiously.

If the aneurysm has ruptured, you may see signs of hemorrhagic shock, such as skin mottling, decreased LOC, diaphoresis, and oliguria. Peripheral pulses may be diminished or absent. The abdomen may be distended and an ecchymosis or hematoma may be present in the abdominal, flank, or groin area.

If a ruptured aneurysm reduces blood flow to your patient's spinal arteries, paraplegia may occur.

Diagnostic test results
The following tests help to confirm a diagnosis of abdominal aortic aneurysm:
• Abdominal ultrasonography and echocardiography may reveal the size, shape, and location of the aneurysm.
• Anteroposterior and lateral X-rays of the abdomen can detect aortic calcification, which outlines 75% of masses that occur.
• Computed tomography may reveal the effect of the aneurysm on nearby organs, especially relative positions of renal arteries to the aneurysm.
• Aortography shows the extent of the aneurysm and conditions of proximal and distal vessels. However, aortography may cause an underestimate of the diameter of the aneurysm because it illustrates only the flow channel, not the surrounding clot.
• Digital subtraction angiography yields information similar to aortography.

NURSING DIAGNOSIS

Common nursing diagnoses for a patient with an abdominal aortic aneurysm include:
• Altered tissue perfusion (cerebral, cardiovascular, peripheral) related to rupture
• Pain related to pressure on surrounding structures or rupture

• Fluid volume deficit related to altered renal function due to rupture, involvement of renal arteries, or shock
• Anxiety related to the diagnosis
• Knowledge deficit related to abdominal aneurysm and cardiovascular risk factors.

PLANNING

Based on the nursing diagnosis *altered tissue perfusion,* develop appropriate patient outcomes. For example, your patient will:
• demonstrate baseline LOC
• exhibit warm, dry skin
• maintain systolic blood pressure within established limits (usually between 90 and 140 mm Hg)
• maintain mean arterial pressure (MAP) within established limits (usually between 80 and 100 mm Hg)
• maintain central venous pressure (CVP), pulmonary artery pressure (PAP), and pulmonary artery wedge pressure (PAWP) at baseline levels
• maintain heart rate less than 100 beats/minute with a regular rhythm
• exhibit palpable, strong, and equal peripheral pulses
• maintain respiratory rhythm and depth at baseline, with respiratory rate within 5 breaths of baseline
• demonstrate adequate breath sounds.

Based on the nursing diagnosis *pain,* develop appropriate patient outcomes. For example, your patient will:
• describe characteristics of pain
• express feelings of comfort or reduced pain.

Based on the nursing diagnosis *fluid volume deficit,* develop appropriate patient outcomes. For example, your patient will:
• maintain urine output greater than 30 ml/hour or 0.5 ml/kg/hour, depending on body size and physical condition.

Based on the nursing diagnosis *anxiety,* develop appropriate patient outcomes. For example, your patient will:

• describe feelings of anxiety
• experience less anxiety, as evidenced by verbal reports and behavior
• express willingness to use support systems to assist with coping.

Based on the nursing diagnosis *knowledge deficit,* develop appropriate patient outcomes. For example, your patient will:

• express understanding of surgical procedures, preoperative and postoperative care measures, and home care measures
• express willingness to take steps to reduce cardiovascular disease risk factors.

IMPLEMENTATION

Treatment for the patient with abdominal aortic aneurysm depends on whether his condition is acute. (See *Medical care of the patient with abdominal aortic aneurysm.*)

Acute care

If the patient requires acute care, perform the following interventions.

• Monitor the patient's vital signs on admission to the intensive care unit (ICU).
• Insert an I.V. line with at least a 14G needle to facilitate blood replacement.
• Obtain ordered blood samples for renal tests such as blood urea nitrogen, creatinine, and electrolyte levels; complete blood count with differential; blood type and crossmatch; and arterial blood gas (ABG) levels.
• Monitor the patient's cardiac rhythm.
• Prepare for inserting an arterial line for continuous blood pressure monitoring.
• Assist with inserting a pulmonary artery line to monitor hemodynamic balance.
• Administer prescribed medications, such as analgesics, antihypertensives, and beta blockers.

• Monitor the patient closely for signs of rupture, such as acute blood loss (which may cause decreasing blood pressure), increasing pulse or respiratory rates, cool or clammy skin, restlessness, or decreased sensorium.
• If rupture occurs, infuse I.V. fluids as prescribed, and immediately transfer the patient to surgery.

Preoperative care

Before surgery, expect to perform the following interventions:
• Weigh the patient.
• Insert an indwelling urinary catheter.
• Establish an I.V. line.
• Assist with insertion of the arterial line and pulmonary artery catheter to monitor hemodynamic balance.
• Insert a nasogastric tube for intestinal decompression. Irrigate the tube frequently to ensure patency.
• Administer prophylactic antibiotics as ordered.

Postoperative care

During the resuscitative period following surgery, your patient may need large amounts of blood. Ischemia may lead to renal failure, requiring possible hemodialysis. The patient will also require mechanical ventilation after surgery.

• Monitor vital signs, intake and hourly output, and ABG levels. Monitor neurologic status by assessing LOC, pupil size, and sensation in the patient's arms and legs.
• Monitor pulse oximetry values and assess the depth, rate, and character of respirations and breath sounds at least every hour.
• Suction the endotracheal tube or instruct the patient to cough to maintain a clear airway.
• If the patient can breathe unassisted 24 hours after surgery and exhibits adequate ABG levels, pulse oximetry readings, tidal volume, vital capacity,

Treatments

Medical care of the patient with abdominal aortic aneurysm

An abdominal aortic aneurysm generally requires resection and replacement of the damaged aortic section with a Dacron graft.

Large aneurysm
Aneurysms 1½″ to 2½″ (4 to 6 cm) in diameter and those that cause symptoms may rupture and, therefore, require immediate repair.

Ruptured aneurysm
An expanding or ruptured abdominal aortic aneurysm requires emergency resection and insertion of a Dacron graft.

Dissecting aneurysm
Emergency preoperative measures include fluid resuscitation and blood transfusion, I.V. propranolol to reduce myocardial contractility, I.V. nitroprusside to reduce and maintain systolic blood pressure at 100 to 120 mm Hg, analgesics to relieve pain, and an arterial line and indwelling urinary catheter to help monitor the patient's condition.

Small aneurysm
If the patient is asymptomatic, regular physical examinations and ultrasound studies may be substituted for surgery.

---

and negative inspiratory force, extubate him and provide oxygen by mask.
• Weigh the patient daily to evaluate fluid status. Watch for evidence of pulmonary edema and volume overload. Replace fluids, if needed, to adequately hydrate the patient.
• Watch for retroperitoneal graft-site bleeding, as evidenced by increased pulse and respiratory rates and hypotension. Severe back pain may indicate a graft tear.
• Check abdominal dressings for excessive bleeding or drainage.
• Check for melena, hematemesis or abdominal pain, and signs of GI hemorrhage from rupture of graft into duodenum.
• Assess the wound site and monitor your patient for evidence of infection, such as temperature elevation or painful or tender groin mass. Use aseptic technique to change dressings.
• Turn the patient frequently and help him walk as soon as possible, usually the second day after surgery.

Patient teaching
If the patient doesn't require acute care, focus on teaching and alleviating his anxiety.
• Allow the patient to express anxiety and fears about his diagnosis and impending surgery. Offer a tour of the ICU to help diminish his anxiety. Offer psychological support to both the patient and family. Answer all questions honestly and provide reassurance as needed.
• Teach your patient and the family about abdominal aortic aneurysm, its causes, symptoms, and complications.
• Explain all diagnostic tests.
• If the patient will not undergo surgery, but instead will be monitored at home, explain the need for adherence to home health care. Instruct the patient to follow the doctor's activity guidelines. (See *Helping your patient live with an aneurysm*, page 264.)
• Emphasize that controlling blood pressure will decrease the risk of rupture. Teach both the patient and the family how to take blood pressure readings.

Helping your patient live with an aneurysm

If your patient with an aneurysm is discharged, give him guidelines to help him adjust to his diagnosis and need for ongoing care. These guidelines apply whether or not the patient is scheduled for surgery. Advise him to contact his doctor if problems or questions arise.

Adjusting lifestyle
Instruct your patient to:
• avoid exertion to keep his blood pressure at a safe and steady level
• maintain an even blood pressure by eating sensibly, restricting salt, following a low-fat diet, and losing weight.

Monitoring blood pressure
Advise your patient to:
• take regular blood pressure readings and record the results
• follow the doctor's guidelines with regard to acceptable blood pressure levels. Contact the doctor if blood pressure is above or below established levels.

Monitoring circulation
Tell the patient to examine his legs each day for:
• changes in color or temperature
• numbness or tingling.

Avoiding infection
Instruct your patient to:
• keep his skin clean, dry, and free of surface scratches

• check his feet daily for cuts, cracks, blisters, or red, swollen areas
• wash his feet in warm, soapy water and dry them thoroughly, especially between the toes, by blotting with a towel
• avoid tight-fitting shoes or clothing that may restrict circulation
• avoid wearing elastic garters, sitting with knees crossed, or walking barefoot.

Taking prescribed drugs
Be sure that your patient understands:
• how and when to take his drugs
• that he should consult with a nurse, doctor, or pharmacist when he has questions about prescription or nonprescription drugs and their possible adverse effects.

Recognizing danger symptoms
Tell the patient to immediately report:
• severe headaches
• severe chest or abdominal pain
• cool, clammy skin
• disorientation or unusual sleepiness
• extreme restlessness or anxiety.

• Review the administration of prescribed medications and advise the patient to carry a list of his medications in case of emergency.
• If indicated, caution the patient to avoid over-the-counter products that contain aspirin, which can hinder clot formation. Also instruct the patient to limit foods and beverages that contain caffeine because it can raise blood pressure.

• Advise the patient and the family to immediately call the doctor if the patient experiences severe abdominal or back pain, syncope, cool or clammy skin, disorientation or unusual sleepiness, sudden restlessness or anxiety, or bloody stools or vomitus.
• If the patient is undergoing abdominal surgery, describe the surgical procedure and expected postoperative measures. Explain the need for I.V. and arterial lines, endotracheal and naso-

Discharge TimeSaver
Ensuring continued care for the patient with an abdominal aortic aneurysm

Review the following topics and referrals to ensure that your patient is adequately prepared for discharge.

Teaching topics
Make sure that the following topics have been covered and that your patient's learning has been evaluated:
☐ explanation of the disorder, associated risk factors, and potential complications
☐ elimination of cardiovascular risk factors or ways to reduce their effects
☐ activity guidelines
☐ antihypertensive drugs, including precautions and possible adverse effects
☐ procedure for monitoring blood pressure
☐ warning signs that should be reported to the doctor
☐ sources of information and support.

Referrals
Make sure that the patient has received appropriate referrals to:
☐ social services
☐ home health care agency
☐ smoking cessation program
☐ dietary consultant
☐ cardiac rehabilitation specialist.

Follow-up appointments
Make sure that the necessary follow-up appointments are scheduled and that the patient is notified:
☐ doctor or cardiologist
☐ diagnostic tests for reevaluation
☐ surgeon.

---

gastric intubation, and mechanical ventilation.
• Instruct the patient in postoperative home care.
• Explain the risk factors for cardiovascular disease, emphasizing that surgical treatment for aneurysm does not arrest the underlying disease. Help your patient develop a plan for risk reduction. (See *Ensuring continued care for the patient with an abdominal aortic aneurysm.*)

EVALUATION

To evaluate the patient's response to your nursing care, gather reassessment data and compare this information with the patient outcomes specified in your plan of care.

Teaching and counseling
Begin by evaluating the effectiveness of patient teaching and counseling. Document statements made by the patient indicating:
• reduced anxiety
• willingness to use available support systems to assist with coping
• understanding of surgical procedures, preoperative and postoperative care measures, and home care steps
• willingness to implement measures to reduce cardiovascular disease risk factors.

Also, talk to the patient and family members to determine the effectiveness of your teaching. Consider the following questions:
• Are they aware of the need for follow-up care and prescribed activity and dietary guidelines?
• Do they understand how to measure blood pressure?

• Are they familiar with the guidelines for administering prescribed medications?
• Do they know all the signs and symptoms that should alert them to call the doctor immediately?

Physical condition
Continue your evaluation by reassessing the patient's physical condition. Consider the following questions:
• Is the patient's skin warm and dry?
• Are his peripheral pulses palpable, strong, and equal?
• Have his LOC and breath sounds returned to baseline?
• In answer to your questions, does he report feeling more comfortable or experiencing less pain?
   Determine if the following target levels are being maintained:
• urine output above 30 ml/hour or 0.5 ml/kg/hour, depending on the patient's body size and physical condition
• systolic blood pressure within established limits (usually between 90 and 140 mm Hg)
• MAP within established limits (usually between 80 and 100 mm Hg)
• CVP, PAP, and PAWP within established limits
• heart rate less than 100 beats/minute with a regular rhythm
• respiratory rate within 5 breaths of baseline with adequate rhythm and depth.

Femoral and popliteal aneurysms

These aneurysms result from abnormal dilation in the two major peripheral arteries. They occur most commonly in men over age 50.
   Patients with femoral and popliteal aneurysms are at risk for thrombosis, embolization, and gangrene. Complications, such as severe ischemia, may

require amputation. The prognosis improves if elective bypass and reconstructive surgery is performed before complications occur.
   Approximately three-fourths of all femoral and popliteal aneurysms are fusiform (spindle-shaped), and the rest are saccular (pouch-shaped). (See *Two types of aneurysms.*) These aneurysms may recur as single or multiple segmental lesions and may affect both legs. They may be accompanied by arterial aneurysms in the abdominal aorta or iliac arteries.

Causes
The most common cause of femoral and popliteal aneurysms is progressive atherosclerotic change in the medial layer of the arterial wall. Less common causes include blunt or penetrating trauma and bacterial infection. A "suture line" or "false" aneurysm may occur after peripheral vascular reconstructive surgery when a blood clot forms a second lumen. Rarely, femoral and popliteal aneurysms result from congenital weakness in the arterial wall.

ASSESSMENT

As part of your assessment, review the patient's medical history for a possible cause of femoral or popliteal aneurysm and for indications of other arterial aneurysms.

Health history
A patient with a femoral or popliteal aneurysm may be asymptomatic or report pain.
   If a *popliteal aneurysm* is large enough to compress the medial popliteal nerve, the patient may report pain in the popliteal space. If the artery is thrombosed, the patient may report feeling a nonpulsating mass.
   With a *femoral aneurysm,* the patient may report feeling a pulsating mass in

Two types of aneurysms

These illustrations show the difference between saccular and fusiform aneurysms. Femoral and popliteal aneurysms occur in one of these two shapes.

Saccular aneurysm
This type of aneurysm occurs as a pouchlike bulge with a narrow neck.

Fusiform aneurysm
This type of aneurysm occurs as a spindle-shaped bulge encompassing the entire diameter of the vessel.

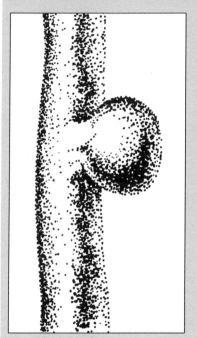

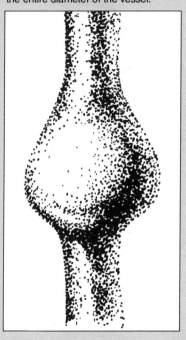

the upper thigh. Later on, thrombosis or embolism may produce symptoms of ischemia.

Physical examination
If the aneurysm compresses a vein, you may note edema and vein distention. In a patient with acute thrombosis, you also may observe distal petechial hemorrhages caused by aneurysmal emboli.

If you suspect a femoral or popliteal aneurysm, perform bilateral palpation to compare the affected leg to the unaffected one. Suspect a popliteal aneurysm when the popliteal pulse is widened and very easily felt. In a patient with a femoral aneurysm, you may detect a pulsating mass above or below the inguinal ligament. In a patient with a popliteal aneurysm, you may feel a pulsating mass behind the knee.

In a patient with acute thrombosis, you may note an absent pulse and a pulsating or nonpulsating mass. The affected leg may be cold and inspection may reveal loss of color or, later on, a gangrenous appearance.

Diagnostic test results
The following tests aid diagnosis of femoral or popliteal aneurysm:
• Arteriography helps confirm the diagnosis and may detect associated aneurysms, especially in the abdominal aorta and iliac arteries.
• Ultrasonography determines the size of femoral and popliteal arteries and shows the aneurysmal dilation.
• A computed tomography scan confirms the size and location of the aneurysm.

NURSING DIAGNOSIS

Common nursing diagnoses for a patient with femoral and popliteal artery aneurysms include:
• Altered peripheral tissue perfusion related to acute thrombosis
• Pain related to ischemia or pressure on nerves
• Anxiety related to the medical diagnosis, diagnostic procedures, or impending surgery
• Knowledge deficit related to aneurysm and its treatment.

PLANNING

Goals of nursing care include relieving the patient's symptoms and teaching him about the disorder and its treatment.

Based on the nursing diagnosis *altered peripheral tissue perfusion,* develop appropriate patient outcomes. For example, your patient will:
• maintain baseline skin color and temperature
• exhibit palpable peripheral pulses.

Based on the nursing diagnosis *pain,* develop appropriate patient outcomes. For example, your patient will:
• describe characteristics of pain
• experience a reduction in pain, as evidenced by verbal reports or behavior.

Based on the nursing diagnosis *anxiety,* develop appropriate patient outcomes. For example, your patient will:
• describe feelings of anxiety
• implement at least two coping mechanisms to alleviate anxiety
• experience reduced anxiety, as evidenced by verbal reports or behavior.

Based on the nursing diagnosis *knowledge deficit,* develop appropriate patient outcomes. For example, your patient will:
• request information concerning surgery or diagnostic procedures
• express his understanding of the need to reduce health risks, for example, by quitting smoking and taking steps to lower cholesterol levels
• describe signs that should immediately be reported to the doctor
• state his understanding of the importance of home care measures.

IMPLEMENTATION

Treatment includes procedures that will be implemented before and after arterial surgery.

Preoperative care
• Assess and record the patient's circulatory status, noting the location and quality of peripheral pulses in the affected leg.
• Administer prophylactic antibiotics, anticoagulants, and analgesics, as prescribed.
• Provide clear and concise information about impending surgery.
• Allow the patient to express fears and anxieties about the disorder and about surgery. Encourage discussion about the impact the disorder will have on his life. Reassure him as needed.

• Ask the patient to describe activities that increase comfort. Encourage him to perform these activities so that he feels a sense of control.

• Encourage family members and friends to provide emotional support to the patient.

Postoperative care

• Carefully monitor your patient for early signs of thrombosis or graft occlusion, including severe pain, loss of pulse, or decreased skin temperature, sensation, and motor function.

• Monitor for signs of infection, such as fever.

• Palpate distal pulses hourly for the first 24 hours and as ordered thereafter. Correlate your findings with those from the preoperative assessment. Mark the pulse sites on the patient's skin for future reference.

• Encourage walking to prevent venous stasis and thrombus formation.

• Administer a plasma volume expander such as dextran, as prescribed, to decrease platelet adhesion and to prevent early graft closure.

• Observe your patient's behavior for nonverbal signs of pain. Administer analgesics, as prescribed, to alleviate pain.

Patient teaching

Before surgery, teach the patient about surgical bypass and reconstruction of the artery. Review expected postoperative procedures and answer your patient's questions directly and honestly.

Postoperative teaching

• Instruct your patient to report any indications of failure of the saphenous vein or prosthetic graft replacement, such as faint or absent pulse, a pale or blue color in the leg or foot, or coldness to the touch in the leg or foot.

• If the patient has atherosclerosis, explain the risk for further arterial occlusions. Tell the patient to report the return of any preoperative symptoms, such as decreased motor function, evidence of leg ulcer or injury, pain in the extremity, or evidence of decreased blood flow to the affected area.

• Instruct the patient in proper incision care. Tell him to monitor the incision and report any drainage, or redness, swelling, or tenderness near the incision.

• Explain that persistent swelling may occur after popliteal artery resection. If antiembolism stockings are ordered, make sure they fit properly and demonstrate how to put them on. Emphasize the need to avoid constrictive clothing.

• If the patient is taking anticoagulants, emphasize the need to prevent bleeding. For example, instruct the patient to use an electric razor for shaving. Explain the importance of follow-up blood studies to monitor anticoagulant therapy. Caution against the use of tobacco and aspirin and urge him to report evidence of bleeding, including bleeding gums, tarry stools, or bruising.

• Discuss the activity level recommended by the doctor. The patient may be allowed to go on daily walks.

• Describe the benefits of using a medical identification bracelet.

• Discuss the benefits of participating in a rehabilitation program to promote reconditioning. (See *Ensuring continued care for the patient with a femoral or popliteal aneurysm,* page 270.)

EVALUATION

To evaluate your patient's response to your nursing care, gather reassessment data and compare this information with the patient outcomes specified in your plan of care.

Teaching and counseling

Begin by evaluating the effectiveness of patient teaching and counseling.

Discharge TimeSaver
Ensuring continued care for the patient with a femoral or popliteal aneurysm

Review the following topics and referrals to ensure that your patient is adequately prepared for discharge.

Teaching topics
Make sure that the following topics have been covered and that your patient's learning has been evaluated:
☐ explanation of the disorder, associated risk factors, and potential complications
☐ life-style modifications to reduce cardiovascular risk factors
☐ exercise program
☐ daily leg and foot care
☐ incision care
☐ signs that should be reported to the doctor
☐ use of antiembolism stockings
☐ prescribed medications, including precautions and potential adverse effects.

Referrals
Make sure that the patient has been provided with appropriate referrals to:
☐ cardiac rehabilitation specialist
☐ social services
☐ home health care agency
☐ smoking cessation program.

Follow-up appointments
Make sure that the necessary follow-up appointments are scheduled and that the patient is notified:
☐ doctor or cardiologist
☐ surgeon
☐ diagnostic testing for reevaluation.

Document statements made by the patient indicating:
• an intention to reduce health risks such as smoking and elevated cholesterol level
• an understanding of signs and symptoms that should be reported to the doctor.

Coping with anxiety
Reevaluate your patient's anxiety level. Consider the following questions:
• Has he demonstrated a willingness to use support systems to enhance coping?
• Has he demonstrated by statements or behavior that he is experiencing less anxiety?

Physical condition
Continue your evaluation by reassessing the patient's physical condition. Consider the following questions:

• Have the color and temperature of the skin on the affected leg returned to baseline range?
• Are the peripheral pulses palpable?
• Has the patient experienced a reduction in pain?

Arterial occlusive disease

In this disorder, the lumen of the aorta and its major branches become obstructed or narrowed, thereby interrupting blood flow. In most cases, restricted blood flow affects the legs and feet. Complications include severe ischemia, skin ulceration, and gangrene.

The prognosis for patients with arterial occlusive disease depends on the location of the occlusion, the development of collateral circulation to counteract reduced blood flow and, in acute cases, the time lapse between development of an occlusion and its removal. (See *Risk factors for arterial occlusive disease.*)

Causes

The most common cause of arterial occlusive disease is atherosclerosis. Occlusion to a major artery may be caused by an embolus, a thrombus, or plaque. Exogenous causes include insertion of an indwelling arterial catheter, use of I.V. drugs, injection of foreign material into a peripheral artery, or direct blunt or penetrating trauma to an artery.

ASSESSMENT

Arterial occlusive disease may be acute or chronic and may affect the carotid, vertebral, innominate, subclavian, mesenteric, and celiac arteries. Assessment findings depend on the vessel involved. (See *Signs and symptoms of arterial occlusive disease,* page 272.)

Obtain a detailed medical, family, social, and drug history to detect risk factors and coexisting diseases. If acute arterial occlusion occurs suddenly, you may not have time to take a detailed health history.

Health history

The patient with peripheral arterial occlusion may report intermittent claudication — pain from exercise, such as walking uphill or climbing stairs, that subsides with rest. The patient may describe his pain in various ways: aches, cramps, fatigue, numbness, or a combination of these symptoms.

To help determine the severity of the condition, ask your patient how much exercise he can tolerate before feeling pain. As ischemia increases, the patient may report constant, aching pain that occurs even without exertion, often

FactFinder

Risk factors for arterial occlusive disease

- Smoking
- Aging
- Hypertension, hyperlipidemia, diabetes mellitus, and other chronic conditions that increase cardiovascular risk
- Family history of vascular disorders, myocardial infarction, or cerebrovascular accident

worsening at night. Pain may be associated with numbness.

Additional indications of possible arterial occlusive disease include cold feet and legs, edema, and trophic changes.

Timesaving tip: To relieve limb pain caused by arterial occlusion, place the foot in a dependent position; limb elevation aggravates the pain. To ease pain caused by venous occlusion, elevate the limb.

Physical examination

In moderate to severe arterial occlusive disease, examination of the patient may reveal postural color changes in involved extremities. To test for presence of the condition, ask the patient to elevate his feet for 1 minute. With elevation, the feet turn pale. When returned to a dependent position, the feet develop a dusky rubor.

During inspection, you may detect edema and trophic changes such as hair loss on the affected limb; thick toenails; dry, shiny, or atrophic skin; or possible ischemic ulcers on toes and heels. You also may see deep purple pregangrenous lesions or gangrenous lesions that are black, shriveled, and hard.

During palpation, you may feel coolness in the involved limb. You also may note diminished or absent pulses

Signs and symptoms of arterial occlusive disease

Site of occlusion	Signs and symptoms
Internal and external carotid arteries	Unilateral sensory or motor dysfunction (such as transient monocular blindness or hemiparesis), aphasia or dysarthria, confusion, decreased mentation, and headache. Signs and symptoms result from transient ischemic attacks (TIAs), which occur secondary to reduced cerebral circulation; episodes may precede a cerebrovascular accident. Other signs include absent or decreased pulsation with an auscultatory bruit over the affected vessels.
Vertebral and basilar arteries	Binocular visual disturbances, vertigo, dysarthria, drop attacks (falling down without loss of consciousness), homonymous hemianopia (loss of vision in both homonymous fields), and sensory deficit in any combination of the extremities. Signs and symptoms result from TIAs of the brain stem and cerebellum.
Innominate (brachiocephalic) artery	Binocular visual disturbances, vertigo, dysarthria, drop attacks, sensory deficit in any combination of the extremities, and homonymous hemianopia. Signs and symptoms result from TIAs of the brain stem and cerebellum. Other signs and symptoms include claudication of the right arm and possible bruit over the right side of the neck.
Subclavian artery	Subclavian steal syndrome (a backflow of blood from the brain through the vertebral artery on the same side as the occlusion and into the subclavian artery distal to the occlusion), binocular visual disturbances, vertigo, dysarthria, drop attacks, sensory deficit in any combination of the extremities, homonymous hemianopia, exercise-induced arm claudication, and gangrene (usually limited to the digits).
Mesenteric artery	Bowel ischemia; infarct necrosis and gangrene; sudden, acute abdominal pain; nausea and vomiting; diarrhea; leukocytosis; and shock due to massive intraluminal fluid and plasma loss.
Aortic bifurcation (saddle block occlusion)	Sensory and motor deficits (muscle weakness, numbness, paresthesia, paralysis) and signs of ischemia in both legs (sudden pain or cold, pale legs with decreased or absent peripheral pulses).
Iliac artery (Leriche's syndrome)	Intermittent claudication of the lower back, buttocks, and thighs, which is relieved by rest; absent or reduced femoral or distal pulses; shiny and scaly skin, subcutaneous tissue loss, and absent body hair on affected limb; nail deformities; increased capillary refill time; blanching of the feet on elevation; possible bruit over femoral arteries; and impotence (in males).
Femoral and popliteal arteries	Intermittent claudication of the calves on exertion; ischemic pain in the feet; pretrophic pain, followed by necrosis and ulceration; leg pallor and coolness, shiny and scaly skin, subcutaneous tissue loss, and absent body hair on the affected limb; nail deformities; increased capillary refill time; blanching of the feet on elevation; gangrene; and absence of palpable pulses distal to the occlusion. Auscultation over the affected area may reveal a bruit.

Assessment TimeSaver

Recognizing acute peripheral arterial occlusions

To quickly recognize signs and symptoms of acute peripheral arterial occlusions, remember the six P's:

1. Pain, the most common symptom, occurs suddenly and locally in the affected arm or leg.
2. Pallor is caused by vasoconstriction distal to the occlusion.
3. Pulse distal to the occlusion is absent.
4. Paralysis in the affected arm or leg

is caused by disturbed nerve endings or disturbed skeletal muscles.
5. Paresthesia may also result from disturbed nerve endings or disturbed skeletal muscles.
6. Poikilothermy, or cool skin, is caused by temperature changes distal to the occlusion.

distal to the occluded artery. Use a Doppler probe for pulses that are difficult to detect.

Pulses can be graded from 0 to + 4:

  0 = absent
  + 1 = weak
  + 2 or + 3 = normal
  + 4 = bounding.

Timesaving tip: Absence of a posterior tibial pulse is the most reliable sign of arterial occlusive disease of the lower extremities.

Check capillary refill time while checking pulses. Refill time of more than 3 seconds may indicate diminished peripheral perfusion.

During auscultation, you may hear bruits over an occluded artery.

During neurologic assessment, you may detect sensory or motor impairments that may create safety risks for the patient. (See *Recognizing acute peripheral arterial occlusions.*)

Diagnostic test results

The following tests help to establish a diagnosis of arterial occlusive disease and to evaluate complications:

• Arteriography discloses type, location, and degree of the obstruction, and status of the patient's collateral circulation. It is most effective for diagnos-

ing chronic disease or for evaluating candidates for reconstructive surgery.

• Digital subtraction angiography helps identify peripheral vascular disease.

• Ultrasonography and plethysmography may show decreased blood flow distal to the occlusion.

• Segmental limb pressures and pulse volume measurements help evaluate the location and extent of the occlusion.

• Ophthalmodynamometry helps determine the degree of obstruction in the internal carotid artery by comparing ophthalmic artery pressure with brachial artery pressure on the affected side. More than a 20% difference between pressures suggests arterial insufficiency.

• Electroencephalography and a computed tomography scan help rule out brain lesions.

NURSING DIAGNOSIS

Common nursing diagnoses for a patient with arterial occlusive disease include:

• Activity intolerance related to pain and ischemia in the lower extremities

• Altered tissue perfusion (peripheral or cerebral) related to reduced blood flow
• High risk for impaired skin integrity related to impaired cellular nutrition
• Pain related to peripheral ischemia in the lower extremities
• High risk for peripheral neurovascular dysfunction related to impaired circulation.

PLANNING

Based on the nursing diagnosis *activity intolerance*, develop appropriate patient outcomes. For example, your patient will:
• maintain muscle strength and joint range of motion
• perform self-care activities to tolerance level
• request assistance with activities, as needed, to prevent tissue injury or trauma.

Based on the nursing diagnosis *altered tissue perfusion,* develop appropriate patient outcomes. For example, your patient will:
• maintain adequate tissue perfusion as evidenced by palpable peripheral pulses
• maintain baseline skin temperature and color in extremities
• maintain capillary refill time of less than 3 seconds
• maintain baseline level of consciousness (LOC)
• express understanding of the rationale for daily assessment of the extremity.

Based on the nursing diagnosis *high risk for impaired skin integrity,* develop appropriate patient outcomes. For example, your patient will:
• agree to perform preventive skin care measures
• maintain intact skin.

Based on the nursing diagnosis *pain,* develop appropriate patient outcomes. For example, your patient will:

• identify factors that cause pain
• express understanding of techniques to reduce pain, including analgesic drug therapy
• experience decreased pain.

Based on the nursing diagnosis *high risk for peripheral neurovascular dysfunction,* develop appropriate patient outcomes. For example, your patient will:
• demonstrate improved circulation in extremities
• agree to adhere to prescribed medication regimen and other measures to improve circulation
• list signs and symptoms of peripheral neurovascular dysfunction that need to be reported to the doctor
• remain free of paralysis or paresthesia.

IMPLEMENTATION

Treatment for the patient with arterial occlusive disease aims to relieve the patient's symptoms and improve circulation to the affected extremity. (See *Medical care of the patient with arterial occlusive disease.*)

Ongoing care
• To increase blood flow to the patient's legs, elevate the head of the bed 30 degrees.
• To prevent trauma to the affected extremity, use a minimal-pressure mattress and heel protectors or a foot cradle to reduce pressure. Keep the arm or leg warm, but do not use a heating pad. Remove socks frequently to examine the patient's skin.
• Avoid using constrictive clothing, such as antiembolism stockings.
• Inspect legs and feet daily for redness, injury, irritation, or other signs of impaired skin integrity.
• Wash the patient's legs and feet daily using warm water and mild soap. Dry well between the toes. Apply mild lotion to dry areas, except between the

Treatments

Medical care of the patient with arterial occlusive disease

In mild, chronic occlusive disease, treatment usually consists of supportive measures, including encouraging the patient to quit smoking, to control hypertension, to reduce dietary cholesterol and saturated fats, to exercise mildly (walking, for instance), and to provide foot and leg care. In more severe cases, drug therapy, surgery, or both may be necessary.

Drug therapy
In carotid artery occlusion, the doctor may prescribe antiplatelet therapy, beginning with dipyridamole and aspirin. For patients with intermittent claudication caused by chronic arterial occlusive disease, pentoxifylline may be prescribed to improve blood flow through the capillaries. This drug is particularly useful for poor surgical candidates. Other prescribed drugs may include heparin to prevent emboli or dextran to reduce platelet adhesion and clot formation.

Thrombolytics, such as urokinase, streptokinase, and alteplase, can dissolve clots and relieve the obstruction caused by a thrombus.

Surgery
Acute arterial occlusive disease usually requires surgery. Types of surgeries for the disease include:
• *Embolectomy.* A balloon-tipped, indwelling urinary catheter is used to remove thrombotic material from the artery. Embolectomy is used mainly for mesenteric, femoral, or popliteal artery occlusion.
• *Thromboendarterectomy.* This procedure involves opening the artery and removing the obstructing thrombus and the medial layer of the arterial wall. Plaque deposits will remain intact. Thromboendarterectomy is usually per-

formed after angiography and is often used in conjunction with autogenous vein or Dacron bypass surgery (femoropopliteal or aortofemoral).
• *Percutaneous transluminal coronary angioplasty (PTCA).* Using fluoroscopy and a special balloon catheter, PTCA dilates the stenotic or occluded artery to a predetermined diameter without overdistending it.
• *Laser surgery.* An excimer or a hot-tipped laser vaporizes the clot and plaque.
• *Patch grafting.* This procedure involves removing the thrombosed arterial segment and replacing it with an autogenous vein or Dacron graft.
• *Bypass graft.* Blood flow is diverted through an anastomosed autogenous or woven Dacron graft to bypass the thrombosed arterial segment.
• *Lumbar sympathectomy.* Depending on the condition of the sympathetic nervous system, this procedure may be an adjunct to reconstructive surgery.
• *Amputation.* If arterial reconstructive surgery fails or if gangrene, uncontrollable infection, or intractable pain develops, amputation may be necessary.
• *Bowel resection.* This procedure may be performed in patients with mesenteric artery occlusion after blood flow has been restored.

toes (to avoid risk of infection and breakdown). Dust the feet with cornstarch if sweating is a problem.
• Administer analgesics as prescribed.
• Take appropriate measures to control diabetes mellitus, when applicable.
• Encourage the patient to express his fears and concerns, and help the patient identify and use effective coping strategies.
• If the patient works in a cold environment or must stand for prolonged periods, provide referrals for occupational counseling for retraining. Also discuss the benefits of participating in a rehabilitation program to promote reconditioning.

Preoperative care
• Assess the patient's circulatory status by checking distal pulses, skin color, and skin temperature.
• Administer analgesics as prescribed.
• Administer heparin or thrombolytics by continuous I.V. drip, as prescribed. Ensure the proper flow rate by using an infusion monitor or pump.
• Wrap the affected foot in soft cotton batting, and reposition it frequently to prevent pressure on a single area. Avoid elevating or applying heat to the affected leg.
• Watch for signs of fluid and electrolyte imbalance, and monitor intake and output for signs of renal failure. Urine output of less than 30 ml/hour or less than 0.5 ml/kg/hour (depending on the patient's body size and physical condition) suggests renal failure.
• If the patient has carotid, innominate, vertebral, or subclavian artery occlusion, monitor for signs of cerebrovascular accident, such as intermittent blindness, limb numbness, or reduced LOC.

Postoperative care
• Monitor vital signs and circulatory function. Assess skin color and temperature, and observe distal pulses.

Compare your findings with the information from the preoperative assessment. Following removal of a thrombus, it usually takes 2 to 6 hours for the extremity to be revascularized.
• Watch closely for signs of hemorrhage, such as tachycardia or hypotension. Check dressings for excessive bleeding.
• In *carotid, innominate, vertebral, or subclavian artery occlusion,* assess neurologic status by checking for changes in LOC, pupil size, and muscle strength.
• In *mesenteric artery occlusion,* connect a nasogastric tube to low intermittent suction. Monitor intake and output. Low urine output may indicate damage to renal arteries during surgery. Check bowel sounds for resumed peristalsis. Increasing abdominal distention and tenderness may indicate extension of bowel ischemia, which may lead to gangrene or peritonitis.
• In *saddle block occlusion* (an occlusion at the aortic bifurcation), check distal pulses for adequate circulation. Watch for signs of renal failure and mesenteric artery occlusion, such as severe abdominal pain and ischemia-induced diarrhea. Because this type of occlusion is associated with cardiac embolization, watch for cardiac arrhythmias, which may precipitate embolus formation.
• In *iliac artery occlusion,* monitor urine output for signs of renal failure due to decreased perfusion to the kidneys after surgery. Provide meticulous catheter care.
• In *femoral and popliteal artery occlusion,* make sure the patient does not sit for extended periods. Help the patient with ambulation following surgery.
• After percutaneous transluminal coronary angioplasty, keep the patient's catheter open by using a heparin infusion. Monitor the insertion site for bleeding. Keep the catheterized leg immobile, and keep the patient on

strict bed rest. Monitor and record pulses in the catheterized leg. Provide analgesics for back pain.

• After limb amputation, check the stump site for drainage. Record the color, amount, and time of drainage. Elevate the stump, as ordered, and provide analgesics. Explain phantom limb pain to your patient.

Patient teaching

• Explain the major causes of reduced arterial blood flow, intermittent claudication, and arterial ulcers.

• Emphasize the importance of daily foot and leg care. Instruct the patient to wash his feet daily and inspect for signs of injury or infection. Advise him to wear sturdy shoes that fit properly. Provide referrals to a podiatrist for foot problems. (See *Foot care guidelines,* page 278.)

• Encourage the patient with mild to moderate arterial occlusive disease without open lesions to participate in a progressive daily exercise program. Explain that regular exercise helps prevent further arterial occlusion and promotes the development of collateral circulation, which reduces intermittent claudication and formation of arterial ulcers. If his physical condition allows it, encourage the patient to walk, swim or bicycle daily until claudication forces him to stop. Advise him to rest, then resume exercising when the pain subsides. Explain that a progressive program will help him gradually increase his exercise tolerance.

• Discuss activity restrictions for the patient with severe arterial occlusive disease or open lesions. If the patient is ambulatory, instruct him to walk for about 10 minutes each hour and to rest for the remainder of the time.

• Discuss prescribed medications. Explain that anticoagulants reduce the blood's ability to clot. Emphasize the need for precautions, such as using an electric razor and avoiding falls and contact with sharp objects, while taking an anticoagulant. Explain that antiplatelet agents, such as aspirin or dipyridamole, reduce clot formation by interfering with platelet formation, and that vasodilators decrease symptoms by dilating the arteries. If the doctor prescribes pentoxifylline, explain that this drug decreases the thickness of blood, which improves flow through the blood vessels.

• Instruct the patient to avoid wearing constrictive clothing (including garters) or crossing his legs. Warn the patient to avoid bumps, jolts, or injuries to affected limbs.

• Teach the patient about the risks associated with using tobacco products, and provide referrals to a smoking cessation program if needed.

• Tell the patient to avoid temperature extremes, dress warmly, and always keep his feet warm.

• Discuss the details of a diet that provides adequate protein, vitamin B_{12}, and vitamin C to help maintain skin integrity and reduce the chance of infection and ulceration. Point out good sources of these nutrients. Warn the patient that meat, dairy products, and eggs are rich in protein, but contain high levels of cholesterol or saturated fats, or both. Inform him about alternative protein sources, such as legumes, nuts, seeds, and grains.

• When appropriate, explain preoperative, postoperative, and home care measures. Following surgery, tell the patient to watch for signs of occlusion of the graft site (or elsewhere), such as pain, pallor, numbness, paralysis, or absence of pulse. (See *Ensuring continued care for the patient with arterial occlusive disease*, page 279.)

EVALUATION

To evaluate the patient's response to your nursing care, gather reassessment data and compare this information

Foot care guidelines

Review the following guidelines with the patient to help safeguard feet from injury or infection.

Daily care
• Instruct the patient to wash his feet daily with mild soap and warm water. To prevent burns, he should use warm — not hot — water. Advise him to dry his feet carefully, especially between the toes.
• Tell him to apply lanolin ointment to dry skin and apply a mild foot powder to feet that sweat. He should dry his feet well before applying powder to avoid caking.
• Instruct him to inspect his feet each day, especially around the nails, between the toes, and the soles. Tell him to look for corns, calluses, redness, swelling, bruises, and breaks in the skin.
• Advise him to treat corns or calluses by soaking the feet, gently patting them dry with a towel, and applying lanolin ointment. Treatment should continue once or twice a day until the condition improves. If the corns or calluses don't improve, refer the patient to a podiatrist.
• Warn him to avoid using over-the-counter corn remedies or cutting corns and calluses with a razor or knife.

Special precautions
• Instruct the patient to cut his toenails flush with the end of the toe and to file them carefully. Explain to him that it is best to cut the toenails after a thorough washing and under good lighting conditions. If toenails are too thick or if they crack when cut, refer the patient to a podiatrist.
• Advise him to wear shoes that fit comfortably and support, protect, and cover the feet completely. New shoes require gradual breaking in.
• Warn him never to go barefoot.
• Tell him to avoid using hot water bottles, heating pads, or ice on his legs or feet. Explain that decreased blood flow to the legs and feet reduces sensation and increases the chances of accidental burns or chills.
• If a foot injury causes a break in the skin, instruct him to immediately wash the affected area with soap and water and to cover it with a dry, sterile gauze bandage. Tell him to change the bandage daily and inspect the area for redness, swelling, and drainage.

Doctor notification
Instruct the patient to call the doctor about any foot injury that does not improve within 72 hours. Also, tell him to call the doctor if any of these signs of impaired circulation appear:
• unusual or persistent warmth or coolness
• numbness or muscle weakness
• swelling that does not resolve after raising the leg.

with the patient outcomes specified in your plan of care.

Teaching and counseling
• Begin by evaluating the effectiveness of your teaching and counseling. Document statements by the patient indicating:

• willingness to ask for assistance when performing activities, to prevent injury or trauma to tissues
• understanding of precautions necessary to prevent tissue damage
• understanding of the need to assess extremities each day

• understanding of how to perform preventive skin measures
• willingness to adhere to a prescribed treatment regimen and to take steps to eliminate cardiovascular risk factors
• understanding of factors that cause pain and willingness to make changes that will help him avoid pain.

Physical condition
Continue your evaluation by reassessing the patient's physical condition. Consider the following questions:
• Does the patient exhibit improved blood flow to the legs and feet?
• Does he maintain muscle strength and joint range of motion?
• Are paralysis and paresthesia absent?
• Does he report decreased pain?
• Can he perform self-care activities?
• Is his skin intact?

Tissue perfusion
Also, reassess tissue perfusion. Consider the following questions:
• Are peripheral pulses palpable?
• Is the patient's skin warm in extremities and has the color returned to baseline?
• Is capillary refill time less than 3 seconds?
• Has LOC returned to baseline?

Raynaud's disease

This circulatory disorder causes numbness and skin color changes; it occurs bilaterally and affects the patient's hands or, less often, the feet. Rarely, it affects the earlobes or tip of the nose. It is five times more common in women than men and begins between adolescence and age 40 in 90% of patients. (See *Key points about Raynaud's disease*.)

Also known as vasospastic arterial disease, Raynaud's disease is one of several primary arteriospastic disorders. Arteriospastic disorders are characterized by episodic vasospasm in the small peripheral arteries and arterioles, which is precipitated by exposure to cold or by stress. Vasospasm occurs independently of vessel disorders.

This disorder usually is benign, requiring no specific treatment. However, severe or persistent vasoconstriction can lead to ischemia, ulceration, or gangrene. Although extremely uncommon, full-thickness tissue necrosis and gangrene necessitate amputation of one or more phalanges.

Raynaud's phenomenon, a separate condition, is a secondary disorder re-

lated to other diseases or conditions, such as collagen vascular disease and other arterial occlusive disorders. Raynaud's phenomenon also may be related to the use of certain drugs, such as beta-adrenergic blocking agents, cisplatin, and vinblastine.

Causes

The precise cause of Raynaud's disease is unknown. Reduced digital blood flow may result from intrinsic vascular wall hypersensitivity to cold and increased vasomotor tone due to sympathetic stimulation, stress, and antigen-antibody immune response.

ASSESSMENT

Your assessment of the patient with Raynaud's disease should include a health history, physical examination, and review of diagnostic test results.

Health history

The patient with Raynaud's disease may report skin color changes induced by cold or stress. The response to cold and stress typically is triphasic, as listed below.

Phase One: The skin of affected areas appears pale due to severe vasoconstriction. Numbness and tingling may be present.

Phase Two: The skin appears cyanotic due to dilation of cutaneous arterioles and venules and to blood oxygen desaturation.

Phase Three: The skin appears red and feels warm due to vasoconstriction and reactive hyperemia. The patient may report throbbing, burning, and pain during phase three.

Physical examination

Affected areas may appear normal if you conduct your examination between attacks, or the skin may be diaphoretic. You may see trophic changes in your patient's fingers, as evidenced by atrophy of skin and nails and loss of hair over the terminal phalanges. In patients whose condition is chronic, you may see sclerodactyly and ulcerations. If decreased peripheral tissue perfusion occurs, you will detect diminished or absent pulses and delayed capillary refill in the affected extremity.

Diagnostic test results

The following tests help confirm a diagnosis of Raynaud's *phenomenon.* (Before Raynaud's *phenomenon* can be diagnosed as Raynaud's *disease*, associated conditions, such as chronic arterial occlusive disease and connective tissue disease, must be ruled out.)

• Doppler ultrasonography measures arm and wrist blood pressures.

• Digital plethysmography helps to differentiate Raynaud's disease from Raynaud's phenomenon.

• Arteriography rules out arterial disease.

• The ice water immersion test measures the body's ability to return to normal temperature. (See *Performing the ice water immersion test.*)

Assessment TimeSaver

Performing the ice water immersion test

To perform the ice water immersion test, take the following steps:
• Measure baseline digital pulp temperature, using a thermistor probe.
• Immerse the patient's hand in ice water for 30 seconds.
• Remove the hand from the ice water, dry it thoroughly, and take pulp temperature readings every 5 minutes until baseline temperature is reached. A healthy patient's baseline temperature will return in 15 minutes or less. In a patient with Raynaud's phenomenon, normal temperature returns in 20 to 25 minutes.

NURSING DIAGNOSIS

Common nursing diagnoses for a patient with Raynaud's disease include:
• Altered peripheral tissue perfusion related to severe arterial vasospasm
• Pain related to vascular hyperemia
• Impaired skin integrity related to diminished cellular nutrition due to extended vasospastic episodes
• Anxiety related to the medical diagnosis
• Knowledge deficit related to effective management of the condition.

PLANNING

Goals of nursing care for the patient with Raynaud's disease include relieving the patient's symptoms and teaching the patient about the disorder and its treatment.

Based on the nursing diagnosis *altered peripheral tissue perfusion*, develop appropriate patient outcomes. For example, your patient will:
• maintain capillary refill time of less than 3 seconds
• maintain full peripheral pulses.

Based on the nursing diagnosis *pain*, develop appropriate patient outcomes. For example, your patient will:
• show evidence that pain is reduced within 30 minutes of a vasoconstriction episode.

Based on the nursing diagnosis *impaired skin integrity*, develop appropriate patient outcomes. For example, your patient will:
• show evidence that baseline skin color is restored within 30 minutes of a vasoconstriction episode.

Based on the nursing diagnosis *anxiety*, develop appropriate patient outcomes. For example, your patient will:
• identify signs of anxiety and describe methods to cope with them
• demonstrate verbally and by behavior that anxiety is reduced.

Treatments

Medical care of the patient with Raynaud's disease

Because the symptoms of Raynaud's disease are usually benign, primary treatments are implemented by the patient. They include avoiding cold, avoiding mechanical or chemical injury, and smoking cessation.

Drug therapy
Drug therapy is reserved for severe cases because adverse reactions to medications, especially vasodilators, can be worse than the disease itself. Drug therapy for a patient with severe Raynaud's disease may call for phenoxybenzamine, nifedipine, diltiazem, reserpine, or guanethidine combined with prazosin.

Surgery
Sympathectomy may help patients whose symptoms are severe when conservative treatment fails to prevent ischemic ulcers. Ischemic ulcers occur in fewer than 25% of patients with Raynaud's disease.

Based on the nursing diagnosis *knowledge deficit,* develop appropriate patient outcomes. For example, your patient will:
• express understanding of the condition
• demonstrate methods to prevent or relieve vasospasms.

IMPLEMENTATION

Treatment for the patient with Raynaud's disease is aimed at alleviating symptoms. (See *Medical care of the patient with Raynaud's disease.*)

Nursing interventions
• If your patient's symptoms are caused by stress, help her identify the stressors and use effective coping strategies. When appropriate, refer your patient to a biofeedback program for help in identifying and controlling symptoms of stress.
• Provide psychological support and reassurance to arrest fears of disfigurement or amputation.
• Evaluate the patient's occupation and environment, and assess their effects on symptom occurrence. Refer

her to an occupational rehabilitation program, as needed.

Patient teaching
• Teach the patient about the disorder, its symptoms, and possible complications.
• Describe the signs and symptoms of vasospastic episodes, and advise the patient to report signs of disease progression or complications.
• If vasoconstriction does occur, suggest immersing the extremities in warm — not hot — water, or drinking a warm beverage. Explain that because vasoconstriction may cause decreased sensation, using hot water may cause burns.
• Instruct the patient to avoid exposure to cold. Advise her to dress warmly and to wear mittens or gloves in cold weather or when handling cold items.
• Advise the patient to stop smoking and provide referral to a smoking cessation program, as needed.
• Review the need for frequent skin inspections, and advise the patient to immediately report signs of skin breakdown or infection.

Discharge TimeSaver

Ensuring continued care for the patient with Raynaud's disease

Review the following topics and referrals to ensure that your patient is adequately prepared for discharge.

Teaching topics
Make sure that the following topics have been covered and that your patient's learning has been evaluated:
☐ explanation of Raynaud's disease, associated risk factors, and potential complications
☐ need to avoid exposure to cold
☐ prescribed medications, including precautions, and adverse effects
☐ need to stop smoking
☐ guidelines for examining and caring for skin
☐ methods to help alleviate symptoms
☐ sources of information and support.

Referrals
Make sure that the patient has been provided with appropiate referrals to:
☐ social services
☐ occupational counseling
☐ smoking cessation program.

Follow-up appointments
Make sure that the necessary follow-up appointments are scheduled and that the patient is notified:
☐ medical doctor
☐ additional diagnostic testing for re-evaluation.

• Tell the patient about prescribed drugs, their proper use, and possible adverse effects. Note that calcium channel blockers often cause adverse reactions. (See *Ensuring continued care for the patient with Raynaud's disease.*)

EVALUATION

To evaluate the patient's response to your nursing care, gather reassessment data and compare this information with the patient outcomes specified in your plan of care.

Teaching and counseling
Begin by evaluating the effectiveness of your teaching and counseling. Document statements by the patient indicating:
• understanding of methods to prevent or relieve vasospasms
• ability to identify signs of stress and appropriate coping methods

• understanding of the purposes of prescribed medications and possible adverse effects.

Physical condition
Continue your evaluation by reassessing the patient's physical condition. Consider the following questions:
• Does the patient's skin color return to baseline within 30 minutes?
• Is capillary refill time less than 3 seconds?
• Does she maintain full peripheral pulses?

Varicose veins

Varicose veins are dilated, tortuous veins that are engorged with blood. Varicose veins eventually may cause venous insufficiency or venous stasis ulcers, especially around the ankles. (See *Key points about varicose veins,* page 284.)

FactFinder
Key points about varicose veins

• Primary varicose veins originate both in veins and in branches of the superficial and saphenous veins.
• Secondary varicose veins occur in deep and perforating veins.
• Primary varicose veins tend to run in families, affect both legs, and occur twice as often in women as in men.
• Usually, secondary varicose veins occur in only one leg.
• Both primary and secondary varicose veins occur most often in middle adulthood.

Causes
Most varicose veins are caused by poorly functioning venous valves. (See *How varicose veins develop.*)

Primary varicose veins may result from congenital weakness of the valves or venous wall or from prolonged venous stasis caused by obesity, pregnancy, tight clothing, or extended periods of standing.

Secondary varicose veins result from disorders of the venous system, such as deep vein thrombophlebitis, trauma, or occlusion.

ASSESSMENT

Because varicose veins often run in families, check for a family history of the disorder. You should also assess for the presence of risk factors for the condition such as pregnancy, wearing tight clothing, or occupations that necessitate standing for long periods.

Health history
A patient with varicose veins may be asymptomatic. Alternatively, she may report mild to severe leg symptoms: a feeling of heaviness that worsens in the evening and in warm weather; muscle cramps and leg fatigue, especially at night; diffuse, dull aching after prolonged periods of sitting, standing, or walking; or pain that is exacerbated during menses or pregnancy.

Physical examination
During inspection of the affected leg, you may see dilated, purplish, ropelike veins, especially on the patient's calf. With chronic venous stasis, the skin of the lower extremities may appear brownish or rust colored. If your patient has valve incompetence in deep veins, you may see orthostatic edema and stasis of the calves and ankles.

During palpation, you may detect nodules along affected veins and valve incompetence. To confirm valve incompetence, use the manual compression test, Trendelenburg's test, or Perthes' test. (See *Testing valve incompetence,* page 286.)

Diagnostic test results
Tests to diagnose varicose vein severity include:
• Plethysmography, a noninvasive test, measures venous capacity and outflow and provides an index of valvular incompetence.
• Doppler ultrasonography quickly and accurately detects venous backflow in deep or superficial veins.
• Venous outflow and reflux plethysmography can detect deep venous occlusion.
• Ascending and descending venography can disclose venous occlusion and patterns of collateral flow. Note that venography is an invasive test that is not routinely used.

NURSING DIAGNOSIS

Common nursing diagnoses for a patient with varicose veins include:
• Impaired tissue integrity related to reduced venous blood flow

How varicose veins develop

Competent venous valves open and close smoothly and completely, allowing blood to flow efficiently from the extremities to the heart. Incompetent venous valves, however, do not close properly, allowing venous blood backflow and pooling. Progressive blood pooling produces the characteristic leg-vein dilation of varicose veins and leads to disturbed tissue oxygenation and nutrient exchange.

Normal venous valves

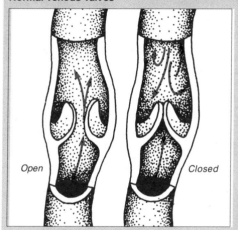

Open   *Closed*

Incompetent venous valve

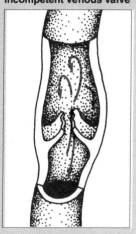

• High risk for impaired skin integrity related to surgery or injection of sclerosing agent
• Pain related to engorged veins
• Body image disturbance related to altered extremity appearance
• Knowledge deficit related to diagnosis and treatment of varicose veins.

PLANNING

Based on the nursing diagnosis *impaired tissue integrity,* develop appropriate patient outcomes. For example, your patient will:
• exhibit evidence of decreased edema and improved blood flow
• demonstrate ability to adhere to the prescribed care regimen, such as elevating legs when sitting in a chair and using proper technique for putting on elastic stockings.

Based on the nursing diagnosis *high risk for impaired skin integrity,* develop appropriate patient outcomes. For example, your patient will:
• exhibit evidence that incisions heal without complications following surgery
• exhibit intact skin without redness, discoloration, or swelling.

Based on the nursing diagnosis *pain,* develop appropriate patient outcomes. For example, your patient will:
• identify activities that cause or increase leg discomfort
• demonstrate measures that reduce pain and improve circulation

Testing valve incompetence

Three techniques for testing valve incompetence are the manual compression test, Trendelenburg's test, and Perthes' test.

Manual compression test
• Palpate the dilated vein with the fingertips of one hand.
• With the other hand, firmly compress the vein at a point 8″ (20 cm) away.
• Feel for an impulse transmitted to your lower hand. No impulse will be detected with competent saphenous valves. A palpable impulse indicates incompetent valves in a vein segment between your hands.

Trendelenburg's test
• While the patient stands, mark distended veins with a felt-tip marker.
• Have the patient lie face up on an examination table, and elevate the affected leg for 1 minute. Elevation allows the veins to drain.
• Have the patient stand, and measure the venous filling time. If valves are competent, veins take at least 30 seconds to fill.
• If the veins fill in less than 30 seconds, return the patient to the examination table, and elevate the leg for 1 minute.
• Apply a tourniquet around the upper thigh. Have the patient stand and remove the tourniquet. If the leg veins begin filling rapidly while the tourniquet is on but return to filling slowly (taking 30 seconds to fill) after the tourniquet is removed, suspect valve incompetence in superficial perforating veins. If the veins fill very rapidly, taking less than a combined time of 30

seconds to fill (with tourniquet on and tourniquet off), suspect valve incompetence in superficial perforating veins and deep veins.

Perthes' test
• Apply a tourniquet at the thigh.
• Have the patient walk. If the varicose veins disappear as the patient walks, both the deep venous system and the superficial perforating veins are competent. If the patient experiences pain while walking, the deep venous system is the source of the obstruction, and the superficial perforating veins provide the major route of venous flow. This information is used to determine if superficial veins can be excised or if disturbed functioning of the deep venous system contraindicates surgery.

Ochsner-Mahorner variation of Perthes' test
If Perthes' test shows the deep veins to be competent, perform the following procedure:
• After testing the patient with the tourniquet at thigh level, move the tourniquet successively downward to increments distal to the initial thigh level, such as above the knee and above the calf.
• Have the patient walk after each tourniquet placement. This will help you identify specific locations of incompetent superficial perforating veins by isolating the obstructed veins of the thigh or calf.

Treatments

Medical care of the patient with varicose veins

Treatment for varicose veins depends on the severity of the disorder.

Mild varicose veins
In mild forms of the disorder, treatment may focus on self-care measures, such as:
• wearing elastic stockings
• avoiding tight clothing and prolonged standing
• walking or other exercise which promotes muscle contraction, minimizes venous pooling, and forces blood through the veins
• elevating the legs.

Moderate varicose veins
In moderate forms of the disorder, the doctor may prescribe antiembolism stockings or elastic bandages, as well as promote self-care measures.

Severe varicose veins
For severe cases, the doctor may order custom-fitted, surgical-weight stockings with graduated pressure (pressure is highest at the ankle, lowest at the top).

Stripping and ligation may be performed if the patient fatigues easily and has pain, heaviness, recurrent superficial thrombophlebitis, and external bleeding. Surgery may also be performed for cosmetic reasons. For patients who are poor surgical risks, the doctor may inject a sclerosing agent into small segments of affected veins.

• experience reduction in pain following administration of postoperative analgesic, as demonstrated by verbal reports or behavior
• report decreased pain following recuperation from stripping and ligation or following injection of a sclerosing agent.

Based on the nursing diagnosis *body image disturbance,* develop appropriate patient outcomes. For example, your patient will:
• express feelings about changes in appearance
• demonstrate techniques for concealing scars and veins
• demonstrate an improved self-image, either verbally or through behavior.

Based on the nursing diagnosis *knowledge deficit,* develop appropriate patient outcomes. For example, your patient will:

• demonstrate willingness to obtain information about varicose veins from appropriate sources
• demonstrate proper care of legs and feet, including frequent skin assessment.

IMPLEMENTATION

Treatment of the patient with varicose veins aims to decrease discomfort during the hospital stay. Teach the patient appropriate home care measures including exercise planning, clothing restrictions, and diet and weight management. (See *Medical care of the patient with varicose veins.*)

Nursing interventions
• If the patient is to undergo surgery, explain stripping and ligation and discuss preoperative, postoperative, and home care measures.

Ensuring continued care for the patient with varicose veins

Review the following topics and referrals to ensure that your patient is adequately prepared for discharge.

Teaching topics
Make sure that the following topics have been covered and your patient's learning has been evaluated:
□ varicose veins, associated risk factors, and potential complications
□ measures to improve venous return, including wearing support stockings
□ foot and leg care.

Referrals
Make sure that the patient has been

provided with appropriate referrals to:
□ social services
□ weight reduction program.

Follow-up appointments
Make sure that the necessary follow-up appointments are scheduled and that the patient is notified:
□ medical doctor
□ surgeon.

• After stripping and ligation or injection of a sclerosing agent, administer analgesics as prescribed.
• Check elastic bandages for signs of incision bleeding. When necessary, rewrap bandages from toe to thigh with the leg elevated.
• Monitor circulation in toes by observing for changes in color and temperature.
• Watch for complications: sensory loss in the leg, indicating saphenous nerve damage; calf pain, indicating thrombophlebitis; or fever, indicating infection.

Patient teaching
Instruct the patient in measures that will promote the return of venous circulation, reduce pain, and minimize progression of the condition.
• Advise the patient to wear nonconstrictive clothing and to sit with her legs elevated.
• Tell the patient to elevate her legs above heart level whenever possible and to avoid prolonged periods of standing or sitting.
• Teach the patient to put on elastic, antiembolism, or compression stock-

ings before getting out of bed, or to elevate the legs for 1 minute before putting on the stockings.
• Strongly encourage the patient to adopt a regular exercise program, such as walking. During exercise, muscle contractions force blood through the veins and minimize venous pooling.
• Advise the obese patient to follow a safe, effective weight reduction program.
• Caution the patient to avoid injury to the lower legs, ankles, and feet and to observe these areas for signs of impaired skin integrity.
• Teach the patient to use proper foot and leg care measures.
• Discuss problems that the patient should report to the doctor, including signs of impaired tissue perfusion.
• Explain that varicosity may recur after surgery.
• Encourage the patient to express feelings about her personal appearance. Suggest ways to conceal varicose veins, such as wearing slacks, long skirts, or dark stockings. (See *Ensuring continued care for the patient with varicose veins.*)

EVALUATION

To evaluate the patient's response to your nursing care, gather reassessment data and compare this information with the patient outcomes specified in your plan of care.

Teaching and counseling
Begin by evaluating the effectiveness of your teaching and counseling. Consider the following questions:

• Has your patient asked for information about varicose veins, treatment of the condition, possible complications, and related topics?

• Is your patient able to conduct skin assessments and demonstrate proper care of the legs and feet?

• Does your patient indicate that she will adhere to the prescribed care regimen, such as elevating her legs while sitting and using the proper technique for putting on elastic stockings?

• Does the patient demonstrate a more positive self-image? Is she able to cope better with changes in appearance caused by varicose veins?

Physical condition
Continue your evaluation by reassessing the patient's physical condition. Consider the following questions:

• Does the patient exhibit decreased swelling and improved blood flow?

• Are incisions properly healed?

• Is the skin intact without redness, discoloration, or swelling?

• Is there evidence of reduced pain and improved circulation following treatment?

Thrombophlebitis

This acute condition is characterized by inflammation and thrombus formation in deep or superficial veins. It usually occurs at valve cusps, where ve-nous stasis fosters accumulation and adherence of platelets and fibrin.

Superficial vein thrombophlebitis is usually self-limiting. Because superficial veins have fewer valves than deep veins, it is less likely to cause complications.

Deep vein thrombophlebitis (DVT) affects small vessels, such as the lesser saphenous vein, and large veins, such as the vena cava and the iliac, femoral, and popliteal veins. Because it affects the veins that carry 90% of the venous outflow from the legs, DVT is more serious than superficial vein thrombophlebitis. Studies indicate that up to 35% of hospitalized patients develop DVT. The incidence of deep subclavian vein thrombophlebitis is increasing as the use of subclavian vein catheters becomes more common.

The major complications of thrombophlebitis are pulmonary embolism and chronic venous insufficiency.

Causes
Three factors — hypercoagulability, venous stasis, and endothelial damage — together cause thrombophlebitis. These factors are known as Virchow's triad.

ASSESSMENT

In both deep vein and superficial vein thrombophlebitis, clinical features vary, depending on the site of inflammation and the length of the affected vein. Your assessment should include a review of the patient's medical history to determine whether risk factors for thrombophlebitis are present. (See *Risk factors for deep vein thrombophlebitis,* page 290.)

Health history
Forty to fifty percent of patients with DVT are asymptomatic. Patients who do develop symptoms most commonly report pain. Your patient may report painful tenderness or a heavy, dull achiness in the involved extremity, com-

FactFinder
Risk factors for deep vein thrombophlebitis

If your patient has one or more of the following conditions, he may be at risk for developing deep vein thrombophlebitis (DVT).
• history of DVT
• infections or cancer
• conditions associated with venous stasis, such as acute myocardial infarction, heart failure, dehydration, immobility due to spinal cord injury, cerebrovascular accident, postoperative convalescence, and incompetent vein valve.
• history of cigarette smoking
• hypercoagulable states, such as disseminated intravascular coagulation, or myeloproliferative disease.
• venipuncture and treatments requiring infusion of irritating I.V. solutions
• abdominal, genitourinary, orthopedic, or thoracic surgery
• traumatic injuries, including fracture of the spine, hip, femur, pelvis, or tibia.
• estrogen use, pregnancy, or postpartum status.

monly the calf. Exercise does not affect the level of pain. Your patient also may report fever, chills, and malaise.

A patient with superficial vein thrombophlebitis may be asymptomatic or may report local pain at the thrombus site.

Physical examination
Examination findings differ between patients with DVT and patients with superficial vein thrombophlebitis.

Deep vein thrombophlebitis
Inspection may reveal redness or swelling of the affected leg or arm. Gentle dorsiflexion of the patient's foot may disclose a positive Homans' sign (pain in the affected calf). However,

the reliability of this sign as an indicator of DVT is questionable. During palpation, you may note that the patient's affected extremity feels warmer than the unaffected extremity.

Superficial vein thrombophlebitis
During inspection, you may see redness and swelling at the site and surrounding area. During palpation, you may feel warmth over the affected area. You also may feel a tender, hard cord along the length of the affected vein.

Diagnostic test results
To confirm a diagnosis of thrombophlebitis, other conditions such as arterial occlusive disease, lymphangitis, cellulitis, and myositis must be ruled out. Diagnosis of superficial vein thrombophlebitis usually is based on the physical examination findings. The following tests will help establish a diagnosis of DVT:
• Doppler ultrasonography identifies reduced blood flow to a specific area and any obstruction to venous flow, particularly in iliofemoral DVT. This test is 80% to 90% accurate.
• Plethysmography shows decreased circulation distal to the affected area and is more sensitive than ultrasonography. This test is approximately 90% accurate for DVT above the knee.
• Phlebography usually confirms the diagnosis and shows filling defects and diverted blood flow.
• Venography visualizes the deep venous system of the legs, detecting obstructions.

NURSING DIAGNOSIS

Common nursing diagnoses for a patient with DVT or superficial vein thrombophlebitis include:
• Pain related to inflammation of the vessel wall

• Altered peripheral tissue perfusion related to inflammation and thrombosis

• High risk for impaired skin integrity related to compromised peripheral circulation

• High risk for injury related to potential for pulmonary emboli

• Knowledge deficit related to the diagnosis, treatment, and complications of thrombophlebitis.

PLANNING

Goals of nursing care for the patient with thrombophlebitis include relieving the patient's symptoms, preventing complications, and teaching him about the disorder and its treatment.

Based on the nursing diagnosis *pain,* develop appropriate patient outcomes. For example, your patient will:

• report or show less pain following treatment

• adhere to a plan for using bed rest and warm compresses to reduce pain and inflammation

• report an absence of pain once thrombophlebitis is eradicated.

Based on the nursing diagnosis *altered peripheral tissue perfusion,* develop appropriate patient outcomes. For example, your patient will:

• maintain baseline color and temperature in the extremities

• demonstrate an absence of edema

• maintain palpable peripheral pulses.

Based on the nursing diagnosis *high risk for impaired skin integrity,* develop appropriate patient outcomes. For example, your patient will:

• maintain intact skin

• demonstrate understanding of appropriate skin care measures

• check skin daily for cuts, cracks, blisters, redness, or swelling.

Based on the nursing diagnosis *high risk for injury,* develop appropriate patient outcomes. For example, your patient will:

• demonstrate willingness to wear support stockings, as prescribed

• remain free of adverse drug reactions such as excessive bleeding

• maintain adequate ventilation

• remain free of pulmonary emboli.

Based on the nursing diagnosis *knowledge deficit,* develop appropriate patient outcomes. For example, your patient will:

• list signs and symptoms of pulmonary emboli or other conditions that should immediately be reported to the doctor

• express understanding of activity guidelines, based on the doctor's recommendations

• express understanding of anticoagulant therapy, including precautions and the need for follow-up testing

• demonstrate proper technique for self-administration of subcutaneous injections of heparin.

IMPLEMENTATION

Treatment of the patient with thrombophlebitis focuses on reducing discomfort and preventing complications. (See *Medical care of the patient with thrombophlebitis,* page 292.)

Nursing interventions

• During an acute episode, enforce bed rest and elevate the affected limb until the episode has passed. When you use pillows to elevate the extremity, position them to support the entire leg and prevent compression of the popliteal space. After an acute episode, increase the patient's activity level according to his tolerance level, and apply anti-embolism stockings.

• Apply warm compresses or a covered aquamatic K pad to increase circulation to the affected area and to relieve pain and inflammation.

• Administer analgesics as prescribed.

• Remind the patient not to rub or massage the calf.

Treatments

Medical care of the patient with thrombophlebitis

Therapy for severe superficial vein thrombophlebitis may include use of an anti-inflammatory drug (such as indomethacin), antiembolism stockings, warm compresses, and leg elevation.

For deep vein thrombophlebitis (DVT), the doctor may prescribe activity restrictions, drug therapy and, in rare cases, surgery.

Activity restrictions
Measures include bed rest with elevation of the affected arm or leg, application of warm, moist compresses to the affected area, and analgesics. After the acute episode subsides, the patient may begin to walk while wearing antiembolism stockings that are applied before he gets out of bed.

Drug therapy
Treatment may include anticoagulants (initially, heparin; later, warfarin) to prolong clotting time. However, the full anticoagulant dose must be discontinued prior to any type of surgery to avoid risk of hemorrhage. After some types of surgery, especially major abdominal or pelvic operations, prophylactic doses of anticoagulants may reduce risk of DVT.

For lysis of acute, extensive DVT, treatment may include streptokinase or urokinase, provided the risk of bleeding does not outweigh the potential benefits of thrombolytic treatment.

Surgery
In rare cases, DVT may cause complete venous occlusion. This complication necessitates venous interruption by simple ligation, vein plication, or clipping. Embolectomy may be indicated if clots are shed to the pulmonary and systemic vasculature and other treatment is unsuccessful. Caval interruption with an umbrella filter placed transvenously can trap emboli, preventing them from traveling to the pulmonary vasculature.

• Place a cradle over the foot of the bed to keep the weight of the linens off the legs, if necessary.

Timesaving tip: To make a homemade foot and leg cradle: remove the top from a cardboard carton, cut an opening on one side of the box, and place the box over the leg and foot.

• Measure and record the circumference of the affected arm or leg daily and compare it to measurements of the unaffected arm or leg. To ensure consistency, mark the skin where the measurement is taken.

• Assess the extremity daily for redness, tenderness, and signs of breakdown.

• Check the presence and status of peripheral pulses every 2 to 4 hours or as dictated by the patient's symptoms.

• Expect to administer heparin I.V. to the patient with DVT. To control flow rate, use an infusion monitor or pump. Switch the patient from I.V. to subcutaneous administration if prescribed.

• For the patient on heparin therapy, regularly measure partial thromboplastin time. For the patient on warfarin, measure the prothrombin time. The therapeutic anticoagulation values for both tests are $1\frac{1}{2}$ to 2 times the control values.

• Watch for signs and symptoms of bleeding, such as tarry stools, coffee-ground vomitus, or ecchymoses.

• Monitor the patient for bleeding at I.V. sites, and check gums for bleeding.
• Be alert for signs of pulmonary emboli, such as crackles, dyspnea, hemoptysis, sudden changes in mental status, restlessness, tachycardia, and hypotension.
• Assist with thrombolytic therapy, if applicable.
• Administer anti-inflammatory drugs, such as indomethacin, as prescribed. Monitor for upper GI bleeding.
• To prevent thrombophlebitis in high-risk patients, perform range-of-motion exercises while the patient is on bed rest, use intermittent pneumatic calf massage during lengthy surgical or diagnostic procedures, apply antiembolism stockings postoperatively, and encourage early ambulation.

Patient teaching
• Teach the patient about the disorder, its causes, symptoms, and complications. Explain all diagnostic tests.
• Counsel the patient about risk factors. Provide referral to a smoking cessation program, as needed.
• Explain the rationale for anticoagulant therapy and instruct the patient to watch for adverse reactions such as bleeding nose or gums, chills, dark blue toes, discolored urine, fatigue, prolonged bleeding from cuts, bruises, red or tarry black stools, or excessive menstrual flow. Emphasize the need for follow-up appointments to monitor anticoagulant therapy. Advise the patient to wear a medical identification bracelet stating that he takes anticoagulant medications.
• If the patient is being discharged on heparin therapy, show him and his family how to give subcutaneous injections. If further assistance is needed, provide referrals to a home health care agency.
• To help prevent bleeding, encourage the patient to use of an electric razor

and advise him to avoid over-the-counter products that contain aspirin.
• Advise the patient to avoid prolonged sitting or standing to help prevent recurrence of thrombophlebitis.
• Encourage the patient to participate in a prescribed exercise program, but caution against excessive physical activity.
• Teach the patient how to inspect and care for the legs and feet.
• Teach the patient how to properly apply and use antiembolism stockings. Have the patient demonstrate the procedure. Urge him to report any complications, such as cold, blue toes.
• Tell the patient to report signs and symptoms of pulmonary emboli, such as sudden shortness of breath, chest pain, and a cough that produces blood-tinged sputum.
• Tell the patient to report signs and symptoms of venous insufficiency, such as leg pain, edema, skin changes (scaling, brown pigmentation), and evidence of leg ulcers or other breaks in the skin.
• Instruct the patient to eat foods high in protein and rich in B complex and C vitamins to minimize complications.
• Teach the patient who must undergo surgery about the procedure, what to expect afterward, and preoperative and postoperative care measures. (See *Ensuring continued care for the patient with thrombophlebitis,* page 294.)

EVALUATION

To evaluate the patient's response to your nursing care, gather reassessment data and compare this information with the patient outcomes specified in your plan of care.

Teaching and counseling
Begin by evaluating the effectiveness of your teaching and counseling. Document statements by the patient indicating:

Discharge TimeSaver

Ensuring continued care for the patient with thrombophlebitis

Review the following topics and referrals to ensure that your patient is adequately prepared for discharge.

Teaching topics
Make sure that the following topics have been covered and that your patient's learning has been evaluated:
☐ disorder, associated risk factors, and potential complications
☐ activity restrictions during acute stages
☐ exercise plan for rehabilitation period
☐ dietary guidelines to promote skin integrity
☐ anticoagulant therapy, including precautions, potential adverse effects, and need for a medical identification bracelet
☐ skin and leg care
☐ warning signs and symptoms to report to the doctor

☐ application of antiembolism stockings.

Referrals
Make sure that the patient has been provided with appropriate referrals to:
☐ social services
☐ home health care agency
☐ smoking cessation program.

Follow-up appointments
Make sure that the necessary follow-up appointments are scheduled and that the patient is notified:
☐ medical doctor
☐ laboratory testing for reevaluation.

• knowledge of signs and symptoms that should be reported immediately to the doctor
• intention to follow appropriate activity guidelines
• understanding of anticoagulant therapy and related precautions
• intention to keep scheduled follow-up appointments for tests
• understanding of skin care measures and the need to check daily for cuts, cracks, blisters, redness, or swelling.

Performing self-care measures
Before the patient leaves the hospital, evaluate his ability to perform necessary self-care measures. Consider the following questions:
• Can he put on support stockings?
• Does he know how to administer subcutaneous injections properly?

Physical condition
Continue your evaluation by reassessing your patient's physical condition. Consider the following questions:
• Does your patient report a reduction in or disappearance of pain and inflammation?
• Does your patient's skin appear intact and has it returned to baseline color and temperature?
• Has edema been eliminated?
• Are the patient's peripheral pulses present and strong?
• Are adverse drug reactions under control?
• Are pulmonary emboli absent?

Chronic venous insufficiency

In this disorder, venous occlusion or valve incompetency causes edema and impairs perfusion, possibly leading to severe venous engorgement. The patient may experience debilitating pain and serious venous ulcers. If pain is dulled, the patient may not detect injury to his feet and legs until it is very pronounced. In many cases, conservative measures, such as exercise and antiembolism stockings, provide effective treatment. More severe cases, however, may require surgical intervention.

Chronic venous insufficiency usually affects the iliac and femoral veins and occasionally the saphenous veins. When veins are unable to drain efficiently, high pressure in the capillary beds results. Fluid migrates into interstitial tissue, causing edema. Erythrocytes leak into surrounding tissue and break down, causing visible hyperpigmentation. Fibrinogen leakage creates a fibrin cuff around the capillaries and impairs tissue perfusion. Inflammation and, ultimately, induration and ulceration occur.

Causes
Chronic venous insufficiency may occur secondary to the following disorders:
• atherosclerosis
• arteriosclerosis
• congestive heart failure
• coronary artery disease
• cardiomyopathy
• pulmonary disease
• hypertension
• diabetes mellitus
• lymphatic disorders
• renal insufficiency.

Postmenopausal women face increased risk for this disorder. Other risk factors include pregnancy, obesity, and occupations that require prolonged standing.

ASSESSMENT

Your assessment should include a review of the patient's medical history for evidence of risk factors such as previous injury, varicosities, thrombophlebitis, or leg ulcers.

Health history
The patient with chronic venous insufficiency may report chronic edema, chronic diffuse leg pain that increases with prolonged standing, nocturnal leg cramps, and possible leg ulcers.

Physical examination
While inspecting the patient's legs and feet, you may observe signs of venous insufficiency. These commonly include an abnormally prominent calf and narrow ankle (champagne bottle leg), edema, varicosities, thickening of the skin, eczema, and hyperpigmentation. You may see brownish discoloration, especially around the ankle or new or healed leg ulcers. (See *How to distinguish between arterial and venous ulcers,* page 296.)

When you palpate the affected limb, you may feel a strong pedal pulse if arterial occlusive disease is not present. The pulse may be difficult to palpate if edema is severe, however. If your patient has venous leg ulcers, you may detect tissue granulation.

Diagnostic test results
The following tests will help establish a diagnosis of chronic venous insufficiency:
• Doppler ultrasonography shows deep vein patency and incompetence and helps you distinguish arterial or venous disease.
• Plethysmography establishes postexercise venous refilling time and may

How to distinguish between arterial and venous ulcers

Chronic arterial occlusive disease can lead to *arterial* ulcers; on the other hand, chronic venous insufficiency causes *venous* ulcers. Each type of ulcer has distinguishing characteristics and requires distinct treatments.

Characteristics	Arterial ulcers	Venous ulcers
Predisposing factors	• Arteriosclerosis • Advancing age • Diabetes	• History of deep vein thrombophlebitis • Valve incompetence in perforating veins
Leg or foot changes	• Thin, shiny, dry skin • Thickened nails • Absence of hair growth • Temperature variations • Pallor on elevation • Dependent rubor	• Firm "brawny" edema • Reddish brown discoloration • Evidence of healed ulcers • Dilated and tortuous superficial veins
Ulcer locations	• Between or at the tips of the toes • Over phalangeal heads • On the heel • Above lateral malleolus • In diabetic patients: over the metatarsal heads or on the side or sole of the foot	• Anteromedial malleolus • Pretibial area
Ulcer attributes	• Well-demarcated edges • Black or necrotic tissue • Deep, pale base • Exceedingly painful	• Uneven edges • Ruddy granulation tissue • Superficial
Nonsurgical treatment	• Moist 0.9% sodium chloride solution dressings, loosely bandaged; no tape on fragile skin • Bed rest to ensure oxygen and nutrients for healing • Topical antibiotic if infected • Immobilization when tendon is exposed; use of a short leg, Fiberglas cast with a window to allow for dressing changes	• Frequent dressing changes with solution, as ordered; tightly bandaged • Limb elevation • Compression bandages to eliminate venous stasis; Unna's boot for walking • Systemic antibiotic for infection or cellulitis • Chemical debridement to dissolve necrotic tissue, if necessary
Surgery	• Vascular reconstruction • Amputation	• Perforating vein ligation • Valvular transposition • Valvuloplasty

reveal deep vein valvular incompetence.

• Venography and color-flow duplex ultrasonography are used to evaluate venous insufficiency in cases for which surgery is a possibility.

NURSING DIAGNOSIS

Common nursing diagnoses for a patient with chronic venous insufficiency include:
• Pain related to increased venous pressure
• Impaired skin integrity related to venous engorgement and high venous pressure in the capillary bed
• Knowledge deficit related to the condition, its treatment, and potential complications.

PLANNING

Based on the nursing diagnosis *pain,* develop appropriate patient outcomes. For example, your patient will:
• comply with measures to reduce pain, such as strict bed rest, occlusive dressings, and analgesic therapy
• express feelings of reduced pain after treatment.

Based on the nursing diagnosis *impaired skin integrity,* develop appropriate patient outcomes. For example, your patient will:
• maintain intact skin
• exhibit evidence of reduced edema
• exhibit decreased or absent leg ulcers.

Based on the nursing diagnosis *knowledge deficit,* develop appropriate patient outcomes. For example, your patient will:
• express understanding of risk factors for venous insufficiency and leg ulcers
• show willingness to adopt life-style changes to improve venous functioning and prevent ulceration
• demonstrate how to change leg ulcer dressings

• implement measures to promote wound healing
• describe postoperative home care measures, as needed
• express understanding of medication regimen and possible adverse effects.

IMPLEMENTATION

Treatment of the patient with chronic venous insufficiency includes measures to relieve the patient's symptoms and teaching about ulcer care. (See *Medical care of the patient with chronic venous insufficiency*, page 298.)

Nursing interventions
• Administer prescribed medications.
• Monitor the patient's legs frequently for signs of improvement or disease progression.
• Clean and debride the ulcer with 0.9% sodium chloride solution. Apply an occlusive or semi-occlusive dressing, as ordered. Expect heavy exudation initially, which should not be confused with infection. Change dressing daily or as needed.

Timesaving tip: To monitor a healing ulcer, place a clear plastic bag over the area and trace the ulcer with a felt-tip marker. Cut out the outline and discard the part that touched the ulcer. Check periodically to see that, as the ulcer heals, it becomes smaller than the cutout. Note that the average time for ulcer healing is about 9 months.

Patient teaching
• Teach the patient about the condition, its causes, treatment, and possible complications. Explain all diagnostic tests.
• Explain the rationale for frequent assessment of legs and for treatment measures. Stress the need for long-term follow-up care.

Treatments

Medical care of the patient with chronic venous insufficiency

First-line treatment for patients with chronic venous insufficiency emphasizes life-style changes, such as walking regularly, losing weight, avoiding prolonged standing, and wearing support stockings. Severe cases may require surgical intervention, such as vein ligation or valvular transposition.

Venous leg ulcers
Treatment for venous leg ulcers may include the following measures:
• debriding the ulcer with 0.9% sodium chloride solution
• applying an occlusive or semi-occlusive dressing and possibly a paste boot, such as Unna's boot, over the dressing
• applying graduated elastic compression from the base of the toes to below the knee to counteract increased venous pressure
• encouraging absolute bed rest and elevating the affected leg to relieve severe pain
• correcting nutritional deficiencies, especially for protein, calories, zinc, iron, and vitamin C.

To help prevent leg ulcers from recurring, steps must be taken to control the underlying disease. Skin grafting may be indicated for intractable ulcers.

Drug therapy
The following medications may be prescribed to treat complications of chronic venous insufficiency:
• systemic antibiotics (such as oral penicillin V) to prevent severe infections, such as osteomyelitis. Topical antibiotics usually are not recommended because of the difficulty of delivering adequate levels of antibiotic to the tissues.
• topical corticosteroids for associated eczema (administered for no longer than 1 week).

• Explain that elevating the leg and wearing support stockings should help alleviate pain.
• For severe pain related to an acute leg ulcer, explain that measures prescribed by the doctor, such as strict bed rest, occlusive dressings, and administration of analgesics, will help alleviate pain.
• Emphasize the importance of keeping follow-up appointments and of complying with therapy, even if the condition improves.
• Discuss prescribed medications, their administration, purpose, and possible adverse effects. Emphasize the importance of completing the full course of antibiotic therapy. Advise the patient that topical corticosteroids should only be used for a short period because pro-

longed treatment may interfere with healing.
• Teach the patient or caregiver how to change dressings. Initially, you made need to supervise this procedure.
• Instruct the patient to recognize and report complications, such as infection or allergic reactions.
• Advise the patient to avoid keeping the leg in a dependent position. Instruct him to elevate the leg when sleeping, either by raising the foot of the bed or by placing a foam rubber wedge under his leg.
• Advise the patient to begin a moderate walking program, as prescribed.
• Encourage the obese patient to lose weight, and provide referral to a dietitian or appropriate self-help group.

Discharge TimeSaver
Ensuring continued care for the patient with chronic venous insufficiency

Review the following topics and referrals to ensure that your patient is adequately prepared for discharge.

Teaching topics
Make sure that the following topics have been covered and that your patient's learning has been evaluated:
☐ how chronic venous insufficiency occurs, its risk factors, and treatment
☐ use of support stockings
☐ prescribed medications and potential adverse effects
☐ foot and leg monitoring and care
☐ leg ulcer care
☐ life-style changes to improve venous return, reduce pain, and help prevent leg ulcers.

Referrals
Make sure that the patient has been provided with appropriate referrals to:
☐ social services
☐ home health care agency
☐ weight reduction program
☐ smoking cessation program
☐ occupational counseling
☐ dietitian.

Follow-up appointments
Make sure that the necessary follow-up appointments are scheduled and that the patient is notified:
☐ medical doctor
☐ vascular surgeon.

• Counsel the patient to stop smoking. Provide referral to a smoking cessation program if needed.
• Show how to properly apply support stockings, if ordered. Ask the patient or a family member to demonstrate the procedure.
• Stress the importance of avoiding leg injuries. Help the patient plan safety measures.
• If the patient's job requires prolonged standing or sitting, provide referral to an occupational counselor, as needed.
• Recommend measures to aid wound healing, such as correcting nutritional deficiencies.
• If surgery is ordered, discuss preoperative, postoperative, and home care measures. (See *Ensuring continued care for the patient with chronic venous insufficiency.*)

EVALUATION
To evaluate the patient's response to your nursing care, gather reassessment data and compare this information to the patient outcomes specified in your plan of care.

Teaching and counseling
Begin by evaluating the effectiveness of your patient teaching and counseling. Document statements by the patient indicating:
• understanding of risk factors for venous insufficiency
• willingness to take steps to improve venous functioning and to promote wound healing
• understanding of the need for surgical treatment, if appropriate
• understanding of the medication regimen.

Also, determine whether your patient has demonstrated an ability to perform necessary self-care skills, such

Evaluation TimeSaver

Evaluating leg ulcer recurrence

If treatment and patient education fail to prevent leg ulcers from recurring, use this checklist to help you evaluate why. You may need to collaborate with other health care professionals when evaluating barriers to successful treatment.

Factors interfering with compliance
☐ Unclear instructions
☐ Failure to provide written instructions
☐ Inadequate patient teaching
☐ Failure to consider need for support programs, such as smoking cessation and weight control programs, or dietary counseling
☐ Failure to include caregiver in patient education
☐ Failure to consider need for occupational counseling
☐ Patient's inability to afford follow-up care, smoking cessation program, weight control program, or compression stockings
☐ Presence of mental impairment, such as a memory deficit, which interferes with patient's cognitive abilities

Conditions that exacerbate venous insufficiency
☐ Arterial component to leg ulcer
☐ Diabetes mellitus
☐ Arteriosclerotic cardiovascular disease
☐ Nutritional deficiencies
☐ Obesity
☐ Excess pain

Factors associated with repeated leg injury
☐ Unsteady gait
☐ Vision impairment
☐ Unsafe environment
☐ Syncope or transient ischemic attacks

as changing ulcer dressings and applying support stockings.

Physical condition
Continue your evaluation by reassessing the patient's physical condition. Consider the following questions:
• Does your patient report a reduction in pain?
• Is his skin intact or is ulcer healing evident? (See *Evaluating leg ulcer recurrence.*)
• Is edema absent or reduced?

CHAPTER 10

Caring for patients with complications and trauma

Hypovolemic shock syndrome

Hypovolemic shock syndrome occurs when reduced intravascular blood volume causes circulatory dysfunction and inadequate tissue perfusion. Tissue anoxia shifts cell metabolism from aerobic to anaerobic pathways, leading to an accumulation of lactic acid and metabolic acidosis.

Hypovolemic shock syndrome calls for quick symptom assessment and prompt, aggressive treatment. Without sufficient blood or fluid replacement, hypovolemic shock may lead to adult respiratory distress syndrome, disseminated intravascular coagulation (DIC), irreversible cerebral and renal damage, cardiac arrest, or death.

Causes

In most cases, hypovolemic shock results from acute massive blood loss caused, for example, by GI bleeding, internal hemorrhage (such as hemothorax or hemoperitoneum), or external bleeding (as from accidental or surgical trauma). Conditions (such as severe burns) that reduce intravascular plasma volume or other body fluids also can cause hypovolemic shock syndrome. Other examples of conditions that can lead to hypovolemic shock syndrome include intestinal obstruction, peritonitis, acute pancreatitis, ascites, or dehydration from excessive perspiration, severe diarrhea, protracted vomiting, diabetes insipidus, diuresis, or inadequate fluid intake.

ASSESSMENT

Hypovolemic shock syndrome is a medical emergency that requires quick assessment and treatment.

Health history

In the early stages of shock, a patient may report thirst or nausea and may experience apprehension and anxiety. A patient with underlying heart disease may report anginal pain because of decreased myocardial perfusion and oxygenation. The patient may have other disorders or conditions that reduce extravascular volume, such as GI hemorrhage, trauma, severe diarrhea, or vomiting.

Physical examination

During inspection of a patient in hypovolemic shock, you may see pale skin, decreased sensorium, and rapid, shallow respirations. When monitoring the patient's urine output, anticipate possible shock if his output is less than 30 ml/hour or 0.5 ml/kg/hour (depending on the patient's body size and physical condition).

Palpation of peripheral pulses may reveal a rapid, thready pulse and cold, clammy skin. Auscultation may disclose tachycardia. While auscultating blood pressure, you usually will detect a mean arterial pressure (MAP) of less than 60 mm Hg in adults and a narrowed pulse pressure. The MAP of a patient with chronic hypotension may fall below 50 mm Hg before signs of hypovolemic shock appear. Central venous pressure (CVP), right atrial pressure, pulmonary artery systolic and diastolic pressures, pulmonary artery wedge pressure (PAWP), and cardiac output usually are reduced.

Checking orthostatic vital signs may help confirm the diagnosis. (See *Checking for impending hypovolemic shock*.)

Diagnostic test results

The following laboratory test findings help establish a diagnosis of hypovolemic shock syndrome:

• Serum potassium, sodium, lactate dehydrogenase, creatinine, and blood urea nitrogen levels are elevated.

• Urine specific gravity is greater than 1.020, with increased urine osmolality.
• Hematocrit and hemoglobin levels, and red blood cell (RBC) and platelet counts are reduced if shock is due to blood loss. However, hematocrit and hemoglobin levels may be increased if shock is due to fluid volume deficit resulting from excessive diuresis, vomiting, diarrhea, or third-space shift.
• Urine creatinine level is decreased.
• Partial pressure of oxygen in arterial blood and pH are decreased. In early hypovolemic shock, partial pressure of carbon dioxide in arterial blood ($PaCO_2$) may be decreased due to hyperventilation. $PaCO_2$ may be increased in later stages of shock, when the patient can no longer maintain hyperventilation.

Additional tests

X-rays, gastroscopy, aspiration of gastric contents through a nasogastric tube, and tests for occult blood may identify internal bleeding sites. Coagulation studies may detect coagulopathy from DIC.

NURSING DIAGNOSIS

Common nursing diagnoses for a patient with hypovolemic shock syndrome include:
• Pain related to decreased myocardial perfusion and oxygenation
• Altered thought processes related to decreased cerebral perfusion
• Altered tissue perfusion (cardiopulmonary, cerebral, renal, gastrointestinal, or peripheral) related to vascular fluid volume loss
• Decreased cardiac output related to decreased preload
• High risk for fluid volume deficit related to vascular fluid volume loss
• Anxiety related to urgency of situation, elevated catecholamine serum levels, and hypoxia.

Assessment TimeSaver

Checking for impending hypovolemic shock

Measuring orthostatic vital signs and performing the tilt test may help assess the possibility of hypovolemic shock.

Orthostatic vital signs
• Measure the patient's blood pressure and pulse rate while he is supine, sitting, and standing. Wait at least 3 minutes between position changes.
• Systolic blood pressure that decreases 20 mm Hg or more between position changes, or pulse rate that increases 20 beats/minute or more between position changes suggests volume depletion and impending hypovolemic shock.

Tilt test
With the patient supine, raise his legs above heart level. If his blood pressure increases significantly, the test is positive, indicating volume depletion and impending hypovolemic shock.

PLANNING

Because hypovolemic shock syndrome is a medical emergency, you may not have time to document a thorough plan of care. Follow your hospital's protocol or prepared plan for treating a patient in hypovolemic shock. After the emergency, you may need to revise the plan of care to reflect your patient's individual needs.

Based on the nursing diagnosis *pain,* develop appropriate patient outcomes. For example, your patient will:
• express a feeling of comfort and relief from pain
• identify pain characteristics
• identify factors that intensify pain and modify his behavior accordingly.

Based on the nursing diagnosis *altered thought processes,* develop appropriate patient outcomes. For example, your patient will:
• maintain baseline level of consciousness (LOC).

Based on the nursing diagnosis *altered tissue perfusion,* develop appropriate patient outcomes. For example, your patient will:
• maintain systolic blood pressure above 90 mm Hg (or baseline level for the patient) and MAP above 80 mm Hg (or baseline level for the patient)
• maintain baseline hemoglobin and hematocrit levels, RBC and platelet counts, electrolyte status, urine specific gravity, and arterial blood gas (ABG) values
• maintain baseline peripheral pulses
• maintain baseline skin color and temperature.

Based on the nursing diagnosis *decreased cardiac output,* develop appropriate patient outcomes. For example, your patient will:
• maintain cardiac output greater than 5 liters/minute
• exhibit cardiac index (CI) greater than 2.5 liters/minute/m²
• maintain baseline heart rate
• maintain baseline PAWP, pulmonary artery systolic and diastolic pressures, and CVP.

Based on the nursing diagnosis *high risk for fluid volume deficit,* develop appropriate patient outcomes. For example, your patient will:
• maintain urine output greater than 30 ml/hour or 0.5 ml/kg/hour (depending on the patient's body size and physical condition)
• exhibit no signs of dehydration
• express understanding of the causes of fluid volume deficit.

Based on the nursing diagnosis *anxiety,* develop appropriate patient outcomes. For example, your patient will:
• experience less anxiety, as evidenced by verbal reports and behavior

• show willingness to adhere to diet and activity guidelines, take prescribed medications, and obtain follow-up medical care for underlying problems.

IMPLEMENTATION

Treatment for the patient with hypovolemic shock syndrome is directed at quickly restoring intravascular volume. (See *Medical care of the patient with hypovolemic shock syndrome.*)

Nursing interventions
• Position the patient supine with his legs elevated.
• Administer oxygen by face mask, airway, or endotracheal intubation and mechanical ventilation to ensure adequate tissue oxygenation.
• Start an I.V. infusion with 0.9% sodium chloride or lactated Ringer's solution, using a large-bore (14G to 18G) catheter, as prescribed, to ease future blood transfusions. If a large-bore needle is used, pressure bags should not be needed during blood transfusions. Excessive pressure may cause some of the RBCs to break apart, leading to hemolysis.

Caution: Do not start an I.V. infusion in the legs of a patient in hypovolemic shock. Peripheral vasoconstriction may cause pooling of the fluid and prevent any improvement in preload.
• Assist with insertion of a CVP line or pulmonary artery catheter for hemodynamic monitoring. Monitor the patient's CVP, pulmonary artery systolic and diastolic pressures, PAWP, and cardiac output.
• Insert an indwelling urinary catheter to measure hourly output. Urine output of less than 30 ml/hour (for the average adult) or less than 0.5 ml/kg/hour (depending on the patient's body size and physical condition) may indicate a problem with renal perfusion.

Treatments

Medical care of the patient with hypovolemic shock syndrome

Emergency treatment measures include replacement of intravascular volume with blood and blood products, crystalloid solutions and, possibly, application of a pneumatic antishock garment.

Blood and fluid replacement

Prompt and adequate blood and fluid replacement helps to restore intravascular volume and to raise and maintain systolic blood pressure above 80 mm Hg.

Infusion of 0.9% sodium chloride solution, lactated Ringer's solution, plasma proteins (albumin), or other plasma expanders may be used. (The choice of fluid is contingent on the cause of fluid loss.) A rapid solution infusion system can provide these crystalloids or colloids at high flow rates.

Pneumatic antishock garment

A pneumatic antishock garment (a MAST suit) is used for moderate to severe shock when symptoms of hypoperfusion of vital organs are present. It is contraindicated in patients with congestive heart failure or pulmonary edema.

Other treatment measures

Treatment also may include administering oxygen, identifying the bleeding site, controlling bleeding directly by applying pressure or elevating extremities, administering dopamine or another inotropic agent and, possibly, performing surgery. To be effective, administration of dopamine or another inotropic agent must be accompanied by vigorous fluid resuscitation.

Timesaving tip: Label each I.V. line close to the lumen with the name of the medication infusing through that port. This will help prevent drug incompatibilities and precipitation in the tubing. Also label each I.V. infusion pump with the name of the medication being delivered. This helps save time if you need to quickly identify a pump associated with a specific medication.

• Administer crystalloid solutions, blood, or blood products, as prescribed, until the patient achieves optimal preload. Optimal preload is indicated by PAWP of 12 to 18 mm Hg and urine output greater than 0.5 ml/kg/minute. (See *Fluid challenge algorithm*, page 306.)

• When fluid resuscitation begins, watch for signs of fluid overload, such as increased PAWP or CVP, crackles, or dyspnea.

• Administer vasopressors, as prescribed, only after achieving adequate fluid replacement; otherwise, cardiac decompensation may result, especially in patients with ischemic heart disease.

• When infusing a vasopressor, titrate the dose to achieve the target effect and carefully monitor the patient for adverse reactions.

• Draw blood samples to measure ABG levels. Adjust the oxygen flow rate as ABG measurements indicate.

• Frequently assess the patient's physical status and hemodynamic parameters. Perform frequent arterial blood pressure readings. Intervene immediately when the patient's systolic blood pressure drops below 80 mm Hg to avoid inadequate coronary artery blood flow, cardiac ischemia, arrhythmias, or further complications of low cardiac output.

Fluid challenge algorithm

To restore intravascular volume and optimal preload, transfusions of balanced crystalloid solutions, blood, or blood products may be required. The flowchart below is a guide to infusion rates for achieving optimal preload.

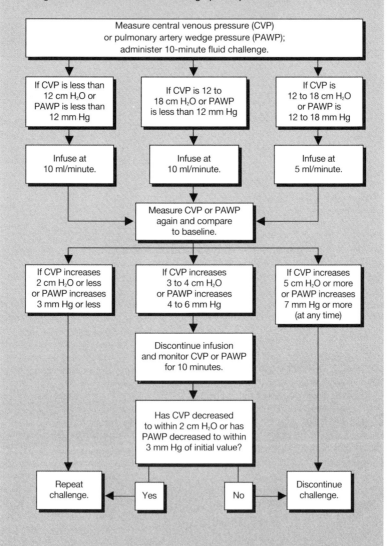

Discharge TimeSaver

Ensuring continued care for the patient with hypovolemic shock syndrome

Review the following teaching topics, referrals, and follow-up appointments to ensure that your patient is adequately prepared for discharge.

Teaching topics
Make sure that the following topics have been covered and that your patient's learning has been evaluated:
□ the condition, its risk factors, and its complications
□ measures to prevent future episodes of hypovolemic shock
□ diet and activity guidelines
□ medications, including precautions and potential adverse effects.

Referrals
Make sure that your patient has been provided with appropriate referrals to:
□ social services
□ home health care agency.

Follow-up appointments
Make sure that your patient has been provided with the times and dates for these necessary follow-up appointments:
□ doctor
□ diagnostic tests for reevaluation.

• Monitor the patient's cardiac rhythm continuously.

• Participate in related care to treat underlying causes of hypovolemic shock.

• Implement measures to ensure that the patient's oxygen and energy needs do not exceed their supply. For example, if anxiety is depleting the patient's oxygen supply and energy level, provide emotional support or administer sedatives, as prescribed.

• Draw venous blood samples for a complete blood count, electrolyte measurements, type and crossmatch, and coagulation studies.

• Watch for signs of impending coagulopathy, such as petechiae, bruising, bleeding, or oozing from gums or venipuncture sites.

• Monitor the patient's LOC by noting his orientation, his response to verbal commands or, if necessary, his response to painful stimuli.

• Provide emotional support to the patient and his family.

Patient teaching
• Explain all procedures to ease the patient's anxiety. Answer his questions honestly.

• Explain blood transfusion risks to the patient and his family.

• Discuss why and how hypovolemic shock occurred.

• Teach measures that will help prevent future episodes of hypovolemic shock syndrome. (See *Ensuring continued care for the patient with hypovolemic shock syndrome.*)

EVALUATION

To evaluate the patient's response to your nursing care, gather reassessment data and compare this information with the patient outcomes specified in your plan of care.

Teaching and counseling
Begin by evaluating the effectiveness of patient teaching and counseling. Document statements from the patient indicating:

FactFinder

Key points about cardiogenic shock

• *Frequency:* Cardiogenic shock is a serious complication in nearly 15% of all patients who are hospitalized with acute myocardial infarction (MI).
• *Pathology:* Cardiogenic shock typically affects patients whose MI involves 40% or more of the left ventricular muscle mass.
• *Mortality:* Most patients in cardiogenic shock die within 24 hours of onset because the body's vital organs cannot overcome the effects of extended hypoperfusion.

• intent to follow diet, activity, and medication guidelines
• intent to seek medical treatment for underlying causes of hypovolemic shock
• reduced anxiety after treatment for hypovolemic shock.

Physical condition

Next, evaluate the patient's physical condition. Consider the following questions:
• Are chest pain, cardiac arrhythmias, and shortness of breath present or absent?
• Does the patient demonstrate strong peripheral pulses, baseline skin color and temperature, baseline heart rate, and baseline LOC?
• Has systolic blood pressure returned to baseline?
• Are blood pressure, hemoglobin and hematocrit levels, RBC and platelet counts, and ABG levels within specified parameters?
• Are electrolyte levels, urine output, and urine specific gravity within specified parameters?
• What are current readings for the patient's cardiac output, CI, PAWP, pulmonary artery systolic and diastolic pressures, and CVP?

Cardiogenic shock

Cardiogenic shock, also known as pump failure, occurs when diminished cardiac output severely impairs tissue perfusion. It usually is fatal.

During cardiogenic shock, left ventricular dysfunction sets off a series of reactions, called compensatory responses, to offset decreased cardiac output and maintain vital organ function. Aortic and carotid baroreceptors activate sympathetic nervous responses. Heart rate, left ventricular filling pressure, and peripheral vascular resistance increase to enhance venous return to the heart. At first, these compensatory responses stabilize the patient. Later, however, they cause deterioration due to increasing oxygen demands on the compromised myocardium. This starts a repeating cycle of low cardiac output, sympathetic compensation, myocardial ischemia, and even lower cardiac output. (See *Key points about cardiogenic shock.*)

Causes

The most common cause of cardiogenic shock is myocardial infarction (MI), but it can be induced by any condition in which left ventricular dysfunction severely reduces cardiac output. Other causes of cardiogenic shock include major cardiac arrhythmias and papillary muscle dysfunction or rupture. Cardiogenic shock also may be caused by myocarditis and depression of myocardial contractility after cardiac arrest and prolonged cardiac surgery, acute acquired ventricular septal defect or ventricular aneurysm, or mechanical abnormalities of the ventricle, such as acute mitral or aortic insufficiency. Congestive heart failure can also progress to cardiogenic shock.

ASSESSMENT

Cardiogenic shock is an emergency situation that requires quick assessment and aggressive treatment. In many cases, the patient's medical history suggests an underlying disorder, such as acute MI, that severely decreases left ventricular function.

Health history

Patients with underlying cardiac disease who are in cardiogenic shock may report anginal pain due to decreased myocardial perfusion and oxygenation. At the onset of cardiogenic shock, the patient may report thirst, nausea, or anxiety.

Physical examination

During your initial inspection, you may note shallow, rapid respirations (exceeding 20 breaths/minute) and severe shortness of breath in patients with alveolar edema. The patient's skin may at first look pale, turning cyanotic and mottled in advanced stages of cardiogenic shock.

Assess the patient for reduced level of consciousness (LOC). In the early stages, he may become restless and agitated, then confused. Usually, the patient can respond to verbal stimuli and follow simple commands in the early stages of cardiogenic shock. As shock progresses, your patient ceases to respond to verbal stimuli but will exhibit flexion in response to painful stimuli, then extension, then flaccidity with no pain response.

Urine output may decrease to less than 30 ml/hour (for the average adult) or 0.5 ml/kg/hour (depending on the patient's body size and physical condition).

During palpation, you may detect rapid, thready peripheral pulses. Skin that feels cool and moist may be an early sign of hypoperfusion.

Auscultation of blood pressure usually reveals systolic blood pressure under 100 mm Hg and mean arterial pressure (MAP) under 80 mm Hg. In the early compensatory stage of cardiogenic shock, systolic pressure usually decreases slightly. Diastolic pressure remains unchanged or increases due to vasoconstriction. This results in a narrow pulse pressure, which indicates a need for prompt intervention. With decompensation, both systolic and diastolic pressures decrease and pulse pressure remains constant.

While auscultating heart sounds, you may hear an S_3 gallop. If cardiogenic shock results from rupture of the interventricular septum or papillary muscles, you will hear a holosystolic murmur.

In the early stages of cardiogenic shock, the heart rate may increase to between 100 and 150 beats/minute. With decompensation, the heart rate may exceed 150 beats/minute. You often will hear an irregular heart rhythm due to ischemic arrhythmias, especially when the heart rate exceeds 150 beats/minute.

When auscultating breath sounds, you may hear bibasilar crackles as pulmonary function worsens and pulmonary edema increases. Auscultation also may reveal hypoactive bowel sounds.

Hemodynamic monitoring

Hemodynamic monitoring may reveal increased left ventricular filling pressure, as reflected in the pulmonary artery wedge pressure (PAWP), which usually rises to more than 18 mm Hg.

Timesaving tip: If the patient has a normal sinus rhythm and his PAWP tracing shows tall v waves, take the PAWP measurement immediately after the a wave.

The patient's cardiac index (CI) may decrease to less than 2.2 liters/minute/m². Cardiac output may decrease to less than 4 liters/minute. Invasive arterial pressure monitoring may reveal systolic arterial pressure less than 80 mm Hg.

Diagnostic test results
The following test results help establish the diagnosis of cardiogenic shock:
• Chest X-ray may reveal an enlarged heart, suggesting congestive heart failure. It also may show pulmonary congestion or pulmonary edema.
• Arterial blood gas (ABG) analysis may show metabolic acidosis, respiratory acidosis, and hypoxia.
• Electrocardiography (ECG) may disclose evidence of acute MI, myocardial ischemia, major arrhythmias (excessively rapid or slow heart rates), or ventricular aneurysm.
• Serum enzyme measurements may reveal elevated levels of creatine kinase (CK), lactate dehydrogenase (LD), aspartate aminotransferase (formerly SGOT), and alanine aminotransferase (formerly SGPT), suggesting MI, myocardial ischemia, heart failure, or shock.
• Echocardiography helps to assess ventricular function, aortic and mitral valve insufficiencies, septal perforation, cardiac tamponade, and pericardial effusions.

NURSING DIAGNOSIS

Common nursing diagnoses for a patient in cardiogenic shock include:
• Decreased cardiac output related to pump failure
• Altered thought processes related to impaired cerebral perfusion
• Altered tissue perfusion (cardiopulmonary, cerebral, renal, gastrointestinal, or peripheral) related to pump failure
• Impaired gas exchange related to hypoxemia due to interstitial and alveolar edema
• Pain related to myocardial ischemia

• Anxiety related to elevated serum catecholamine levels, hypoxia, and the medical diagnosis.

PLANNING

Direct your plan of care for the cardiogenic shock patient toward enhancing cardiovascular status and improving myocardial perfusion.

Based on the nursing diagnosis *decreased cardiac output*, develop appropriate patient outcomes. For example, your patient will:
• maintain cardiac output at more than 5 liters/minute and CI at more than 2.5 liters/minute/m^2
• maintain baseline heart rate, respiratory rate, and breath sounds
• maintain pulmonary artery diastolic pressure (PADP) below 18 mm Hg
• maintain PAWP below 18 mm Hg
• maintain MAP of 80 mm Hg or higher
• maintain systolic blood pressure at 90 mm Hg or higher.

Based on the nursing diagnosis *altered thought processes*, develop appropriate patient outcomes. For example, your patient will:
• maintain baseline LOC.

Based on the nursing diagnosis *altered tissue perfusion*, develop appropriate patient outcomes. For example, your patient will:
• demonstrate strong peripheral pulses
• maintain baseline skin color and temperature.

Based on the nursing diagnosis *impaired gas exchange*, develop appropriate patient outcomes. For example, your patient will:
• maintain baseline ABG levels.

Based on the nursing diagnosis *pain,* develop appropriate patient outcomes. For example, your patient will:
• remain free from chest pain, cardiac arrhythmias, and shortness of breath.

Treatments

Medical care of the patient with cardiogenic shock

The goal of treatment for the patient with cardiogenic shock is to enhance cardiovascular status by increasing cardiac output, improving myocardial perfusion, and decreasing cardiac work load. Treatment procedures call for combinations of cardiovascular drugs and mechanical-assist techniques. Emergency surgery may be warranted.

Drug therapy
The following I.V. drugs are used to treat cardiogenic shock patients:
• *Dopamine:* A vasopressor that increases cardiac output, blood pressure, and renal perfusion.
• *Amrinone and dobutamine:* Inotropic agents that increase myocardial contractility.
• *Norepinephrine:* A potent vasoconstrictor.
  Nitroglycerin or nitroprusside may be used with a vasopressor to further improve cardiac output by reducing left ventricular end-diastolic pressure (preload) and decreasing peripheral vascular resistance (afterload). However, the patient's blood pressure must be adequate to support nitroglycerin or nitroprusside therapy and must be monitored closely.

Mechanical-assist techniques
The doctor may order insertion of an intra-aortic balloon pump (IABP) to improve coronary artery perfusion and decrease cardiac work load. The inflatable balloon pump is inserted through the femoral artery and passed into the descending thoracic aorta. The balloon inflates during diastole (to increase coronary artery perfusion pressure) and deflates before systole and before the aortic valve opens (to reduce resistance to ejection and lessen cardiac work load). Improved cardiac output and subsequent vasodilation in the peripheral vessels lead to lower preload volume.
  When drug therapy and IABP insertion fail, a ventricular assist pump may be used.

Based on the nursing diagnosis *anxiety,* develop appropriate patient outcomes. For example, your patient will:
• show willingness to use support systems to help reduce anxiety
• demonstrate reduced anxiety, either verbally or through behavior.

IMPLEMENTATION

Treatment for cardiogenic shock seeks to enhance the patient's cardiovascular status. An intra-aortic balloon pump (IABP) may be inserted to reduce the patient's cardiac work load. (See *Medical care of the patient with cardiogenic shock.*)

Nursing interventions
Care for the patient in cardiogenic shock is provided in the intensive care unit (ICU).
• The prognosis for surviving cardiogenic shock is poor. Therefore, provide emotional support to help the patient and family members prepare for possible emergency surgery or death.
• Secure the patient's airway and administer oxygen. A nonrebreather mask with a reservoir bag can provide 90% to 100% oxygen.
• Anticipate endotracheal intubation if the patient's partial pressure of oxygen in arterial blood is 60 mm Hg or lower when administering 100% oxygen; if oxygen saturation cannot be main-

tained at more than 90% with 100% oxygen administration; if your patient shows signs of decreasing LOC, such as restlessness, agitation, or confusion; or if you see signs of increasing acidosis and increasing partial pressure of carbon dioxide in arterial blood.

• In addition to endotracheal intubation and mechanical ventilation, some patients may require 5 to 15 cm H_2O of positive end-expiratory pressure or continuous positive airway pressure.

• Start an I.V. infusion with a large-bore catheter for fluid and drug administration. If your patient has profound hypotension and there is no evidence of pulmonary congestion, administer 0.9% sodium chloride or lactated Ringer's solution, as prescribed, to increase blood pressure. If the patient has pulmonary congestion, expect to administer dextrose 5% in water, as prescribed, at a keep-vein-open rate.

Timesaving tip: Label each I.V. line close to the lumen with the name of the medication infusing through that port. This will help to avoid drug incompatibilities and precipitation in the tubing. Also label each I.V. infusion pump with the name of the medication being delivered. This helps save time if you need to quickly identify a pump associated with a specific medication.

• Obtain a 12-lead ECG, assist with chest X-ray, and connect the patient to a cardiac monitor.

• Obtain blood samples for ABG analysis and other prescribed tests.

• Insert an indwelling urinary catheter to measure urine output. Output less than 30 ml/hour (for the average adult) or 0.5 ml/kg/hour (depending on the patient's body size and physical condition) usually indicates decreased renal perfusion.

• Assist with arterial line insertion for continuous blood pressure monitoring. A systolic blood pressure of less than 80 mm Hg often causes inadequate cor-

onary artery blood flow, resulting in myocardial ischemia, arrhythmia, or other complications of low cardiac output.

• Assist with inserting a pulmonary artery catheter. Closely monitor the patient's pulmonary artery pressure (PAP), PAWP, and CI. Increasing PAP and PAWP with decreasing cardiac output and CI indicate worsening of the patient's condition.

• If PADP is within 2 to 4 mm Hg of PAWP, monitor PADP instead of PAWP.

• When measuring intracardiac pressures, keep in mind that frequent balloon inflation may lead to balloon rupture and possible air embolism.

• When monitoring hemodynamic parameters, assess the patient and take appropriate action. For example, if PAWP is greater than 20 mm Hg and you detect increased dyspnea, frothy sputum, and crackles, administer a diuretic, such as furosemide, to reduce fluid volume and pulmonary edema.

• Administer medications, as prescribed, to improve the heart's pumping effectiveness. Titrate vasoactive and inotropic medications to achieve desired systolic blood pressure, MAP, PAWP, PADP, and CI.

• Monitor the patient for adverse reactions to medications and watch for signs of increasing hypoxemia or inadequate organ perfusion.

• Administer morphine in 2- to 5-mg increments at intervals of 30 minutes to 1 hour, as prescribed, to reduce pain and anxiety.

• Administer sedatives, as prescribed, according to the patient's status.

• If pharmacologic therapy fails to restore the balance between oxygen supply and demand, anticipate insertion of an IABP.

Intra-aortic balloon pump

• After an IABP is in place, move the patient as little as possible. Do not flex the catheterized leg at the hip, which could displace or rupture the catheter. Never place the patient in a sitting position or raise the head of the bed more than 30 degrees for any reason, including the need to obtain chest X-rays, while the balloon is inflated. Immediate death can result if a balloon tears through the aorta.

• If you're responsible for monitoring the pump's console, you will usually use an arterial waveform to synchronize inflation and deflation of the balloon (alternatively, you may use an ECG). Balloon inflation should begin when the aortic valve closes, as indicated by the dicrotic notch on the arterial waveform. Deflation should occur just before systole. Proper timing is crucial. Early inflation may damage the aortic valve by forcing it closed, whereas late inflation permits most of the blood emerging from the ventricle to flow past the balloon, reducing pump effectiveness. Late deflation increases the resistance against which the left ventricle must pump, possibly causing cardiac arrest.

• Evaluate circulation to the patient's leg by checking pedal pulses, skin temperature, and color.

• Frequently check the dressing at the insertion site for signs of bleeding, hematoma, or infection. Culture any drainage. Change dressings according to hospital protocol.

• Once the patient achieves hemodynamic stability, gradually decrease the frequency of balloon inflation. While weaning the patient, carefully monitor for chest pain or other signs of recurring myocardial ischemia and cardiogenic shock.

• Prepare the patient for emergency surgery, cardiac catheterization, emergency percutaneous transluminal coronary angioplasty, or administration of an intravenous thrombolytic agent, if necessary.

• Take steps to alleviate the patient's anxiety. Anxiety stimulates the release of catecholamines and further increases myocardial consumption. Encourage the patient to express his fears. Provide frequent rest periods and as much privacy as possible for the patient. Allow family members to visit and comfort the patient. Provide prescribed sedatives, as needed.

Patient teaching
Answer all questions from the patient and family members regarding equipment used in the ICU, drug therapy, IABP therapy, or other procedures. (See *Ensuring continued care for the patient with cardiogenic shock*, page 314.)

EVALUATION

To evaluate the patient's response to your nursing care, gather reassessment data and compare this information with the patient outcomes specified in your plan of care. Because of the gravity of cardiogenic shock, the patient's status may change rapidly or dramatically, requiring revisions of your plan of care, nursing diagnoses, and interventions. Also, be aware that the patient may not regain effective cardiac pumping action despite the best clinical efforts.

Physical condition
Consider the following questions:
• Has the patient experienced a reduction in chest pain, cardiac arrhythmias, and shortness of breath?
• Is LOC at or near baseline?
• Does the patient maintain adequate urine output?
• Are his peripheral pulses palpable and strong?
• Do skin color and temperature appear to remain at baseline?

Discharge TimeSaver
Ensuring continued care for the patient with cardiogenic shock

If your patient recovers from cardiogenic shock, review the following teaching topics, referrals, and follow-up appointments to ensure that he's adequately prepared for discharge.

Teaching topics
Make sure that the following topics have been covered and that your patient's learning has been evaluated:
☐ the condition, its risk factors, and its complications
☐ measures that will help prevent future episodes of cardiogenic shock
☐ diet and activity restrictions
☐ medications, including precautions and potential adverse effects.

Referrals
Make sure that your patient has been

provided with appropriate referrals to:
☐ social services
☐ home health care agency.

Follow-up appointments
Make sure that your patient has been provided with the times and dates for these necessary follow-up appointments:
☐ doctor
☐ surgeon
☐ diagnostic tests for reevaluation.

Cardiac output
Check the patient for evidence of improved cardiac output. Assess his heart rate, respiratory rate, breath sounds, and ABG levels. Determine whether the following parameters are maintained:
• PADP and PAWP below 18 mm Hg
• systolic blood pressure at 90 mm Hg or higher
• MAP greater than 80 mm Hg.

Anxiety
Continue your evaluation by assessing whether the patient exhibits less anxiety. Does he use available support systems to help reduce anxiety?

Ventricular aneurysm

A ventricular aneurysm is a non-contractile outpouching of a ventricle. It almost always affects the heart's left ventricle. Ventricular aneurysms may

become enlarged but seldom rupture. Ventricular aneurysm can lead to potentially life-threatening conditions, such as ventricular arrhythmia, cerebral embolization, or heart failure.

Aggressive management of acute myocardial infarction (MI) with thrombolytic therapy may decrease the incidence of ventricular aneurysm. When ventricular failure or ventricular arrhythmias do occur in patients with ventricular aneurysm, resection improves the prognosis.

Causes
Ventricular aneurysm is a complication of MI. It occurs in about 8% to 15% of MI cases. An aneurysm may develop days, weeks, or years after MI occurs. The condition usually is associated with transmural infarction and involves the anterior or apical wall in 80% of cases. (See *Looking at ventricular aneurysm.*)

Looking at ventricular aneurysm

When myocardial infarction destroys a large, muscular section of the left ventricle, necrosis reduces the ventricular wall to a thin layer of fibrous tissue. The thin wall stretches under intracardiac pressure and forms a ventricular aneurysm.

Blood is diverted to the distended muscle wall of the aneurysm, which does not contract. To maintain stroke volume and cardiac output, the remaining normally functioning myocardial fibers increase contractile force.

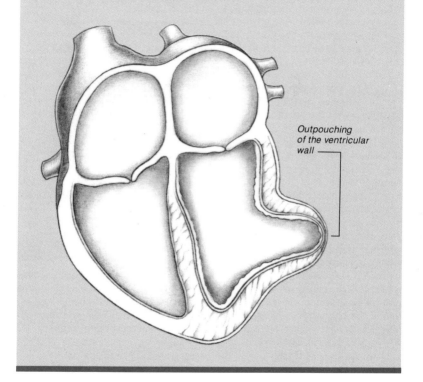

Outpouching of the ventricular wall

ASSESSMENT

During your assessment, check the patient's medical history for MI. Keep in mind that the patient may have experienced a silent MI that was never diagnosed and, consequently, not documented.

Health history

The patient with ventricular aneurysm may report palpitations and anginal pain. If aneurysm causes heart failure, the patient may report dyspnea, fatigue, and peripheral edema.

Physical examination

During inspection, you may observe a systolic precordial bulge, which may be palpable. If the patient is experiencing heart failure, you may observe distended neck veins.

Palpation of the patient's peripheral pulses may reveal arrhythmias, such as premature ventricular contractions or ventricular tachycardia. You may detect pulsus alternans.

When palpating the patient's chest, you may detect a double, diffuse, or displaced apical impulse.

During auscultation, you may hear an irregular or gallop heart rhythm. If your patient is experiencing heart failure, you may note crackles and rhonchi.

Diagnostic test results

The following test results may confirm the diagnosis of ventricular aneurysm:

• Two-dimensional echocardiography reveals abnormal motion in the left ventricular wall, left ventricular enlargement, and decreased ejection fraction.

• Left ventriculography shows left ventricular enlargement with an area of akinesia or dyskinesia (during cardiac catheterization) and reveals diminished cardiac function.

• Electrocardiography may show persistent ST-T segment elevations at rest.

• Chest X-rays may disclose an abnormal bulge distorting the heart's contour if the aneurysm is large. X-rays may not reveal a small aneurysm.

• Myocardial perfusion imaging may indicate the site of MI and suggest the area of aneurysm.

NURSING DIAGNOSIS

Common nursing diagnoses for ventricular aneurysm include:

• Decreased cardiac output related to reduced stroke volume

• Fluid volume excess related to heart failure

• Anxiety related to the medical diagnosis and risk of complications.

PLANNING

Based on the nursing diagnosis *decreased cardiac output,* develop appropriate patient outcomes. For example, your patient will:

• maintain hemodynamic stability

• maintain adequate tissue perfusion

• agree to comply with prescribed treatments to increase cardiac output

• list signs and symptoms of heart failure

• express understanding of the need to immediately report signs and symptoms of heart failure or angina.

Based on the nursing diagnosis *fluid volume excess,* develop appropriate patient outcomes. For example, your patient will:

• regain fluid balance following treatment for heart failure.

Based on the nursing diagnosis *anxiety,* develop appropriate patient outcomes. For example, your patient will:

• identify signs of anxiety

• describe two methods for coping with anxiety

• exhibit signs of reduced anxiety.

IMPLEMENTATION

Depending on the severity of the condition, treatment for a ventricular aneurysm ranges from routine to aggressive. (See *Medical care of the patient with ventricular aneurysm.*)

Nursing interventions

• For the patient with heart failure, closely monitor his vital signs, heart sounds, intake and output, fluid and electrolyte balance, and blood urea nitrogen and serum creatinine levels.

• Watch for sudden changes in sensorium, which may indicate cerebral embolization.

• Monitor the patient for signs of renal failure or MI.

• Arrhythmia may require elective cardioversion. If the patient is conscious,

Treatments

Medical care of the patient with ventricular aneurysm

Depending on the size of the aneurysm and the complications that occur, treatment ranges from routine medical examinations to monitor the condition to more aggressive measures. Surgery may be warranted for patients with intractable ventricular arrhythmias, heart failure, worsening angina, and ventricular thrombus formation and emboli.

Emergency measures
Emergency treatment for a patient with ventricular arrhythmia may include administration of I.V. antiarrhythmics. Cardioversion or defibrillation may be required. Emergency measures for a patient experiencing heart failure with pulmonary edema include oxygen administration, digoxin I.V., furosemide I.V., potassium replacement, morphine I.V., and, when necessary, nitroprusside I.V. and endotracheal intubation.

Drug therapy for complications of ventricular aneurysm
Treatment for a patient with ventricular aneurysm and arrhythmia may include administering oral antiarrhythmics, such as procainamide or quinidine. Maintenance drug therapy following emergency treatment for congestive heart failure may consist of oral nitrates, captopril, and hydralazine.

Additional treatments
Anticoagulants or embolectomy may be warranted for the patient with systemic embolization. Surgery also may be required for a patient with refractory ventricular tachycardia, heart failure, recurrent arterial embolization, and persistent angina with coronary artery occlusion. The most effective surgery in such cases is aneurysmectomy with myocardial revascularization.

---

administer diazepam by I.V. infusion, as prescribed, before cardioversion.

• If the patient is receiving antiarrhythmics, check appropriate laboratory test results. For example, if the patient takes procainamide, check antinuclear antibody levels because the drug may induce signs and symptoms that mimic lupus erythematosus.

• If the patient is scheduled for resection, describe preoperative and postoperative care measures and explain intensive care unit procedures and equipment, such as endotracheal tubes, ventilators, and chest tubes.

• After surgery, monitor the patient's vital signs, intake and output, heart sounds, and hemodynamic parameters. Watch for signs of infection, such as fever or drainage from the incision.

• Provide psychological support for the patient and his family as needed.

Patient teaching
• Teach the patient how to check for pulse irregularities and rate changes.

• Advise the patient to adhere to the prescribed medication regimen and to report adverse reactions. Tell him to keep doses evenly spaced, even if this requires taking medication at night.

• Refer the patient to a cardiac rehabilitation program for activity and diet instructions.

• Refer family members to a cardiopulmonary resuscitation training program. (See *Ensuring continued care for the patient with ventricular aneurysm,* page 318.)

Discharge TimeSaver
Ensuring continued care for the patient with ventricular aneurysm

Review the following teaching topics, referrals, and follow-up appointments to ensure that your patient is adequately prepared for discharge.

Teaching topics
Make sure that the following topics have been covered and that your patient's learning has been evaluated:
□ causes of ventricular aneurysm
□ method of taking a pulse
□ prescribed medications, especially precautions and possible adverse effects
□ warning signs and symptoms of heart failure, cerebral emboli, arrhythmias, and angina
□ possible elective cardioversion.

Referrals
Make sure that your patient has been provided with appropriate referrals to:

□ cardiac rehabilitation program
□ social services
□ home health care agency
□ community-based cardiopulmonary resuscitation training program for family.

Follow-up appointments
Make sure that your patient has been provided with the times and dates for these necessary follow-up appointments:
□ doctor
□ surgeon
□ diagnostic tests for reevaluation.

EVALUATION

To evaluate the patient's response to your nursing care, gather reassessment data and compare this information with the patient outcomes specified in your plan of care.

Teaching and counseling
Begin by evaluating the effectiveness of your teaching and counseling. Consider the following questions:
• Can the patient identify signs of anxiety and is he willing to use coping methods to reduce anxiety?
• Can he identify early signs of heart failure and does he understand the need for immediate medical treatment if such signs occur?
• Is he willing to comply with prescribed treatment measures?

Physical condition
Consider the following questions:

• Does the patient demonstrate evidence of hemodynamic stability?
• Is tissue perfusion adequate?
• Is he able to maintain fluid balance?

Cardiac tamponade

In this disorder, a rapid or drastic rise in intrapericardial pressure impairs diastolic filling of the heart. The rise in pressure usually results from blood or fluid accumulation in the pericardial sac. (See *Key points about cardiac tamponade*.)

Causes
Cardiac tamponade may be idiopathic (Dressler's syndrome). It may also result from:
• effusion secondary to cancer, bacterial infections, tuberculosis or, in rare cases, acute rheumatic fever

- hemorrhage from trauma, such as gunshot or stab wounds of the chest, perforation by a catheter during cardiac or central venous catheterization, or postcardiac surgery
- hemorrhage from a nontraumatic cause, such as rupture of an aneurysm, aortic dissection, or anticoagulant therapy for pericarditis
- viral, postirradiation, or idiopathic pericarditis
- acute myocardial infarction
- chronic renal failure during dialysis
- drug reaction, possibly to procainamide, hydralazine, minoxidil, isoniazid, penicillin, methysergide, or daunorubicin
- connective tissue disorders, such as rheumatoid arthritis, systemic lupus erythematosus, rheumatic fever, vasculitis, or scleroderma.

ASSESSMENT

Your patient assessment should include a review of the patient's medical history for disorders that can lead to cardiac tamponade. You will need to pay close attention to physical examination findings and diagnostic test results.

Health history
The patient may report acute pain and dyspnea.

Physical examination
The clinical presentation of cardiac tamponade depends on how rapidly it develops. If cardiac tamponade develops slowly, the patient will not look as critically ill as a patient with rapidly developing tamponade.

During inspection, you may note that your patient is orthopneic, diaphoretic, anxious, and restless. He may need to sit upright and lean forward to breathe more easily and to reduce pain. The patient's skin may look pale or cyanotic. Neck vein distention may occur

FactFinder
Key points about cardiac tamponade

- *Pathophysiology:* The pericardial sac normally holds 30 to 50 ml of fluid. Any increase in fluid may cause a rise in intrapericardial pressure. However, the rate of accumulation is more important than the volume in determining if cardiac tamponade will occur. If fluid accumulates slowly, the pericardial fibers stretch to accommodate 1 to 2 liters of fluid. However, if fluid accumulates rapidly, the addition of 200 ml of fluid in the pericardial sac may lead to a medical emergency.
- *Complications:* If cardiac tamponade is not treated, pressure from fluid in the pericardium impairs ventricular filling and cardiac output. Cardiogenic shock and death may result.
- *Treatment:* The major treatment for cardiac tamponade is pericardiocentesis (the removal of pericardial fluid through a needle, cannula, or catheter, or by open drainage).

secondary to increased venous pressure. If the patient is hypovolemic, however, neck vein distention may not occur.

Palpation may reveal rapid, weak peripheral pulses. Palpation of the right upper quadrant of the abdomen may reveal hepatomegaly.

When performing chest percussion, you may detect a widening area of flatness across the patient's anterior chest wall, indicating a large effusion.

Auscultation of blood pressure may reveal decreased arterial blood pressure and narrow pulse pressure. Pulsus paradoxus (an abnormal inspiratory drop in systemic blood pressure greater than 15 mm Hg) is usually present and is an important finding because most patients with slowly developing

Assessment TimeSaver

Understanding clinical findings in cardiac tamponade

Clinical findings	Cause
Chest pain, dyspnea, fullness in the chest, distant heart sounds, pulsus paradoxus	Increased pressure in the pericardial sac resulting from accumulation of pericardial fluid
Anxiety, restlessness	Epinephrine release in response to stress
Tachycardia, hypotension, narrow pulse pressure	Decreased cardiac output secondary to reduced blood volume entering the heart
Jugular vein distention, elevated central venous pressure	Impaired filling of the right side of the heart leading to venous distention
Decreased consciousness or loss of consciousness	Decreased cardiac output leading to decreased cerebral perfusion (in severe tamponade)

tamponade do not exhibit classic physical signs and symptoms.

Heart sounds may be muffled. During severe tamponade — occurring after cardiac rupture or trauma, for example — you may note a quiet heart with faint sounds. This finding usually appears within minutes of the onset of cardiac tamponade. The combination of muffled heart sounds, narrowed pulse pressure, and neck vein distention is commonly referred to as Beck's triad. Breath sounds are clear. (See *Understanding clinical findings in cardiac tamponade.*)

Diagnostic test results
The following test results help establish the diagnosis of cardiac tamponade:
• Chest X-rays may show a slightly widened mediastinum and enlargement of the cardiac silhouette.
• Electrocardiography (ECG) helps rule out other cardiac disorders. The QRS amplitude may be reduced, and electrical alternans of the QRS complex may be present. In severe cardiac tamponade, you may see alternans of the P wave,

QRS complex, and T wave. Generalized ST-segment elevation is noted in all leads.
• Pulmonary artery pressure monitoring reveals increases in right atrial pressure (RAP), right ventricular end-diastolic pressure (RVEDP), and pulmonary artery wedge pressure (PAWP).
• Echocardiography provides a record of the presence and magnitude of pericardial effusion. It also detects diastolic right ventricular and atrial compression, an early sign of cardiac tamponade.

NURSING DIAGNOSIS

Common nursing diagnoses for a patient with cardiac tamponade include:
• Decreased cardiac output related to increased intrapericardial pressure
• Altered tissue perfusion (cerebral, renal, or cardiopulmonary) related to decreased cardiac output
• Pain related to ineffective breathing patterns
• Anxiety related to the medical diagnosis.

PLANNING

Direct your plan of care for the patient with cardiac tamponade toward relieving the patient's symptoms, preventing complications, and teaching the patient about the disorder and expected treatments.

Based on the nursing diagnosis *decreased cardiac output,* develop appropriate patient outcomes. For example, your patient will:
• regain baseline intracardiac pressures, including RAP, RVEDP, and PAWP.
• maintain normal renal function, as evidenced by urine output of at least 30 ml/hour or 0.5 ml/kg/hour, depending on the patient's body size and physical condition
• have no cardiac arrhythmias that threaten hemodynamic stability
• maintain baseline ABG levels.

Based on the nursing diagnosis *altered tissue perfusion,* develop appropriate patient outcomes. For example, your patient will:
• maintain pulse rate and blood pressure within specified ranges
• maintain baseline level of consciousness (LOC)
• maintain respiratory rate within 5 breaths of baseline.

Based on the nursing diagnosis *pain,* develop appropriate patient outcomes. For example, your patient will:
• report being able to breathe more comfortably.

Based on the nursing diagnosis *anxiety,* develop appropriate patient outcomes. For example, your patient will:
• express feelings of anxiety
• identify causes of anxiety
• exhibit fewer signs of anxiety after interventions.

IMPLEMENTATION

Focus your nursing interventions on providing care before and after pericardiocentesis or thoracotomy. If your patient is not already in the intensive care unit, arrange for transfer. (See *Medical care of the patient with cardiac tamponade,* page 322.)

Nursing interventions
• Check for signs of increasing tamponade, as evidenced by increasing dyspnea, tachycardia, and diminished (distant) heart sounds.
• Administer oxygen therapy as needed.
• Prepare the patient for pericardiocentesis, pericardotomy, or pericardiectomy, as indicated. Help alleviate anxiety by explaining procedures and allowing the patient to voice concerns. Provide emotional support as needed for the patient and his family.
• Infuse I.V. solutions and possibly an inotropic drug, such as dopamine, as prescribed, to maintain the patient's blood pressure.
• Assist with the insertion of a pulmonary arterial catheter. Closely monitor the patient's hemodynamic status.

Pericardiocentesis care
• Place at the patient's bedside a pericardiocentesis tray, an ECG machine, and an emergency cart with a defibrillator. Make sure the equipment is turned on and ready for immediate use.
• Use an ECG to monitor the aspiration needle's placement. Position the patient at a 45- to 60-degree angle. Connect the precordial ECG lead to the hub of the aspiration needle to monitor for ST-segment changes. Assist with fluid aspiration. When the needle touches the myocardium, you will observe an ST-segment elevation or premature ventricular contractions on the rhythm strip. Note that some doctors may use echocardiography to monitor needle placement.
• Monitor the patient's cardiac rhythm, pulse rate, LOC, and respiratory status during and after the procedure.

Treatments

Medical care of the patient with cardiac tamponade

The goal of treatment is to relieve intrapericardial pressure and cardiac compression by removing accumulated blood or fluid.

Draining pericardial fluid
To remove accumulated fluid, the doctor may do one of the following:
• perform pericardiocentesis (needle aspiration of the pericardial cavity)
• surgically create an opening in the pericardial sac (a pericardial window)
• surgically place a drain in the pericardial sac to remove the effusion.
  This dramatically improves systemic arterial pressure and cardiac output (even if as little as 25 ml of fluid is aspirated). A drain may be left in place until the effusion process stops or until another corrective action, such as opening a pericardial window, is performed. If infection develops, antibiotics can be instilled through the drain, which is clamped, and later drained off.

Maintaining cardiac output
For a hypotensive patient, trial volume loading with I.V. 0.9% sodium chloride solution with albumin, and perhaps an inotropic drug such as dopamine, is necessary to maintain cardiac output.

Additional treatments
Depending on what causes the tamponade, additional treatments may include:
• blood transfusion or a thoracotomy to drain accumulating fluid or to repair bleeding sites if caused by traumatic injury
• protamine (a heparin antagonist) in case of heparin-induced tamponade
• vitamin K in case of warfarin-induced tamponade.

• Monitor the patient's blood pressure, RAP, pulmonary artery pressure (PAP), and PAWP during and after pericardiocentesis. A decrease in RAP and PAP and an increase in blood pressure indicate relief of intrapericardial pressure. Be aware that cardiac tamponade can recur, however, and continue to monitor the patient carefully.

Complications
Notify the doctor immediately if you detect complications of pericardiocentesis.
• Arrhythmias may result from the needle touching the myocardium.
• If the myocardium or a coronary artery is lacerated, the patient may experience hemorrhage, increased heart rate, and decreased blood pressure. Signs, however, may be masked. Check aspirated fluids for clots, anoth-

er possible indication of laceration. If you see clots, prepare for immediate surgical repair and resuscitation.
• Needle perforation of the lung, liver, or stomach may cause sudden chest or epigastric pain, dyspnea, or decreased blood pressure. If the needle punctures a lung, the patient may develop pneumothorax and require immediate chest tube insertion. If the needle punctures the liver or stomach, he may require surgical repair of the tear.
• An elevated white blood cell count, fever, chills, and drainage or redness at the insertion site may indicate infection.

Thoracotomy care
• Prepare the patient for surgery. Administer antibiotics, protamine, and vitamin K, as prescribed.

Discharge TimeSaver

Ensuring continued care for the patient with cardiac tamponade

Review the following teaching topics, referrals, and follow-up appointments to ensure that your patient is adequately prepared for discharge. Keep in mind that you will need to individualize the discharge plan for your patient depending on the underlying cause of cardiac tamponade.

Teaching topics
Make sure that the following topics have been covered and that your patient's learning has been evaluated:
☐ causes of cardiac tamponade and its risk factors and complications
☐ home care measures including activity guidelines and incisional care
☐ follow-up treatment for underlying conditions
☐ warning signs and symptoms that should be reported to the doctor.

Referrals
Make sure that your patient has been provided with appropriate referrals to:
☐ social services
☐ home health care agency.

Follow-up appointments
Make sure that your patient has been provided with the times and dates for these necessary follow-up appointments:
☐ medical doctor
☐ surgeon
☐ diagnostic tests for reevaluation.

• After surgery, monitor your patient's vital signs and ABG levels. Assess his heart and breath sounds.

• Administer prescribed pain medication.

• Maintain the patient's chest drainage system and watch for signs of complications, such as hemorrhage and arrhythmias.

Patient teaching
• Describe the condition, its cause, and treatments.

• Explain what the patient may expect after surgery, such as the use of chest tubes, drainage bottles, and oxygen.

• Before surgery, teach the patient how to turn, breathe deeply, and cough.

• Instruct the patient to immediately alert the nurse if his symptoms worsen.

• Discuss the details of home care measures, including activity guidelines and possible incision care.

• Emphasize the importance of complying with follow-up care measures and keeping appointments.

• List warning signs and symptoms to immediately report to the doctor. (See *Ensuring continued care for the patient with cardiac tamponade.*)

EVALUATION

To evaluate your patient's response to nursing care, gather reassessment data and compare this information with the patient outcomes specified in your plan of care.

Teaching and counseling
Evaluate the effectiveness of your teaching and counseling by considering the following questions:

• Does the patient express feelings of anxiety?

• Does he exhibit fewer signs of anxiety following interventions?

• Does he demonstrate understanding of the importance of follow-up care?

Physical condition
Consider the following questions:
• Does the patient maintain baseline LOC and does he breathe comfortably?
• Are his pulses and blood pressure readings within specified ranges?
• Has respiratory rate returned to within 5 breaths of baseline?
• Have ABG measurements returned to baseline levels?
• Does the patient's urine output indicate normal renal function?
• Do cardiac rhythm strips indicate that arrhythmias are present or absent?

Appendices and index

Quick reference to cardiovascular treatments

Treatment	Indications	Complications
Arterial bypass grafting in the lower extremities This surgical procedure involves grafting of an autogenous vein or a synthetic graft to bypass an arterial occlusion and restore continuous blood flow in the extremity.	• Arterial occlusive disease	• Thrombosis, narrowing, dilation, or rupture of graft • Infection • Hemorrhage • Embolism • Compartment syndrome • Lymphocele
Atherectomy In this procedure, a special catheter is threaded into a plaque-narrowed artery. In directional coronary atherectomy, the catheter has a rotating cutting blade that cuts the plaque. A balloon is used to stabilize the catheter without dilating the stenotic area. In transluminal extraction atherectomy, an investigational procedure, the catheter has a rotating abrasive tip that grinds plaque into fine particles. Atherectomy may be performed with or without percutaneous transluminal coronary angioplasty (PTCA).	In coronary artery disease (CAD), atherectomy may be performed to: • decrease residual stenosis, restenosis, and early and late abrupt closure • minimize dissection or intervene when dissection causes abrupt closure • treat lesions that are unapproachable by conventional angioplasty • treat lesions when balloon methods have failed	• Restenosis • Embolization • Bleeding from catheter entry site • Arrhythmia • Myocardial infarction (MI) • Coronary dissection or perforation • Coronary artery spasm
Use of implantable cardioverter defibrillator This procedure involves surgical implantation of a pulse generator and lead system to monitor the heart's electrical activity and treat tachyarrhythmias. When the implantable cardioverter defibrillator senses a ventricular tachyarrhythmia, it discharges a small shock (25 to 30 joules) to defibrillate the heart automatically.	• Detection and treatment of tachycardias in patients who have survived one episode of cardiac arrest • Detection and treatment of tachycardias in patients who, in the absence of previous arrest, can be induced into sustained hypotensive ventricular tachycardia or ventricular fibrillation despite drug treatment	• Infection • Arrhythmias • Device failure or malfunction, including inadvertent shocks, inadvertent deactivation of device, or malfunction of unit or lead system
Cardioversion, synchronized Cardioversion delivers an electrical current to the heart through paddles applied to the patient's chest, in an effort to restore normal rhythm. This procedure differs from defibrillation in two ways: much lower energy levels are used (typi-	• Unstable ventricular tachycardia with a pulse • Unstable supraventricular tachycardia • Stable atrial arrhythmias (elective procedure)	• Induction of ventricular fibrillation • Induction of pulseless ventricular tachycardia • Electrical burns • Marked bradycardia • Embolic episodes

Quick reference to cardiovascular treatments *(continued)*

Treatment	Indications	Complications
Cardioversion, synchronized *(continued)* cally 25 to 100 joules), and the burst of electricity is precisely timed to coincide with the peak of the R wave. It may be performed as an emergency or elective procedure.		
Carotid sinus massage This vagal maneuver, used to slow the heart rate, is performed by applying manual pressure for 3 to 5 seconds to the left or right carotid sinus.	• Atrial tachycardias • Junctional tachycardias • Supraventricular tachycardias • Diagnostic aid for certain arrhythmias	• Ventricular fibrillation • Ventricular tachycardia • Bradycardia that may advance to complete heart block or asystole • Cerebrovascular accident (CVA)
Coronary artery bypass grafting (CABG) This surgical procedure circumvents an occluded or stenosed coronary artery with an autogenous graft (usually a segment of the saphenous vein or internal mammalian artery), thereby restoring blood flow to the myocardium. CABG techniques vary according to the patient's condition and the number of arterial bypasses.	• Unstable angina from atherosclerosis despite medical therapy • Acute MI • Some uncontrollable ventricular arrhythmias • CAD with a high MI risk • Coronary lesions not treatable with PTCA and other procedures • Significant left main CAD	• CVA • Pulmonary embolism • Wound infection • Hemorrhage • Hypertension • Shock • Perioperative MI • Myocardial injury • Electrolyte imbalances • Atelectasis • Arrhythmias • Cardiac tamponade • Heart failure • Hypotension • Hypovolemia • Postpericardiotomy syndrome
Defibrillation In this advanced cardiac life support procedure, a defibrillator delivers a strong burst of electrical current to the heart through paddles applied to the patient's chest. This brief electric shock completely depolarizes the myocardium, allowing the heart's natural pacemaker to regain control of cardiac rhythm.	• Ventricular fibrillation • Pulseless ventricular tachycardia	• Electrical burns • Possible induction of ventricular fibrillation if used in patients with supraventricular tachyarrhythmias
Heart transplantation This procedure involves the surgical replacement of a diseased heart with a healthy one from a brain-dead donor.	End-stage cardiac disease after more conventional therapies have failed. Candidates may have a history of:	• Hemorrhage • Cardiac tamponade • Heart failure • MI • Hypertension

(continued)

Quick reference to cardiovascular treatments *(continued)*

Treatment	Indications	Complications
Heart transplantation *(continued)*	• Severe CAD or widespread left ventricular dysfunction • Idiopathic hypertrophic subaortic stenosis • Myotonic muscular dystrophy • Cardiomyopathy caused by viral infection	• Fluid and electrolyte imbalances • Infection • Rejection • Arrhythmia • Pneumothorax • Atelectasis • Thrombus formation and embolization • Renal failure • Postcardiotomy psychosis • Cardiac arrest • Graft atherosclerosis • Accelerated CAD
Intra-aortic balloon counter-pulsation (IABC) The IABC device consists of a single-chamber or multichamber polyurethane balloon (inserted via the femoral artery into the descending aorta) attached to an external pump console by a large-lumen catheter. The external pump works in precise counterpoint to the left ventricle, inflating the balloon early in diastole and deflating it just before systole. Balloon inflation forces blood toward the aortic valve, augmenting diastolic pressure and improving coronary artery perfusion. Balloon deflation reduces aortic volume and pressure and the work load of the left ventricle in opening the aortic valve.	• Left ventricular failure and cardiogenic shock caused by acute MI • Unstable or preinfarction angina • Support with high-risk cardiac surgery • Support before cardiac surgery • Acute mitral regurgitation and ventricular septal defect • Angina after infarction • Septic shock • Pulmonary embolism • Myocardial contusion	• Aortic or femoral artery dissection or perforation • Thrombocytopenia • Ischemia or loss of pulses in extremities • Thrombus formation and subsequent pulmonary embolism or CVA • Gas embolus from balloon rupture • Infection at balloon insertion site
Laser angioplasty In this procedure, which may be performed with or in place of PTCA, a laser-containing catheter is threaded into a plaque-narrowed coronary artery. Laser bursts then almost instantly vaporize the fatty, fibrous, and calcified plaque and restore blood flow.	• CAD, including patients with lesions not ideal for PTCA, such as lesions longer than 20 mm or involving the ostium • Diffuse CAD, including removal of calcified lesions • Restenotic lesions • Highly degenerated or thrombotic vein grafts • Lesions that can't be dilated with a balloon	• Dissection or perforation of coronary artery • MI • Restenosis of involved artery • CVA • Hematoma at femoral puncture site • Coronary embolism

Quick reference to cardiovascular treatments *(continued)*

Treatment	Indications	Complications
Use of a pacemaker These battery-operated generators emit timed electrical impulses that trigger heart-muscle contraction and control the heart rate. Fixed-rate pacemakers fire continuously; demand pacemakers, if the intrinsic heart rate drops below a preset limit. Demand pacemakers may be single chamber (with the pacing wire located in the right atria or ventricle) or dual chamber (with two pacing wires, one in each right chamber). A rate-responsive pacemaker can be programmed to respond to increased demand by increasing its firing rate. These pacemakers have an activity sensor that can detect electromuscular acceleration. Temporary pacemakers come in four types: *transcutaneous* (completely noninvasive); *transvenous* (inserted via the subclavian or jugular vein into the right ventricle); *transthoracic* (needle insertion of leads into the heart); and *epicardial* (implanted during open-heart surgery). A permanent pacemaker may be implanted through a thoracotomy but most doctors use the transvenous approach.	For permanent pacemaker: • Symptomatic sinus bradycardia • Advanced second-degree atrioventricular (AV) block • Complete AV block • Sick sinus syndrome • Bradycardia-tachycardia syndrome For temporary pacemaker: • During cardiopulmonary resuscitation • Before or during open-heart surgery • During catheterization on the right side of the heart or during PTCA in patients with preexisting bundle-branch block • After cardiac surgery • Symptomatic arrhythmias, such as second-degree and complete AV block brought on by acute MI • Tachyarrhythmias unresponsive to medications • Before permanent pacemaker insertion	Complications of permanent pacemaker: • Bleeding at insertion site • Intrathoracic bleeding • Transvenous lead-related thrombosis • Embolus • Infection • Pneumothorax • Hemothorax • Pacer-induced muscle stimulation • Arrhythmias • Cardiac tamponade • Abnormal pacemaker operation with lead dislodgment or fracture, including failure to capture, failure to sense, firing loss, pacemaker rejection, pacemaker syndrome, and pacemaker-mediated tachycardia Complications of temporary pacemaker: • Bleeding at insertion site • Ventricular arrhythmias • Pneumothorax • Hemothorax • Infection • Pacemaker malfunction
Percutaneous balloon valvuloplasty This procedure is an alternative for patients who are poor candidates for valvular surgery to repair mitral or aortic stenosis. Performed under local anesthesia, it involves insertion of a catheter into an artery or vein in the groin and advancement to the involved mitral or aortic valve, where balloon inflation is used to enlarge the valve orifice.	• Mitral stenosis • Aortic stenosis	In aortic stenosis: • Cardiac tamponade • Fatal arrhythmias • CVA • Sepsis • Ventricular perforation and tamponade • Massive aortic insufficiency • Vascular injury • Embolic events In mitral stenosis: • Thrombotic episodes (transient) • Mitral insufficiency • Transient heart block • Pericardial tamponade *(continued)*

Quick reference to cardiovascular treatments *(continued)*

Treatment	Indications	Complications
Percutaneous transluminal coronary angioplasty A nonsurgical alternative to CABG, PTCA is usually performed in the cardiac catheterization laboratory under a local anesthetic. A balloon-tipped catheter is introduced through a guide wire into the occluded coronary artery. Repeated balloon inflations dilate the occluded area and improve blood flow.	• Symptomatic CAD • Asymptomatic CAD (severe ischemia on low-level exercise despite medical therapy) • Acute MI	• Recurrent chest pain • Restenosis of treated artery • Coronary occlusion • Coronary dissection • Coronary artery spasm • MI • Prolonged angina • Vascular access site hematoma • Infection • AV fistula • Pseudoaneurysm
Pericardiocentesis This procedure involves needle aspiration of the pericardial sac to remove blood or other fluid that has accumulated in the sac, thereby relieving pressure on the heart.	• Cardiac tamponade	• Cardiac arrhythmias • Hemorrhage • Infection • Laceration to the heart, coronary arteries, or lung
Valsalva's maneuver This maneuver is used to increase vagal tone and slow the heart rate. To perform the procedure, the patient forcefully exhales, then holds his breath and bears down for 10 to 15 seconds (if possible), as if having a bowel movement.	• Supraventricular tachyarrhythmias	• Bradycardia with decreased cardiac output
Use of a ventricular assist device (VAD) A temporary life-sustaining treatment for a failing heart, the VAD diverts systemic blood flow from a diseased ventricle into a centrifugal pump. Used most commonly to assist (not replace) the left ventricle, a VAD may also assist the right ventricle or both ventricles. The pumping chambers usually are not implanted in the patient. However, a permanent VAD may be used, which is implanted in the patient's chest cavity.	Ventricular failure associated with: • Massive MI • Irreversible cardiomyopathy • Acute myocarditis • Valvular disease • Bacterial endocarditis May also be used if: • Heart transplant is rejected • Awaiting heart transplant • Unable to wean from cardiopulmonary bypass • Cardiogenic shock arises after MI	• Bleeding • Renal failure • Biventricular failure • Respiratory failure • Infection

Quick reference to cardiovascular drugs

Drug	Indications & dosage	Adverse reactions
Acebutolol Monitan, Sectral Pharmacologic classification: cardioselective beta-adrenergic blocker Therapeutic classification: antihypertensive, Class II antiarrhythmic	*Hypertension* **Adults:** 400 mg P.O. either as a single daily dosage or divided b.i.d. Patients may receive as much as 1,200 mg daily. *Ventricular arrhythmias* **Adults:** 400 mg P.O. daily divided b.i.d. Dosage is then increased to provide an adequate clinical response. Usual dosage is 600 to 1,200 mg daily.	**CNS:** *fatigue,* headache, dizziness, insomnia **CV:** chest pain, edema, bradycardia, ***congestive heart failure (CHF),*** *hypotension* **GI:** nausea, constipation, diarrhea, dyspepsia **Metabolic:** hypoglycemia without tachycardia **Respiratory:** dyspnea, ***bronchospasm*** **Skin:** rash **Other:** fever
Adenosine Adenocard Pharmacologic classification: nucleoside Therapeutic classification: antiarrhythmic	*Conversion of paroxysmal supraventricular tachycardia (PSVT) to sinus rhythm* **Adults:** 6 mg I.V. by rapid bolus injection (over 1 to 2 seconds). If PSVT is not eliminated in 1 to 2 minutes, give 12 mg by rapid I.V. push. Repeat 12-mg dose if necessary. Single doses over 12 mg are not recommended.	**CNS:** apprehension, back pain, blurred vision, burning sensation, dizziness, heaviness in arms, light-headedness, neck pain, numbness, tingling in arms **CV:** chest pain, *facial flushing,* headache, hypotension, marked bradycardia, palpitations, sweating **GI:** metallic taste, nausea **Respiratory:** *chest pressure, dyspnea, shortness of breath,* hyperventilation **Other:** *tightness in throat, groin pressure*
Alteplase (tissue plasminogen activator, recombinant; t-PA) Activase Pharmacologic classification: thrombolytic enzyme Therapeutic classification: thrombolytic enzyme	*Lysis of thrombi obstructing coronary arteries in acute MI* **Adults:** 100 mg I.V. infusion over 3 hours as follows: 60 mg in the first hour, of which 6 to 10 mg is given as a bolus over the first 1 to 2 minutes. Then 20 mg/hour infusion for 2 hours. Smaller adults (weighing under 143 lb [65 kg]) should receive a dose of 1.25 mg/kg in a similar fashion (60% in the first hour, with 10% as a bolus; then 20% of the total dose per hour for 2 hours).	**Blood:** ***severe, spontaneous bleeding (cerebral, retroperitoneal, GU, GI)*** **CNS:** ***cerebral hemorrhage,*** fever **CV:** hypotension, arrhythmias **GI:** nausea, vomiting **Local:** bleeding at puncture sites **Other:** ***hypersensitivity,*** urticaria
Amiloride hydrochloride Midamor Pharmacologic classification: potassium-sparing diuretic	*Hypertension; edema associated with left ventricular failure, usually in patients who are also taking thiazide or other potassium-wasting diuretics*	**CNS:** headache, weakness, dizziness **CV:** orthostatic hypotension **GI:** *nausea, anorexia, diarrhea, vomiting,* abdominal pain, constipation *(continued)*

Common adverse reactions in *italics;* life-threatening, in ***bold italics.***

Quick reference to cardiovascular drugs (continued)

Drug	Indications & dosage	Adverse reactions
Amiloride hydro-chloride *(continued)* Therapeutic classification: diuretic, antihypertensive	**Adults:** usual dosage is 5 mg P.O. daily. Dosage may be increased to 10 mg daily if necessary. As much as 20 mg daily can be given.	**GU:** impotence **Metabolic:** hyperkalemia
Amiodarone hydrochloride Cordarone Pharmacologic classification: iodinated benzofuran derivative Therapeutic classification: ventricular and supraventricular antiarrhythmic (Class III)	*Ventricular and supraventricular arrhythmias, including recurrent supraventricular tachycardia (Wolff-Parkinson-White syndrome), atrial fibrillation and flutter, and ventricular tachycardia refractory to other antiarrhythmics* **Adults:** loading dose is 5 to 10 mg/kg by I.V. infusion via central line, followed by I.V. infusion of 10 mg/kg/day for 3 to 5 days. (*Note:* I.V. use of amiodarone is investigational.) Or, give loading dose of 800 to 1,600 mg P.O. daily for 1 to 3 weeks until initial therapeutic response occurs. Maintenance dosage is 200 to 600 mg P.O. daily.	**CNS:** peripheral neuropathy, extrapyramidal symptoms, headache, *malaise, fatigue* **CV:** bradycardia, hypotension, ***arrhythmias, CHF*** **EENT:** *corneal microdeposits,* visual disturbances **Endocrine:** hypothyroidism, hyperthyroidism, gynecomastia **GI:** *nausea, vomiting,* constipation **Hepatic:** *altered liver enzymes,* hepatic dysfunction **Respiratory:** ***severe pulmonary toxicity (pneumonitis, alveolitis)*** **Skin:** *photosensitivity,* blue-gray skin pigmentation **Other:** muscle weakness
Amlodipine Norvasc Pharmacologic classification: calcium channel blocker Therapeutic classification: antihypertensive, antianginal	*Hypertension* **Adults:** initially, 5 mg P.O. once daily. Small, frail, or elderly patients; patients currently receiving other antihypertensive medications; or patients with hepatic insufficiency should begin therapy at 2.5 mg daily. Adjust dosage according to patient response and tolerance. Maximum dosage is 10 mg daily. *Chronic stable angina; vasospastic angina (Prinzmetal's or variant angina)* **Adults:** initially, 10 mg P.O. once daily. Small, frail, or elderly patients or patients with hepatic insufficiency should begin at 5 mg daily. Most patients require 10 mg daily for adequate therapy.	**Blood:** decreased platelet aggregation **CNS:** *headache,* fatigue, somnolence **CV:** *edema,* dizziness, flushing, palpitations **EENT:** epistaxis **GI:** nausea, abdominal pain, constipation **Other:** micturition, increased nocturia

Common adverse reactions in *italics;* life-threatening, in ***bold italics.***

Quick reference to cardiovascular drugs (continued)

Drug	Indications & dosage	Adverse reactions
Amrinone lactate Inocor Pharmacologic classification: bipyridine derivative Therapeutic classification: inotropic agent, vasodilator	*Short-term management of CHF* **Adults:** initially, 0.75 mg/kg I.V. bolus over 2 to 3 minutes. Then begin maintenance infusion of 5 to 10 mcg/kg/minute. Additional bolus of 0.75 mg/kg may be given 30 minutes after start of therapy. Total daily dosage should not exceed 10 mg/kg.	**Blood:** thrombocytopenia (dose dependent) **CV:** *arrhythmias*, hypotension **GI:** nausea, vomiting, cramps, dyspepsia, diarrhea **Hepatic:** elevated enzymes, rarely hepatotoxicity **Local:** burning at site of injection **Other:** hypersensitivity reactions (pericarditis, ascites, myositis vasculitis, pleuritis)
Anistreplase (anisoylated plasminogen-streptokinase activator complex; APSAC) Eminase Pharmacologic classification: enzyme Therapeutic classification: thrombolytic enzyme	*Lysis of coronary artery thrombi after acute MI* **Adults:** 30 units I.V. over 2 to 5 minutes. Administer by direct injection.	**Blood:** *bleeding,* eosinophilia **CNS:** *intracranial hemorrhage* **CV:** arrhythmias, conduction disorders, hypotension **EENT:** hemoptysis, gum and mouth hemorrhage **GI:** *bleeding* **GU:** hematuria **Skin:** hematomas, urticaria, itching, flushing, delayed (2 weeks after therapy) purpuric rash **Local:** bleeding at puncture sites **Other:** *anaphylactoid reactions* (rare)
Aspirin (acetylsalicylic acid) ASA, Bayer Aspirin, Ecotrin, Empirin, ZORprin Pharmacologic classification: salicylate Therapeutic classification: antipyretic, anti-inflammatory, antiplatelet	*Thromboembolic disorders* **Adults:** 325 to 650 mg P.O. daily or b.i.d. *Transient ischemic attacks in men* **Adults:** 650 mg P.O. b.i.d. or 325 mg q.i.d. *To reduce the risk of heart attack in patients with previous MI or unstable angina or to prevent graft closure after coronary artery bypass grafting (CABG)* **Adults:** several protocols have been studied; most employ doses of 80 to 325 mg P.O. daily or 325 mg every other day.	**Blood:** *prolonged bleeding time* **EENT:** *tinnitus, hearing loss* **GI:** *nausea, vomiting, GI distress, occult bleeding* **Hepatic:** abnormal liver function studies, hepatitis **Skin:** *rash*, bruising **Other:** *hypersensitivity manifested by anaphylaxis, asthma, or both*
Atenolol Tenormin Pharmacologic classification: cardio-selective beta-adrenergic blocker	*Hypertension* **Adults:** initially, 50 mg P.O. daily as a single dose. Dosage may be increased to 100 mg daily after 7 to 14 days. Dosages greater than 100 mg	**CNS:** fatigue, lethargy **CV:** *bradycardia, hypotension, CHF,* peripheral vascular disease **GI:** nausea, vomiting, diarrhea *(continued)*

Common adverse reactions in *italics;* life-threatening, in **bold italics.**

Quick reference to cardiovascular drugs *(continued)*

Drug	Indications & dosage	Adverse reactions
Atenolol *(continued)* Therapeutic classification: antihypertensive, antianginal, antiarrhythmic	are unlikely to produce further benefit. Dosage adjustment is necessary in patients with creatinine clearance below 35 ml/minute. *Angina pectoris* **Adults:** 50 mg P.O. once daily. May increase to 100 mg daily after 7 days for optimal effect. May give as much as 200 mg daily. *To reduce cardiovascular mortality and risk of reinfarction in patients with acute MI* **Adults:** 5 mg I.V. over 5 minutes, followed by another 5 mg 10 minutes later. After an additional 10 minutes, administer 50 mg P.O., followed by 50 mg in 12 hours. Thereafter, give 100 mg P.O. daily (as a single dose or 50 mg b.i.d.) for at least 7 days. *To reduce the incidence of supraventricular tachycardia in patients undergoing CABG* **Adults:** 50 mg P.O. daily starting 3 days before surgery.	**Respiratory:** dyspnea, ***bronchospasm*** **Skin:** rash **Other:** fever
Atropine sulfate Pharmacologic classification: anticholinergic, belladonna alkaloid Therapeutic classification: antiarrhythmic, vagolytic	*Symptomatic bradycardia, bradyarrhythmia (junctional or escape rhythm), bradyarrhythmias with atrioventricular (AV) block, or bradycardia-related ventricular ectopy* **Adults:** usually 0.5 to 1 mg I.V. push; repeat q 5 minutes, to maximum of 2 mg. Lower doses (less than 0.5 mg) or slow administration can cause bradycardia.	**Blood:** leukocytosis **CNS:** *headache, restlessness,* ataxia, disorientation, hallucinations, delirium, coma, *insomnia, dizziness;* excitement, agitation, and confusion (especially in elderly patients) **CV:** 1 to 2 mg — *tachycardia, palpitations;* more than 2 mg — ***extreme tachycardia, angina*** **EENT:** 1 mg — *slight mydriasis,* photophobia; 2 mg — *blurred vision, mydriasis* **GI:** *dry mouth* (common even at low doses) **GU:** urine retention **Skin:** hotness, flushing
Bretylium tosylate Bretylol Pharmacologic classification: adrenergic blocker	*Ventricular fibrillation* **Adults:** 5 mg/kg by I.V. push over 1 minute. If necessary, increase dose to 10 mg/kg and	**CNS:** *vertigo, dizziness, lightheadedness, syncope* (usually secondary to hypotension)

Common adverse reactions in *italics;* life-threatening, in ***bold italics.***

Quick reference to cardiovascular drugs (continued)

Drug	Indications & dosage	Adverse reactions
Bretylium tosylate *(continued)* Therapeutic classification: ventricular antiarrhythmic	repeat q 15 to 30 minutes until 30 mg/kg have been given. *Other ventricular arrhythmias* **Adults:** initially, 500 mg diluted to 50 ml with dextrose 5% in water (D_5W) or 0.9% sodium chloride solution and infused I.V. over more than 8 minutes at 5 to 10 mg/kg. Dose may be repeated in 1 to 2 hours. Thereafter, repeat q 6 to 8 hours. *I.V. maintenance* — infuse in diluted solution of 500 ml D_5W or 0.9% sodium chloride solution at 1 to 2 mg/minute. *I.M. injection* — 5 to 10 mg/kg undiluted. Repeat in 1 to 2 hours if needed. Thereafter, repeat q 6 to 8 hours.	**CV:** *severe hypotension (especially orthostatic), bradycardia,* anginal pain, transient arrhythmias, transient hypertension **GI:** severe nausea, vomiting (with rapid infusion)
Bumetanide Bumex Pharmacologic classification: loop diuretic Therapeutic classification: diuretic	*Edema in left ventricular failure* **Adults:** 0.5 to 2 mg P.O. once daily. If diuretic response not adequate, a second or third dose may be given at 4- to 5-hour intervals. Maximum dosage is 10 mg/day. May be administered parenterally when P.O. not feasible. Usual initial dose is 0.5 to 1 mg I.V. or I.M. If response is not adequate, a second or third dose may be given at 2- to 3-hour intervals. Maximum dosage is 10 mg/day.	**CNS:** dizziness, headache **CV:** volume depletion and dehydration, orthostatic hypotension, ECG changes **EENT:** transient deafness **GI:** nausea **Metabolic:** hypokalemia; hypochloremic alkalosis; asymptomatic hyperuricemia; fluid and electrolyte imbalances, including dilutional hyponatremia, hypocalcemia, and hypomagnesemia; hyperglycemia and impaired glucose tolerance **Skin:** rash **Other:** muscle pain and tenderness
Captopril Capoten Pharmacologic classification: angiotensin-converting enzyme (ACE) inhibitor, antihypertensive Therapeutic classification: antihypertensive, adjunctive treatment of CHF	*Hypertension* **Adults:** 25 mg P.O. b.i.d. or t.i.d. initially. If blood pressure isn't satisfactorily controlled in 1 to 2 weeks, dosage may be increased to 50 mg t.i.d. If not satisfactorily controlled after another 1 to 2 weeks, a diuretic should be added to regimen. If further blood pressure reduction is necessary, dosage may be raised to as high as 150 mg t.i.d. while continuing the diuretic. Maximum dosage is	**Blood:** *leukopenia, agranulocytosis, pancytopenia* **CNS:** dizziness, fainting **CV:** *tachycardia, hypotension,* angina pectoris, *CHF,* pericarditis **EENT:** *loss of taste (dysgeusia)* **GI:** anorexia **GU:** *proteinuria, nephrotic syndrome, membranous glomerulopathy, renal failure* (patients with preexisting renal

(continued)

Common adverse reactions in *italics;* life-threatening, in ***bold italics.***

Quick reference to cardiovascular drugs *(continued)*

Drug	Indications & dosage	Adverse reactions
Captopril *(continued)*	450 mg daily. Daily dose may also be administered b.i.d. *CHF* **Adults:** 6.25 to 12.5 mg P.O. t.i.d. initially. May be gradually increased to 50 mg t.i.d. Maximum dosage is 450 mg daily.	disease or patients receiving high dosages), urinary frequency **Metabolic:** hyperkalemia **Skin:** *urticarial rash, maculopapular rash,* pruritus **Other:** fever, angioedema (face and extremities), transient increases in liver enzymes, persistent cough
Chlorothiazide Diachlor, Diurigen, Diuril **Chlorothiazide sodium** Diuril Sodium Pharmacologic classification: thiazide diuretic Therapeutic classification: diuretic, antihypertensive	*Edema, hypertension* **Adults:** 500 mg to 2 g P.O. or I.V. daily or in two divided doses.	**Blood: *aplastic anemia, agranulocytosis,*** leukopenia, thrombocytopenia **CV:** volume depletion and dehydration, orthostatic hypotension **GI:** anorexia, nausea, pancreatitis **Hepatic:** hepatic encephalopathy **Metabolic:** hypokalemia, asymptomatic hyperuricemia, hyperglycemia and impaired glucose tolerance, fluid and electrolyte imbalances including dilutional hyponatremia and hypochloremia, metabolic alkalosis, hypercalcemia, gout **Skin:** dermatitis, photosensitivity, rash **Other:** hypersensitivity reactions, such as pneumonitis and vasculitis
Cholestyramine Cholybar, Questran Pharmacologic classification: anion exchange resin Therapeutic classification: antilipemic, bile acid sequestrant	*Reduction of elevations in lowdensity lipoprotein (LDL) levels or treatment of type IIa hyperlipidemia; as adjunctive therapy for the reduction of elevated serum cholesterol in patients with primary hypercholesterolemia; to reduce the risks of atherosclerotic CAD and MI* **Adults:** 4 g before meals and h.s., not to exceed 32 g daily. Each scoop or packet of Questran contains 4 g of cholestyramine. Also available as Cholybar, a chewable candy bar (raspberry or caramel flavored) containing 4 g of cholestyramine.	**GI:** *constipation,* fecal impaction, hemorrhoids, *abdominal discomfort,* flatulence, *nausea,* vomiting, steatorrhea **Skin:** *rashes;* irritation of skin, tongue, and perianal area **Other:** *vitamin A, D, and K deficiency from decreased absorption;* hyperchloremic acidosis with long-term use or very high dosage; hypertriglyceridemia

Common adverse reactions in *italics;* life-threatening, in ***bold italics.***

Quick reference to cardiovascular drugs (continued)

Drug	Indications & dosage	Adverse reactions
Clofibrate Atromid-S, Novo-fibrate Pharmacologic classification: fibric acid derivative Therapeutic classification: antilipemic	*Hyperlipidemia and xanthoma tuberosum; type III hyperlipidemia; treatment of patients with very high serum triglyceride levels (type IV or V hyperlipidemia)* **Adults:** 2 g P.O. daily in two to four divided doses. Some patients may respond to lower doses as assessed by serum lipid monitoring.	**Blood:** leukopenia **CNS:** fatigue, weakness **CV:** *arrhythmias* **GI:** *nausea, diarrhea, vomiting,* stomatitis, *dyspepsia,* flatulence **GU:** impotence and decreased libido, acute renal failure **Hepatic:** gallstones, *transient and reversible elevations of liver function tests* **Skin:** rashes, urticaria, pruritus, dry skin and hair **Other:** myalgia and arthralgia (resembling a flulike syndrome), *weight gain, polyphagia,* fever, decreased libido
Clonidine hydrochloride Catapres, Catapres-TTS Pharmacologic classification: centrally acting antiadrenergic Therapeutic classification: antihypertensive	*Essential, renal, and malignant hypertension* **Adults:** initially, 0.1 mg P.O. b.i.d. Then increase by 0.1 to 0.2 mg daily on a weekly basis. Usual dosage range is 0.2 to 0.8 mg daily in divided doses; infrequently, dosages as high as 2.4 mg daily. Or apply transdermal patch to a hairless area of intact skin on the upper arm or torso once every 7 days.	**CNS:** *drowsiness,* dizziness, fatigue, sedation, nervousness, headache, vivid dreams **CV:** orthostatic hypotension, bradycardia, *severe rebound hypertension* **GI:** *constipation, dry mouth* **GU:** urine retention, impotence **Metabolic:** transient glucose intolerance (after large doses) **Skin:** *pruritus, dermatitis* (from transdermal patch)
Colestipol hydrochloride Colestid Pharmacologic classification: anion exchange resin Therapeutic classification: antilipemic	*Primary hypercholesterolemia and xanthomas; type IIa hyperlipidemia* **Adults:** 5 to 30 g P.O. daily in two to four divided doses.	**CNS:** headache, dizziness **GI:** *constipation (common, may require decreasing the dosage),* fecal impaction, hemorrhoids, abdominal discomfort, flatulence, nausea, vomiting, steatorrhea **Skin:** rashes; irritation of skin, tongue, and perianal area **Other:** vitamin A, D, and K deficiency from decreased absorption; hyperchloremic acidosis with long-term use or very high dosage
Cyclandelate Cyclan, Cyclospasmol Pharmacologic classification: mandelic acid derivative Therapeutic classification: antispasmodic, vasodilator	*Adjunct in intermittent claudication, arteriosclerosis obliterans, vasospasm and muscular ischemia associated with thrombophlebitis, Raynaud's phenomenon* **Adults:** initially, 1.2 to 1.6 g P.O. daily, in divided doses before meals and h.s. For	**CNS:** *headache, tingling of the extremities, dizziness* **CV:** *mild flushing,* tachycardia **GI:** pyrosis, eructation, nausea, heartburn **Other:** *sweating* *(continued)*

Common adverse reactions in *italics;* life-threatening, in ***bold italics.***

Quick reference to cardiovascular drugs (continued)

Drug	Indications & dosage	Adverse reactions
Cyclandelate *(continued)*	maintenance, decrease dosage by 200 mg/day to the lowest effective level. Maintenance dosage is usually 400 to 800 mg daily in two to four divided doses.	
Digitoxin Crystodigin Pharmacologic classification: digitalis glycoside Therapeutic classification: antiarrhythmic, inotropic agent	*CHF, PSVT, atrial fibrillation and flutter* **Adults:** loading dose is 1.2 to 1.6 mg P.O. in divided doses over 24 hours; average maintenance dosage is 0.15 mg daily (range: 0.05 to 0.3 mg daily)	*Note:* The following are signs of toxicity that may occur with all digitalis glycosides. **CNS:** *fatigue, generalized muscle weakness, agitation, hallucinations,* headache, malaise, dizziness, vertigo, stupor, paresthesia **CV:** *increased severity of CHF, arrhythmias (most commonly conduction disturbances with or without AV block, premature ventricular contractions, and supraventricular arrhythmias),* hypotension *Note:* Toxic effects on heart may be life-threatening and require immediate attention. **EENT:** *yellow-green halos around images, blurred vision,* light flashes, photophobia, diplopia **GI:** *anorexia, nausea,* vomiting, diarrhea
Digoxin Lanoxicaps, Lanoxin, Novodigoxin Pharmacologic classification: digitalis glycoside Therapeutic classification: antiarrhythmic, inotropic agent	*CHF, PSVT, atrial fibrillation and flutter* **Adults:** loading dose is 0.5 to 1 mg I.V. or P.O. in divided doses over 24 hours; maintenance dosage is 0.125 to 0.5 mg I.V. or P.O. daily (average 0.25 mg). Larger doses are often needed for treatment of arrhythmias, depending on patient response. Smaller loading and maintenance doses should be given in patients with impaired renal function. **Adults over age 65:** 0.125 mg P.O. daily as maintenance dose. Frail or underweight elderly patients may require only 0.0625 mg daily or 0.125 mg every other day.	*Note:* The following are signs of toxicity that may occur with all digitalis glycosides. **CNS:** *fatigue, generalized muscle weakness, agitation, hallucinations,* headache, malaise, dizziness, vertigo, stupor, paresthesia **CV:** *increased severity of CHF, arrhythmias (most commonly conduction disturbances with or without AV block), premature ventricular contractions, and supraventricular arrhythmias),* hypotension *Note:* Toxic effects on heart may be life-threatening and require immediate attention. **EENT:** *yellow-green halos around images, blurred vision,*

Common adverse reactions in *italics;* life-threatening, in ***bold italics.***

Quick reference to cardiovascular drugs *(continued)*

Drug	Indications & dosage	Adverse reactions
Digoxin *(continued)*		light flashes, photophobia, diplopia **GI:** *anorexia, nausea,* vomiting, diarrhea
Digoxin immune FAB (ovine) Digibind Pharmacologic classification: antibody fragment Therapeutic classification: digitalis antidote	*Potentially life-threatening digitalis toxicity* **Adults and children:** the I.V. dosage varies according to the amount of digoxin or digitoxin to be neutralized. Each vial binds about 0.6 mg digoxin or digitoxin. Average dosage is 10 vials (400 mg). However, if the toxicity resulted from acute digoxin ingestion and neither a serum digoxin level nor an estimated ingestion amount is known, 20 vials (800 mg) should be administered. See package insert for complete, specific dosage instructions.	**CV: *CHF,*** rapid ventricular rate (both caused by reversal of the digitalis glycoside's therapeutic effects) **Metabolic:** hypokalemia **Other: *hypersensitivity***
Diltiazem hydrochloride Cardizem, Cardizem CD, Cardizem SR, Dilacor XR Pharmacologic classification: calcium channel blocker Therapeutic classification: antianginal, antihypertensive, antiarrhythmic	*Management of vasospastic angina (Prinzmetal's or variant angina) and classic chronic stable angina pectoris* **Adults:** initially, 30 mg P.O. q.i.d. before meals and h.s. Dosage may be gradually increased to a maximum of 360 mg/day, in divided doses. Sustained-release use: initially, 120 or 180 mg once daily. Titrate to a maximum of 480 mg daily. *Hypertension* **Adults:** 60 mg P.O. b.i.d. (sustained-release capsule [SR]). Titrate dosage to effect. Maximum recommended dosage is 360 mg/day. Alternatively, initially use 180 to 240 mg daily (extended-release capsule [CD]). Maximum effect is seen within 14 days. Adjust dosage as necessary. There is limited experience with doses above 360 mg/day. *Atrial fibrillation or flutter* **Adults:** for direct I.V. injection (bolus), initial dose is 0.25 mg/kg, administered over 2	**CNS:** *headache, fatigue, drowsiness,* dizziness, nervousness, depression, insomnia, confusion **CV:** *edema,* **arrhythmias,** flushing, bradycardia, hypotension, conduction abnormalities, ***CHF*** **GI:** *nausea,* vomiting, diarrhea **GU:** nocturia, polyuria **Hepatic:** transient elevation of liver enzymes **Skin:** *rash,* pruritus **Other:** photosensitivity

(continued)

Common adverse reactions in *italics;* life-threatening, in ***bold italics.***

Quick reference to cardiovascular drugs *(continued)*

Drug	Indications & dosage	Adverse reactions
Diltiazem hydrochloride *(continued)*	minutes. If response is inadequate, a second bolus dose may be administered after 15 minutes. The second bolus dose is 0.35 mg/kg, administered over 2 minutes. Subsequent I.V. boluses must be individualized. Continuous I.V. infusion: if necessary, start continuous I.V. infusion after bolus. Initial infusion rate is 5 mg/hour. Infusion rate may be increased in increments of 5 mg/hour, up to 15 mg/hour, as needed. Maintain infusion for up to 24 hours.	
Dipyridamole Apo-Dipyridamole, Persantine Pharmacologic classification: pyrimidine analogue Therapeutic classification: coronary vasodilator, platelet aggregation inhibitor	*Inhibition of platelet adhesion in prosthetic heart valves, in combination with warfarin or aspirin; after CABG* **Adults:** 75 to 100 mg P.O. q.i.d. *As an alternative to exercise in the evaluation of coronary artery disease during thallium myocardial perfusion imaging* **Adults:** 0.57 mg/kg as an I.V. infusion at a constant rate over 4 minutes (0.142 mg/kg/minute). Do not give more than 60 mg.	**CNS:** *headache, dizziness,* weakness **CV:** flushing, fainting, *hypotension; chest pain,* **ECG abnormalities,** *blood pressure lability, hypertension* (with I.V. infusion) **GI:** *nausea,* vomiting, diarrhea **Local:** irritation (with undiluted injection) **Skin:** rash
Disopyramide Rythmodan **Disopyramide phosphate** Norpace, Norpace CR, Rythmodan LA Pharmacologic classification: pyridine derivative antiarrhythmic Therapeutic classification: ventricular antiarrhythmic, supraventricular antiarrhythmic, atrial antitachyarrhythmic	*Premature ventricular contractions (unifocal, multifocal, or coupled); ventricular tachycardia not severe enough to require electrocardioversion; to convert atrial fibrillation or flutter to normal sinus rhythm* **Adults:** usual maintenance dosage is 150 to 200 mg P.O. q 6 hours; for patients who weigh less than 50 kg or those with renal, hepatic, or cardiac impairment, 100 mg P.O. q 6 hours. May give sustained-release capsule q 12 hours. Recommended dosages in advanced renal insufficiency: if creatinine clearance is 30 to 40 ml/minute, dosing interval is q 8	**CNS:** dizziness, agitation, depression, fatigue, muscle weakness, syncope **CV:** *hypotension,* **CHF, heart block,** edema, weight gain, **arrhythmias** **EENT:** *blurred vision, dry eyes, dry nose* **GI:** nausea, vomiting, anorexia, bloating, abdominal pain, *constipation, dry mouth* **GU:** urine retention, urinary hesitancy **Hepatic:** cholestatic jaundice **Metabolic:** hypoglycemia **Skin:** rash in 1% to 3% of patients

Common adverse reactions in *italics;* life-threatening, in ***bold italics.***

Quick reference to cardiovascular drugs *(continued)*

Drug	Indications & dosage	Adverse reactions
Disopyramide *(continued)*	hours; if creatinine clearance is 15 to 30 ml/minute, dosing interval is q 12 hours; if creatinine clearance is below 15 ml/minute, dosing interval is q 24 hours.	
Dobutamine hydrochloride Dobutrex Pharmacologic classification: adrenergic, beta$_1$ agonist (some beta$_2$ effects) Therapeutic classification: inotropic agent	*To increase cardiac output in treatment of cardiac decompensation caused by depressed contractility* **Adults:** 2.5 to 10 mcg/kg/minute as an I.V. infusion. Rarely, infusion rates up to 40 mcg/kg/minute may be needed. Titrate dosage carefully to patient response.	**CNS:** headache **CV:** *increased heart rate,* **hypertension, premature ventricular contractions,** angina, nonspecific chest pain **GI:** nausea, vomiting **Other:** shortness of breath
Dopamine hydrochloride Intropin, Revimine Pharmacologic classification: adrenergic Therapeutic classification: inotropic agent, vasopressor	*To treat shock and correct hemodynamic imbalances, to improve perfusion to vital organs, to increase cardiac output, to correct hypotension* **Adults:** 2 to 5 mcg/kg/minute I.V. infusion, up to 50 mcg/kg/minute. Titrate the dosage to the desired hemodynamic or renal response.	**CNS:** headache **CV:** *arrhythmias,* ectopic beats, tachycardia, anginal pain, palpitations, hypotension. Less frequently, bradycardia, widening of QRS complex, conduction disturbances, vasoconstriction **GI:** nausea, vomiting **Local:** necrosis and tissue sloughing with extravasation **Other:** piloerection, dyspnea
Enalaprilat Vasotec I.V. **Enalapril maleate** Vasotec Pharmacologic classification: ACE inhibitor Therapeutic classification: antihypertensive	*Hypertension* **Adults:** initially, 5 mg P.O. once daily, then adjust according to response. Usual dosage range is 10 to 40 mg daily as a single dose or two divided doses. Alternatively, give by I.V. infusion 1.25 mg q 6 hours over 5 minutes. To convert from I.V. therapy to oral therapy: initially, 5 mg P.O. once daily. Adjust dosage to response. To convert from oral therapy to I.V. therapy: 1.25 mg I.V. over 5 minutes q 6 hours. Higher doses have not demonstrated greater efficacy. *Adjunctive treatment of heart failure (with diuretics and digitalis glycosides)* **Adults:** initially, 2.5 mg P.O. b.i.d. Adjust dosage based on clinical or hemodynamic	**Blood:** **neutropenia, agranulocytosis** **CNS:** *headache, dizziness, fatigue,* insomnia **CV:** *hypotension* **GI:** diarrhea, nausea **GU:** decreased renal function (patients with bilateral renal artery stenosis or CHF) **Skin:** rash **Other:** persistent cough, *angioedema*

(continued)

Common adverse reactions in *italics;* life-threatening, in ***bold italics.***

Quick reference to cardiovascular drugs *(continued)*

Drug	Indications & dosage	Adverse reactions
Enalaprilat **Enalapril maleate** *(continued)*	response. Usual range is 5 to 20 mg daily in two divided doses; maximum dosage is 40 mg/day.	
Esmolol hydrochloride Brevibloc Pharmacologic classification: cardioselective beta₁-adrenergic blocker Therapeutic classification: antiarrhythmic	*Supraventricular tachycardia, hypertensive crisis* **Adults:** loading dose is 500 mcg/kg/minute by I.V. infusion over 1 minute, followed by a 4-minute maintenance infusion of 50 mcg/kg/minute. If adequate response does not occur within 5 minutes, repeat the loading dose followed by a maintenance infusion of 100 mcg/kg/minute for 4 minutes. Maximum maintenance infusion is 200 mcg/kg/minute.	**CNS:** dizziness, somnolence, headache, agitation, fatigue **CV:** *arrhythmias,* hypotension (sometimes with diaphoresis) **GI:** *nausea,* vomiting **Local:** inflammation and induration at infusion site **Respiratory: *bronchospasm***
Ethacrynate sodium Edecrin sodium **Ethacrynic acid** Edecrin Pharmacologic classification: loop diuretic Therapeutic classification: diuretic	*Acute pulmonary edema* **Adults:** 50 to 100 mg of ethacrynate sodium I.V. slowly over several minutes. *Edema* **Adults:** 50 to 200 mg P.O. daily. Refractory cases may require up to 200 mg b.i.d.	**Blood: *agranulocytosis,*** neutropenia, thrombocytopenia **CV:** volume depletion and dehydration, orthostatic hypotension **EENT:** transient deafness with too rapid an I.V. injection **GI:** abdominal discomfort and pain, diarrhea **Metabolic:** hypokalemia; hypochloremic alkalosis; asymptomatic hyperuricemia; fluid and electrolyte imbalances including dilutional hyponatremia, hypocalcemia, hypomagnesemia; hyperglycemia and impaired glucose tolerance **Skin:** dermatitis
Felodipine Plendil Pharmacologic classification: dihydropyridine-derivative calcium channel blocker Therapeutic classification: antihypertensive	*Hypertension* **Adults:** initially, 5 mg P.O. daily. Adjust dosage according to patient response, generally at intervals of not less than 2 weeks. The usual dose is 5 to 10 mg daily; the maximum recommended dose is 20 mg daily. **Elderly patients and patients with impaired hepatic function:** 5 mg P.O. daily; adjust dosage as for adults. Maximum recommended dose is 10 mg daily.	**CNS:** headache, dizziness, paresthesia, asthenia **CV:** *peripheral edema,* chest pain, palpitations, increased heart rate **EENT:** cough, rhinorrhea **GI:** dyspepsia, abdominal pain, nausea, constipation, diarrhea **Respiratory:** upper respiratory infection, pharyngitis **Skin:** rash, flushing **Other:** muscle cramps, back pain, gingival hyperplasia

Common adverse reactions in *italics;* life-threatening, in ***bold italics.***

Quick reference to cardiovascular drugs *(continued)*

Drug	Indications & dosage	Adverse reactions
Flecainide acetate Tambocor Pharmacologic classification: benzamide derivative local anesthetic (amide) Therapeutic classification: ventricular antiarrhythmic	*Symptomatic life-threatening ventricular arrhythmias, such as sustained ventricular tachycardia* **Adults:** 100 mg P.O. q 12 hours. May be increased in increments of 50 mg b.i.d. q 4 days until efficacy is achieved. Maximum dosage is 400 mg daily for most patients. Initial dosage for patients with CHF is 50 mg q 12 hours. *I.V.* (where available)—2 mg/kg I.V. push over not less than 10 minutes; or the dose may be diluted with D_5W and administered as an infusion. Do not use any other solutions for infusion.	**CNS:** *dizziness, headache,* fatigue, tremor **CV:** *new or worsened arrhythmias,* chest pain, *CHF, cardiac arrest* **EENT:** *blurred vision and other visual disturbances* **GI:** nausea, constipation, abdominal pain **Other:** *dyspnea,* edema, skin rash
Fosinopril sodium Monopril Pharmacologic classification: ACE inhibitor Therapeutic classification: antihypertensive	*Hypertension* **Adults:** initially, 10 mg P.O. daily. Adjust dosage based on blood pressure response at peak and trough levels. Usual dose is 20 to 40 mg, up to 80 mg. Dose may be divided.	**CNS:** headache, dizziness, fatigue, light-headedness, syncope, memory disturbances, mood change, paresthesia, sleep disturbance, drowsiness, weakness **CV:** *cerebrovascular accident (CVA),* chest pain, angina, *MI, hypertensive crisis,* rhythm disturbances, palpitations, hypotension, flushing, claudications, orthostatic hypotension **EENT:** tinnitus, vision disturbances, eye irritation, epistaxis **GI:** nausea, vomiting, diarrhea, pancreatitis, hepatitis, dysphagia, abdominal distention, abdominal pain, flatulence, constipation, heartburn, appetite change, weight change, dry mouth **GU:** sexual dysfunction, decreased libido, urinary frequency, renal insufficiency, acute renal failure **Respiratory:** cough, *bronchospasm,* pharyngitis, sinusitis, rhinitis, laryngitis, hoarseness **Skin:** urticaria, rash, photosensitivity, pruritus **Other:** *angioedema,* fever, arthralgia, musculoskeletal pain, myalgia, jaundice, gout

(continued)

Common adverse reactions in *italics;* life-threatening, in ***bold italics.***

Quick reference to cardiovascular drugs *(continued)*

Drug	Indications & dosage	Adverse reactions
Furosemide (frusemide) Apo-Furosemide, Furomide M.D., Furoside, Lasix, Lasix Special, Myrosemide, Novosemide, Uritol Pharmacologic classification: loop diuretic Therapeutic classification: diuretic, antihypertensive	*Acute pulmonary edema* **Adults:** 40 mg I.V. injected slowly; then 40 mg I.V. in 1 to 1½ hours if needed. *Edema* **Adults:** 20 to 80 mg P.O. daily in morning; second dose can be given in 6 to 8 hours; carefully titrate up to 600 mg daily if needed; or 20 to 40 mg I.M. or I.V. Increase by 20 mg q 2 hours until desired response is achieved. I.V. dose should be given slowly over 1 to 2 minutes. *Hypertension* **Adults:** 40 mg P.O. b.i.d. Adjust dose according to response. *Hypertensive crisis* **Adults:** 100 to 200 mg I.V. over 1 to 2 minutes.	**Blood:** *agranulocytosis, leukopenia, thrombocytopenia* **CV:** volume depletion and dehydration, orthostatic hypotension **EENT:** transient deafness with too rapid an I.V. injection **GI:** abdominal discomfort and pain, diarrhea (with oral solution) **Metabolic:** hypokalemia; hypochloremic alkalosis; asymptomatic hyperuricemia, fluid and electrolyte imbalances, including dilutional hyponatremia, hypocalcemia, and hypomagnesemia; hyperglycemia and impaired glucose tolerance **Skin:** dermatitis
Gemfibrozil Lopid Pharmacologic classification: fibric acid derivative Therapeutic classification: antilipemic	*Type IV hyperlipidemia (hypertriglyceridemia) and hypercholesterolemia unresponsive to diet and other drugs; type III, type IIb, and type V hyperlipidemias; to reduce the risk of coronary heart disease in patients intolerant of or refractory to treatment with bile acid sequestrants or niacin* **Adults:** 1,200 mg P.O. administered 30 minutes before meals in two divided doses. Usual dosage range is 900 to 1,500 mg daily.	**Blood:** anemia, leukopenia **CNS:** blurred vision, headache, dizziness **GI:** *abdominal and epigastric pain, diarrhea, nausea,* vomiting, flatulence **Hepatic:** bile duct obstruction, elevated enzymes **Skin:** rash, dermatitis, pruritus **Other:** painful extremities
Guanfacine hydrochloride Tenex Pharmacologic classification: centrally acting antiadrenergic Therapeutic classification: antihypertensive	*Mild to moderate hypertension* **Adults:** initially, 0.5 to 1 mg P.O. daily, h.s. Average dose is 1 to 3 mg daily.	**CNS:** *drowsiness, dizziness,* fatigue, headache, insomnia. **CV:** bradycardia, orthostatic hypotension, rebound hypertension. **GI:** *constipation,* diarrhea, nausea, dry mouth **Skin:** dermatitis, pruritus
Heparin calcium Calcilean, Calciparine **Heparin sodium** Hepalean, Heparin Lock Flush Solution (Tubex), Hep Lock, Liquaemin Sodium	*Treatment of deep vein thrombosis, MI* **Adults:** initially, 5,000 to 7,500 units I.V. push, then adjust dose according to prothrombin time (PT) results and give dose I.V. q 4 hours (usually 4,000 to 5,000 units); or 5,000 to 7,500	**Blood:** *hemorrhage with excessive dosage,* overly prolonged clotting time, *thrombocytopenia* **Local:** irritation, mild pain, hematoma, ulceration, cutaneous or subcutaneous necrosis. **Other:** *"white clot" syn-*

Common adverse reactions in *italics;* life-threatening, in ***bold italics.***

Quick reference to cardiovascular drugs *(continued)*

Drug	Indications & dosage	Adverse reactions
Heparin calcium **Heparin sodium** *(continued)* Pharmacologic classification: anticoagulant Therapeutic classification: anticoagulant	units I.V. bolus, then 1,000 units/hour by I.V. infusion pump. Wait 8 hours following bolus dose, and adjust hourly rate according to PT. *Prophylaxis of embolism, venous thrombosis, pulmonary embolism, atrial fibrillation with embolism, postoperative deep vein thrombosis* **Adults:** 5,000 units S.C. q 12 hours. In surgical patients, give first dose 2 hours before procedure; follow with 5,000 units S.C. q 8 to 12 hours for 5 to 7 days or until patient is fully ambulatory. *Open-heart surgery* **Adults:** (total body perfusion) 150 to 300 units/kg by continuous I.V infusion.	*drome,* hypersensitivity reactions (including chills, fever, pruritus, rhinitis, burning of feet, conjunctivitis, lacrimation, arthralgia, and urticaria)
Hydralazine **hydrochloride** Alazine, Apresoline, Novo-Hylazin Pharmacologic classification: peripheral vasodilator Therapeutic classification: antihypertensive	*Essential hypertension (oral, alone or in combination with other antihypertensives); to reduce afterload in severe CHF (with nitrates); severe essential hypertension (parenteral to lower blood pressure quickly)* **Adults:** initially, 10 mg P.O. q.i.d.; gradually increased to 50 mg q.i.d. Maximum recommended dosage is 200 mg daily, but some patients may require 300 to 400 mg daily. Can be given b.i.d. for CHF. *I.V.:* 10 to 20 mg given slowly and repeated as necessary, generally q 4 to 6 hours. Switch to oral antihypertensives as soon as possible. *I.M.:* 20 to 40 mg repeated as necessary, generally q 4 to 6 hours. Switch to oral antihypertensives as soon as possible.	**Blood:** neutropenia, leukopenia **CNS:** peripheral neuritis, *headache, dizziness* **CV:** orthostatic hypotension, *tachycardia,* arrhythmias, angina, palpitations, sodium retention **GI:** *nausea, vomiting, diarrhea, anorexia* **Skin:** rash **Other:** *lupus erythematosus– like syndrome (especially with high doses), weight gain*
Hydrochlorothia- **zide** Esidrix, HydroDIURIL, Novohydrazide, Or-etic, Urozide Pharmacologic clas-	*Edema* **Adults:** initially, 25 to 100 mg P.O. daily or intermittently for maintenance dosage. *Hypertension* **Adults:** 25 to 100 mg P.O. daily or in divided dosage. Daily	**Blood:** ***aplastic anemia, agranulocytosis,*** leukopenia, thrombocytopenia **CV:** volume depletion and dehydration, orthostatic hypotension **GI:** anorexia, nausea, pancreatitis *(continued)*

Common adverse reactions in *italics;* life-threatening, in ***bold italics.***

Quick reference to cardiovascular drugs *(continued)*

Drug	Indications & dosage	Adverse reactions
Hydrochlorothiazide *(continued)* sification: thiazide diuretic Therapeutic classification: diuretic, antihypertensive	dosage increased or decreased according to blood pressure.	**Hepatic:** hepatic encephalopathy **Metabolic:** hypokalemia, asymptomatic hyperuricemia, hyperglycemia and impairment of glucose tolerance, fluid and electrolyte imbalances including dilutional hyponatremia and hypochloremia, metabolic alkalosis, hypercalcemia, gout **Skin:** dermatitis, photosensitivity, rash **Other:** hypersensitivity reactions, such as pneumonitis and vasculitis
Isoproterenol Aerolone, Dey-Dose Isoproterenol, Isuprel, Vapo-Iso **Isoproterenol hydrochloride** Isuprel, Norisodrine Aerotrol **Isoproterenol sulfate** Medihaler-Iso Pharmacologic classification: beta-adrenergic agonist Therapeutic classification: bronchodilator, cardiac stimulant	*Heart block and ventricular arrhythmias* **Adults:** (hydrochloride) initially, 0.02 to 0.06 mg I.V. Subsequent doses 0.01 to 0.2 mg I.V. or 5 mcg/minute I.V.; or 0.2 mg I.M. initially, then 0.02 to 1 mg, p.r.n. *Shock* **Adults:** (hydrochloride) 0.5 to 5 mcg/minute by continuous I.V. infusion. Usual concentration is 1 mg (5 ml) in 500 ml D_5W. Adjust rate according to heart rate, central venous pressure, blood pressure, and urine flow.	**CNS:** *headache,* mild tremor, weakness, dizziness, nervousness, insomnia **CV:** *palpitations, tachycardia, ventricular arrhythmias, anginal pain; blood pressure may rise and then fall* **GI:** nausea, vomiting **Metabolic:** hyperglycemia. **Other:** sweating, flushing of face, ***bronchial edema and inflammation***
Isosorbide dinitrate Apo-ISDN, Cedocard-SR, Coronex, Dilatrate-SR, Iso-Bid, Isonate, Isorbid, Isordil, Isotrate, Novosorbide, Sorbitrate, Sorbitrate SA **Isosorbide mononitrate** Ismo Pharmacologic classification: nitrate Therapeutic classification: antianginal, vasodilator	*Acute anginal attacks (sublingual and chewable tablets of isosorbide dinitrate only); prophylaxis in situations likely to cause anginal attacks; treatment of CHF* **Adults:** *Sublingual form*—2.5 to 10 mg under the tongue for prompt relief of anginal pain, repeated q 5 to 10 minutes (maximum of three doses per 30-minute period). For prophylaxis, 2.5 to 10 mg under the tongue q 2 to 3 hours. *Chewable form*—5 to 10 mg p.r.n. for acute attack or q 2 to 3 hours for prophylaxis but only	**CNS:** *headache, sometimes with throbbing; dizziness;* weakness **CV:** *orthostatic hypotension, tachycardia, palpitations, ankle edema,* fainting **GI:** nausea, vomiting **Skin:** cutaneous vasodilation, *flushing* **Local:** sublingual burning **Other:** hypersensitivity reactions, nitrate tolerance

Common adverse reactions in *italics;* life-threatening, in ***bold italics.***

Quick reference to cardiovascular drugs *(continued)*

Drug	Indications & dosage	Adverse reactions
Isosorbide dinitrate **Isosorbide mononitrate** *(continued)*	after initial test dose of 5 mg to determine risk of severe hypotension. *Oral form* (dinitrate)—5 to 30 mg P.O. q.i.d. for prophylaxis only (use smallest effective dose); 40 mg P.O. (sustained-release form) q 6 to 12 hours. *Oral form* (mononitrate)—20 mg P.O. b.i.d., usually 7 hours apart (the first dose upon awakening). *Topical form* (where available) — initially, 2 sprays to the chest in the morning from a distance of about 20 cm. Rub solution in. Dosage is gradually increased as needed to 2 to 5 sprays, daily or b.i.d. (in the morning and h.s.).	
Isradipine DynaCirc Pharmacologic classification: calcium channel blocker Therapeutic classification: antihypertensive	*Essential hypertension* **Adults:** initially, 2.5 mg P.O. b.i.d. given alone or with a thiazide diuretic. Adjust dosage based on tolerance and response, to a maximum of 20 mg daily.	**CNS:** dizziness **CV:** edema, flushing, palpitations, increased heart rate **GI:** nausea, diarrhea **GU:** frequent urination **Skin:** rash **Other:** dyspnea
Labetalol hydrochloride Normodyne, Trandate Pharmacologic classification: nonselective alpha- and beta-adrenergic blocker Therapeutic classification: antihypertensive	*Hypertension* **Adults:** 100 mg P.O. b.i.d. with or without a diuretic. Dose may be increased to 200 mg b.i.d. after 2 days. Further dose increases may be made q 1 to 3 days until optimum response is reached. Usual maintenance dosage is 200 to 400 mg b.i.d. *Severe hypertension and hypertensive emergencies* **Adults:** dilute 200 mg to 200 ml with D_5W. Infuse at 2 mg/minute until satisfactory response is obtained. Then stop the infusion. May repeat q 6 to 8 hours. Alternative administration by repeated I.V. injection: initially, give 20 mg I.V. slowly over 2 minutes. May repeat injections of 40 to 80 mg q 10 minutes until maximum dose of 300 mg is reached.	**CNS:** vivid dreams, fatigue, headache **CV:** *orthostatic hypotension and dizziness,* peripheral vascular disease, bradycardia, ***CHF*** **EENT:** nasal stuffiness **Endocrine:** hypoglycemia without tachycardia **GI:** nausea, vomiting, diarrhea **GU:** sexual dysfunction, urine retention **Respiratory: *bronchospasm*** **Skin:** rash **Other:** increased airway resistance, transient scalp tingling

(continued)

Common adverse reactions in *italics;* life-threatening, in ***bold italics.***

Quick reference to cardiovascular drugs (continued)

Drug	Indications & dosage	Adverse reactions
Lidocaine hydrochloride (lignocaine hydrochloride) Lido Pen Auto-Injector, Xylocaine, Xylocard Pharmacologic classification: amide derivative Therapeutic classification: ventricular antiarrhythmic, local anesthetic	*Ventricular arrhythmias from MI, cardiac manipulation, or digitalis glycosides; ventricular tachycardia* **Adults:** 50 to 100 mg (1 to 1.5 mg/kg) I.V. bolus at 25 to 50 mg/minute. Give half this amount to elderly patients or patients under 110 lb (50 kg), and to those with CHF or hepatic disease. Repeat bolus q 3 to 5 minutes until arrhythmias subside or adverse reactions develop. Don't exceed 300-mg total bolus during a 1-hour period. Simultaneously, begin constant infusion of 20 to 50 mg/kg/minute (1 to 4 mg/minute). If single bolus has been given, repeat smaller bolus 15 to 20 minutes after start of infusion to maintain therapeutic serum level. When completed, discontinue; no need to wean patient from drug. *I.M. administration*—200 to 300 mg in deltoid muscle only.	**CNS:** *confusion, tremor,* lethargy, somnolence, *stupor, restlessness,* slurred speech, euphoria, depression, *lightheadedness,* paresthesia, muscle twitching, ***seizures*** **CV:** *hypotension,* bradycardia, ***new or worsened arrhythmias*** **EENT:** *tinnitus, blurred or double vision* **Other:** ***anaphylaxis,*** soreness at injection site, sensations of cold, diaphoresis
Lisinopril Prinivil, Zestril Pharmacologic classification: ACE inhibitor Therapeutic classification: antihypertensive	*Mild to severe hypertension* **Adults:** initially, 10 mg P.O. daily. Most patients are well controlled on 20 to 40 mg daily as a single dose.	**Blood:** neutropenia **CNS:** *dizziness, headache, fatigue,* depression, somnolence, paresthesia **CV:** hypotension, *orthostatic hypotension,* chest pain **EENT:** *nasal congestion* **GI:** *diarrhea,* nausea, dyspepsia, dysgeusia **GU:** impotence **Metabolic:** hyperkalemia **Skin:** rash **Other:** *upper respiratory symptoms, cough, muscle cramps,* ***angioedema,*** decreased libido
Lovastatin Mevacor Pharmacologic classification: lactone Therapeutic classification: 3-hydroxy-3-methylglutaryl-coenzyme A (HMG-CoA) reductase inhibitor	*Reduction of LDL and total cholesterol levels in patients with primary hypercholesterolemia (types IIa and IIb)* **Adults:** initially, 20 mg P.O. once daily with the evening meal. For patients with severely elevated cholesterol levels (for example, over 300 mg/dl), the initial dose should be 40 mg.	**CNS:** headache, dizziness **EENT:** blurred vision, dysgeusia **GI:** constipation, diarrhea, dyspepsia, flatus, abdominal pain or cramps, heartburn, nausea **Metabolic:** elevated serum transaminase levels, abnormal liver test results

Common adverse reactions in *italics;* life-threatening, in ***bold italics.***

Quick reference to cardiovascular drugs *(continued)*

Drug	Indications & dosage	Adverse reactions
Lovastatin *(continued)*	The recommended range is 20 to 80 mg in single or divided doses.	**Skin:** rash, pruritus **Other:** peripheral neuropathy, muscle cramps, myalgia, myositis
Metaraminol bitartrate Aramine Pharmacologic classification: adrenergic Therapeutic classification: vasopressor	*Prevention of hypotension* **Adults:** 2 to 10 mg I.M. or S.C. *Severe shock* **Adults:** 0.5 to 5 mg direct I.V. followed by I.V. infusion. *Treatment of hypotension caused by shock* **Adults:** 15 to 100 mg in 500 ml 0.9% sodium chloride solution or D_5W I.V. infusion. Adjust rate to maintain blood pressure.	**CNS:** apprehension, restlessness, dizziness, headache, tremor, weakness; with excessive use, **seizures** **CV:** hypertension; hypotension; precordial pain; palpitations; **arrhythmias,** including sinus or **ventricular tachycardia;** bradycardia; premature supraventricular contractions; AV dissociation **GI:** nausea, vomiting **GU:** decreased urine output **Metabolic:** hyperglycemia **Skin:** flushing, pallor, sweating **Local:** abscess, necrosis, and sloughing upon extravasation **Other:** *metabolic acidosis in hypovolemia,* increased body temperature, **respiratory distress**
Methyldopa Aldomet, Apo-Methyldopa, Dopamet, Novomedopa **Methyldopate hydrochloride** Aldomet Pharmacologic classification: centrally acting antiadrenergic Therapeutic classification: antihypertensive	*Sustained mild to severe hypertension; shouldn't be used for acute treatment of hypertensive emergencies* **Adults:** initially, 250 mg P.O. b.i.d. to t.i.d. in first 48 hours. Then increase as needed q 2 days. May give entire daily dosage in the evening or h.s. Dosages may need adjustment if other antihypertensives are added to or deleted from therapy. Maintenance dosage is 500 mg to 2 g daily in two to four divided doses. Maximum recommended daily dosage is 3 g. *I.V.*—250 to 500 mg q 6 hours, diluted in D_5W and administered over 30 to 60 minutes. Maximum dosage is 1 g q 6 hours. Switch to oral antihypertensives as soon as possible.	**Blood:** *hemolytic anemia,* reversible granulocytopenia, thrombocytopenia **CNS:** *sedation,* headache, asthenia, weakness, dizziness, *decreased mental acuity,* involuntary choreoathetotic movements, psychic disturbances, depression, nightmares **CV:** bradycardia, *orthostatic hypotension,* aggravated angina, **myocarditis,** *edema, weight gain* **EENT:** *nasal stuffiness* **GI:** *dry mouth,* diarrhea, pancreatitis **Hepatic:** *hepatic necrosis* **Other:** gynecomastia, lactation, rash, **drug-induced fever,** impotence

(continued)

Common adverse reactions in *italics;* life-threatening, in ***bold italics.***

Quick reference to cardiovascular drugs *(continued)*

Drug	Indications & dosage	Adverse reactions
Metolazone Diulo, Mykrox, Zaroxolyn Pharmacologic classification: quinazoline derivative (thiazide-like) diuretic Therapeutic classification: diuretic, antihypertensive	*Edema in CHF* **Adults:** 5 to 10 mg P.O. daily. *Hypertension* **Adults:** 2.5 to 5 mg (Diulo or Zaroxolyn) P.O. daily. Maintenance dosage determined by patient's blood pressure. Or 0.5 mg (Mykrox) once daily in the morning. Increase to 1 mg P.O. daily as needed. If response is inadequate, add another antihypertensive.	**Blood:** *aplastic anemia, agranulocytosis,* leukopenia, thrombocytopenia **CV:** volume depletion and dehydration, orthostatic hypotension **GI:** anorexia, nausea, pancreatitis **Hepatic:** hepatic encephalopathy **Metabolic:** hypokalemia, asymptomatic hyperuricemia, hyperglycemia and impaired glucose tolerance, fluid and electrolyte imbalances including dilutional hyponatremia and hypochloremia, metabolic alkalosis, hypercalcemia, gout **Skin:** dermatitis, photosensitivity, rash **Other:** hypersensitivity reactions, such as pneumonitis and vasculitis
Metoprolol tartrate Apo-Metoprolol, Lopresor, Lopresor SR, Lopressor **Metoprolol succinate** Toprol-XL Pharmacologic classification: beta-adrenergic blocker Therapeutic classification: antihypertensive, adjunctive treatment of acute MI	*Hypertension; may be used alone or in combination with other antihypertensives* **Adults:** initially, 50 mg b.i.d. or 100 mg once daily P.O. Up to 200 to 400 mg daily in two or three divided doses. *Early intervention in acute MI* **Adults:** three injections of 5-mg I.V. boluses q 2 minutes. Then, 15 minutes after last dose, administer 50 mg P.O. q 6 hours for 48 hours. Maintenance dosage is 100 mg P.O. b.i.d.	**CNS:** fatigue, lethargy, dizziness **CV:** *bradycardia, hypotension, CHF,* peripheral vascular disease **GI:** nausea, vomiting, diarrhea **Skin:** rash **Respiratory:** dyspnea, *bronchospasm* **Other:** fever, arthralgia
Mexiletine hydrochloride Mexitil Pharmacologic classification: lidocaine analogue, sodium channel blocker Therapeutic classification: ventricular antiarrhythmic (class Ib)	*Refractory ventricular arrhythmias, including ventricular tachycardia and premature ventricular contractions* **Adults:** 200 to 400 mg P.O. followed by 200 mg q 8 hours. May increase dose to 400 mg q 8 hours if satisfactory control is not obtained. Some patients may respond well to a q-12-hour schedule. May give up to 450 mg q 12 hours. *I.V.* (where available) — **Adults:** following a loading dose of	**CNS:** *tremor, dizziness,* blurred vision, ataxia, diplopia, confusion, nystagmus, nervousness, headache **CV:** hypotension, bradycardia, widened QRS complex, *new or worsened arrhythmias* **GI:** nausea, vomiting, indigestion **Skin:** rash

Common adverse reactions in *italics;* life-threatening, in ***bold italics.***

Quick reference to cardiovascular drugs *(continued)*

Drug	Indications & dosage	Adverse reactions
Mexiletine hydro-chloride *(continued)*	100 to 250 mg I.V. at a rate of 12.5 to 25 mg/minute, prepare an infusion solution of 250 mg mexiletine in 500 ml D$_5$W. Administer the first 120 ml (60 mg) over 1 hour. If clinical response is inadequate, give another bolus of 200 mg over 10 to 20 minutes. Maintenance dose is 0.5 mg/minute (1 ml/minute of prepared solution).	
Minoxidil Loniten, Minodyl Pharmacologic classification: peripheral vasodilator Therapeutic classification: antihypertensive	*Severe hypertension* **Adults:** 5 mg P.O. initially as a single dose. Effective dosage range is usually 10 to 40 mg daily. Maximum dosage is 100 mg daily.	**CV:** *edema, tachycardia, pericardial effusion and tamponade, **CHF**,* ECG changes **Skin:** rash, ***Stevens-Johnson syndrome*** **Other:** *hypertrichosis* (elongation, thickening, and enhanced pigmentation of fine body hair), profuse hirsutism, breast tenderness
Nadolol Corgard Pharmacologic classification: nonselective beta-adrenergic blocker Therapeutic classification: antihypertensive, antianginal	*Management of angina pectoris* **Adults:** 20 to 40 mg P.O. once daily, initially. Dosage may be increased in 40- to 80-mg increments until optimum response occurs. Usual maintenance dosage range is 40 to 240 mg daily. *Treatment of hypertension* **Adults:** 40 mg P.O. once daily, initially. Dosage may be increased in 40- to 80-mg increments until optimum response occurs. Usual maintenance dosage range is 40 to 320 mg daily.	**CNS:** fatigue, lethargy **CV:** *bradycardia, hypotension, **CHF**,* peripheral vascular disease **GI:** nausea, vomiting, diarrhea **Metabolic:** hypoglycemia without tachycardia (in diabetic patients) **Respiratory:** ***bronchospasm*** **Skin:** rash **Other:** *increased airway resistance,* fever
Nicardipine Cardene Pharmacologic classification: calcium channel blocker Therapeutic classification: antianginal, antihypertensive	*Chronic stable angina; used alone or in combination with beta blockers* **Adults:** initially, 20 mg P.O. t.i.d. Titrate dosage according to patient response. Usual dosage range is 20 to 40 mg P.O. t.i.d. *Hypertension* **Adults:** initially, 20 to 40 mg P.O. t.i.d. Increase dosage according to patient response.	**CNS:** dizziness or lightheadedness, headache, paresthesia, drowsiness, asthenia **CV:** peripheral edema, palpitations, angina, tachycardia **GI:** nausea, abdominal discomfort, dry mouth **Skin:** rash, flushing

(continued)

Common adverse reactions in *italics;* life-threatening, in ***bold italics.***

Quick reference to cardiovascular drugs *(continued)*

Drug	Indications & dosage	Adverse reactions
Nifedipine Adalat, Adalat P.A., Apo-Nifed, Novo-Nifedin, Procardia, Procardia XL Pharmacologic classification: calcium channel blocker Therapeutic classification: antianginal, antihypertensive	*Management of vasospastic angina (Prinzmetal's or variant angina) and classic chronic stable angina pectoris; Raynaud's disease* **Adults:** starting dose is 10 mg P.O. t.i.d. Usual effective dose range is 10 to 20 mg t.i.d. Some patients may require up to 30 mg q.i.d. Maximum daily dosage is 180 mg. *Hypertension* **Adults:** 30 to 90 mg P.O. (sustained-release form only) once daily. Titrate over a 7- to 14-day period.	**CNS:** *light-headedness, flushing, headache, dizziness,* weakness, syncope **CV:** peripheral edema, hypotension, palpitations **EENT:** nasal congestion **GI:** *nausea, heartburn,* diarrhea **Metabolic:** hypokalemia **Other:** muscle cramps, dyspnea
Nitroglycerin (glyceryl trinitrate) Nitrodisc, Nitro-Dur, Nitrol, Nitrolingual, Nitrong, Nitrostat, Nitrostat I.V., Transderm-Nitro Pharmacologic classification: nitrate Therapeutic classification: antianginal, vasodilator	*Prophylaxis in chronic anginal attacks* **Adults:** 2.5 mg sustained-release (capsule) q 8 to 12 hours; or 2% ointment. Start with ½″ ointment, increasing by ½″ increments until headache occurs, then decreasing to previous dose. Range of dosage with ointment is 2″ to 5″. Usual dose is 1″ to 2″. Alternatively, transdermal disk or pad (Nitrodisc, Nitro-Dur, or Transderm-Nitro) may be applied to hairless site once daily for 12 hours. *Relief of acute angina pectoris; prophylaxis to prevent or minimize anginal attacks when taken immediately before stressful events* **Adults:** 1 sublingual tablet (gr 1/400, 1/200, 1/150, 1/100) dissolved under tongue or in buccal pouch immediately upon indication of anginal attack. May repeat q 5 minutes for 15 minutes. Alternatively, using Nitrolingual spray, spray one or two doses onto the tongue. May repeat q 3 to 5 minutes to a maximum of three doses within a 15-minute period. Do not shake container. Or, transmucosally, 1 to 3 mg q 3 to 5 hours during waking hours.	**CNS:** *headache (sometimes with throbbing, dizziness),* weakness **CV:** *orthostatic hypotension, tachycardia, flushing, palpitations,* fainting **GI:** nausea, vomiting **Skin:** cutaneous vasodilation **Local:** sublingual burning **Other:** hypersensitivity reactions, nitrate tolerance

Common adverse reactions in *italics;* life-threatening, in ***bold italics.***

Quick reference to cardiovascular drugs *(continued)*

Drug	Indications & dosage	Adverse reactions
Nitroglycerin (glyceryl trinitrate) *(continued)*	*To control hypertension associated with surgery; to treat CHF associated with MI; to relieve angina in acute situations* **Adults:** initial infusion rate is 5 mcg/minute. May be increased by 5 mcg/minute q 3 to 5 minutes until a response is noted. If a 20 mcg/minute rate doesn't produce a response, dosage may be increased by as much as 20 mcg/minute q 3 to 5 minutes.	
Nitroprusside sodium Nipride, Nitropress Pharmacologic classification: balanced vasodilator Therapeutic classification: antihypertensive	*To rapidly reduce blood pressure in hypertensive emergencies; to control hypotension during anesthesia; to reduce preload and afterload in cardiac pump failure or cardiogenic shock; may be used with or without dopamine* **Adults:** 50-mg vial diluted with 2 to 3 ml of D_5W I.V. and then added to 250, 500, or 1,000 ml D_5W. Infuse at 0.5 to 10 mcg/kg/minute. Average dose is 3 mcg/kg/minute. Maximum infusion rate is 10 mcg/kg/minute. Patients taking other antihypertensives along with nitroprusside are very sensitive to this drug. Adjust dosage accordingly.	*Note:* The following adverse reactions usually indicate overdosage or accumulation of toxic metabolites. **CNS:** *headache, dizziness,* ataxia, loss of consciousness, ***coma,*** weak pulse, absent reflexes, widely dilated pupils, *restlessness, muscle twitching, diaphoresis* **CV:** distant heart sounds, palpitations, dyspnea, shallow breathing, angina **GI:** *vomiting, nausea, abdominal pain* **Metabolic:** acidosis **Skin:** pink color
Norepinephrine injection (levarterenol bitartrate) Levophed Pharmacologic classification: adrenergic (direct acting) Therapeutic classification: vasopressor	*To restore blood pressure in acute hypotension* **Adults:** initially, 8 to 12 mcg/minute I.V. infusion, then adjust to maintain normal blood pressure. Average maintenance dosage is 2 to 4 mcg/minute.	**CNS:** *headache,* anxiety, weakness, dizziness, tremor, restlessness, insomnia **CV:** bradycardia, ***severe hypertension,*** marked increase in peripheral resistance, decreased cardiac output, ***arrhythmias, ventricular tachycardia, fibrillation,*** bigeminal rhythm, AV dissociation, precordial pain **GU:** decreased urine output **Metabolic:** metabolic acidosis, hyperglycemia, increased glycogenolysis **Local:** irritation with extravasation **Other:** fever, respiratory difficulty

(continued)

Common adverse reactions in *italics;* life-threatening, in ***bold italics.***

Quick reference to cardiovascular drugs (continued)

Drug	Indications & dosage	Adverse reactions
Papaverine hydro-chloride Cerespan, Pavabid, Pavarine Spancaps, Pavasule, Pavatine, Pavatym, Paverolan Lanacaps Pharmacologic classification: benzylisoquinoline derivative; opiate alkaloid Therapeutic classification: peripheral vasodilator	*Relief of cerebral and peripheral ischemia associated with arterial spasm and myocardial ischemia; treatment of smooth muscle spasm (coronary occlusion, angina pectoris)* **Adults:** 60 to 300 mg P.O. one to five times daily, or 150 to 300 mg sustained-release preparations q 8 to 12 hours; 30 to 120 mg I.M. or I.V. q 3 hours, as indicated.	**CNS:** *headache* **CV:** *increased heart rate, increased blood pressure* (with parenteral use), depressed AV and intraventricular conduction, hypotension, ***arrhythmias*** **GI:** constipation, *nausea* **Other:** *sweating, flushing,* malaise, ***hepatic damage,*** increased depth of respiration, worsening of glaucoma
Penbutolol sulfate Levatol Pharmacologic classification: nonselective beta-adrenergic blocker Therapeutic classification: antihypertensive	*Mild to moderate hypertension* **Adults:** 10 to 20 mg P.O. once daily. Usually given with other antihypertensives, such as thiazide diuretics.	**CNS:** syncope, *dizziness,* vertigo, headache, fatigue, mental depression, paresthesia, hypoesthesia or hyperesthesia, lethargy, anxiety, nervousness, diminished concentration, sleep disturbances, nightmares, bizarre or frequent dreams, sedation, changes in behavior, reversible mental depression, catatonia, hallucinations, alteration of time perception, memory loss, emotional lability, light-headedness **CV:** *bradycardia,* chest pain, ***CHF,*** asymptomatic hypotension, peripheral ischemia, worsening of angina or arterial insufficiency, peripheral vascular insufficiency, claudication, edema, ***pulmonary edema,*** vasodilation, symptomatic postural hypotension, tachycardia, palpitations, ***conduction disturbances,*** first-degree heart block, ***third-degree heart block***, intensification of AV block **GI:** dry mouth, gastric pain, flatulence, nausea, constipation, heartburn, vomiting, taste alteration **GU:** impotence, nocturia, urine retention **Metabolic:** hyperglycemia, hypoglycemia **Respiratory:** pharyngitis, laryngospasm, respiratory distress,

Common adverse reactions in *italics;* life-threatening, in ***bold italics.***

Quick reference to cardiovascular drugs *(continued)*

Drug	Indications & dosage	Adverse reactions
Penbutolol sulfate *(continued)*		shortness of breath, ***broncho-spasm*** **Skin:** pallor, flushing, rash **Other:** allergic reactions, eye discomfort, decreased libido
Pentoxifylline Trental Pharmacologic classification: xanthine derivative Therapeutic classification: hemorrheologic agent	*Intermittent claudication caused by chronic occlusive vascular disease* **Adults:** 400 mg P.O. t.i.d. with meals.	**CNS:** headache, dizziness **GI:** dyspepsia, nausea, vomiting
Phenoxybenzamine hydrochloride Dibenzyline Pharmacologic classification: alpha-adrenergic blocker Therapeutic classification: antihypertensive for pheochromocytoma; cutaneous vasodilator	*To control hypertension and sweating secondary to pheochromocytoma; may be used in combination with propranolol to control excessive tachycardia* **Adults:** initially, 10 mg P.O. daily. Increase by 10 mg daily q 4 days. Maintenance dosage is 20 to 60 mg daily. *To control Raynaud's phenomenon, acrocyanosis* **Adults:** initially, 10 mg P.O., then increase by 10 mg q 4 days to a maximum of 60 mg daily.	**CNS:** lethargy, drowsiness **CV:** *orthostatic hypotension, tachycardia,* shock **EENT:** *nasal stuffiness, miosis* **GI:** vomiting, abdominal distress, dry mouth **Other:** *impotence, inhibition of ejaculation*
Phenylephrine hydrochloride Neo-Synephrine Pharmacologic classification: adrenergic Therapeutic classification: vasoconstrictor	*Mild to moderate hypotension* **Adults:** 2 to 5 mg S.C. or I.M.; repeat in 1 to 2 hours as needed and tolerated. Initial dose should not exceed 5 mg. Alternatively, give 0.1 to 0.5 mg I.V., not to be repeated more often than 10 to 15 minutes. *Paroxysmal supraventricular tachycardia* **Adults:** initially, 0.5 mg rapid I.V.; subsequent doses should not exceed the preceding dose by more than 0.1 to 0.2 mg and should not exceed 1 mg. *Severe hypotension and shock (including drug-induced)* **Adults:** 10 mg in 500 ml D$_5$W. Start 100 to 180 drops/minute I.V. infusion, then 40 to 60 drops/minute. Adjust according to patient response.	**CNS:** *headache, restlessness, light-headedness, weakness* **CV:** palpitations, bradycardia, ***arrhythmias,*** hypertension, anginal pain **EENT:** blurred vision **Skin:** goose bumps, feeling of coolness **Local:** tissue sloughing with extravasation **Other:** tachyphylaxis (with continued use) *(continued)*

Common adverse reactions in *italics;* life-threatening, in ***bold italics.***

Quick reference to cardiovascular drugs *(continued)*

Drug	Indications & dosage	Adverse reactions
Pindolol Visken Pharmacologic classification: nonselective beta-adrenergic blocker Therapeutic classification: antihypertensive	*Hypertension* **Adults:** initially, 5 mg P.O. b.i.d. Dosage may be increased by 10 mg/day q 2 to 3 weeks to a maximum of 60 mg/day.	**CNS:** *insomnia, fatigue, dizziness, nervousness,* vivid dreams, hallucinations, lethargy **CV:** *edema,* bradycardia, ***CHF,*** peripheral vascular disease, hypotension **EENT:** visual disturbances **GI:** *nausea,* vomiting, diarrhea **Metabolic:** hypoglycemia without tachycardia **Respiratory:** ***bronchospasm*** **Skin:** rash **Other:** *increased airway resistance, muscle pain, joint pain,* chest pain
Pravastatin sodium Pravachol Pharmacologic classification: lactone Therapeutic classification: HMG-CoA reductase inhibitor	*Reduction of LDL and total cholesterol levels in patients with primary hypercholesterolemia (types IIa and IIb)* **Adults:** initially, 5 to 10 mg daily h.s. Adjust dosage q 4 weeks based on patient tolerance and response; maximum daily dosage is 40 mg. Most elderly patients respond to a daily dosage of 20 mg or less.	**CNS:** headache, fatigue, dizziness **CV:** chest pain **EENT:** rhinitis **GI:** vomiting, diarrhea, heartburn, nausea **Respiratory:** cough **Skin:** rash **Other:** influenza, localized muscle pain, myalgia, cold
Prazosin hydrochloride Minipress Pharmacologic classification: alpha-adrenergic blocker Therapeutic classification: antihypertensive	*Mild to moderate hypertension (used alone or in combination with a diuretic or other antihypertensives), also used to decrease afterload in severe chronic CHF* **Adults:** P.O. test dose is 1 mg given before bedtime to prevent "first-dose syncope." Initial dose is 1 mg t.i.d. Increase dosage slowly. Maximum daily dosage is 20 mg. Maintenance dosage is 3 to 20 mg daily in three divided doses. A few patients have required dosages larger than this (up to 40 mg daily). If other antihypertensives or diuretics are added to this drug, decrease prazosin dosage to 1 to 2 mg t.i.d. and retitrate.	**CNS:** *dizziness,* headache, drowsiness, weakness, *"first-dose syncope,"* depression **CV:** orthostatic hypotension, *palpitations* **EENT:** blurred vision **GI:** vomiting, diarrhea, abdominal cramps, constipation, *nausea,* dry mouth **GU:** priapism, impotence

Common adverse reactions in *italics;* life-threatening, in ***bold italics.***

Quick reference to cardiovascular drugs (continued)

Drug	Indications & dosage	Adverse reactions
Probucol Lorelco Pharmacologic classification: bis-phenol derivative Therapeutic classification: cholesterol lowering agent	*Primary hypercholesterolemia* **Adults:** 500 mg P.O. b.i.d. with morning and evening meals. Do not exceed 1 g/day.	**CV:** prolonged QT interval, arrhythmias **GI:** *diarrhea, flatulence, abdominal pain, nausea, vomiting* **Other:** *hyperhidrosis,* fetid sweat, ***angioneurotic edema,*** transient increases in concentrations of liver enzymes (AST, ALT, alkaline phosphatase), bilirubin, blood urea nitrogen (BUN), and serum glucose
Procainamide hydrochloride Procan SR, Promine, Pronestyl, Pronestyl-SR, Rhythmin Pharmacologic classification: procaine derivative Therapeutic classification: ventricular antiarrhythmic, supraventricular antiarrhythmic	*Premature ventricular contractions, ventricular tachycardia, atrial arrhythmias unresponsive to quinidine, paroxysmal atrial tachycardia* **Adults:** 100 mg q 5 minutes slow I.V. push, no faster than 25 to 50 mg/minute until arrhythmias disappear, adverse reactions develop, or 1 g has been given. (Usual effective dose is 500 to 600 mg.) When arrhythmias disappear, give continuous infusion of 2 to 6 mg/minute. If arrhythmias recur, repeat bolus as above and increase infusion rate. Alternatively, give 0.5 to 1 g I.M. q 4 to 8 hours until oral therapy begins. *Loading dose for atrial fibrillation or paroxysmal atrial tachycardia* **Adults:** 1 to 1.25 g P.O. If arrhythmias persist after 1 hour, give additional 750 mg. If no change occurs, give 500 mg to 1 g q 2 hours until arrhythmias disappear or adverse reactions occur. *Loading dose for ventricular tachycardia* **Adults:** 1 g P.O. Maintenance dosage is 50 mg/kg daily q 3 hours; average is 250 to 500 mg q 3 hours. *Note:* Sustained-release tablet may be used for maintenance dosing when treating ventricular	**Blood:** thrombocytopenia, ***neutropenia*** (especially with sustained-release forms), ***agranulocytosis,*** hemolytic anemia, *increased antinuclear antibodies titer* **CNS:** hallucinations, confusion, ***seizures,*** depression **CV:** ***severe hypotension,*** *bradycardia,* AV block, ***ventricular fibrillation*** (after parenteral use) **GI:** *nausea, vomiting, anorexia, diarrhea, bitter taste* **Skin:** *maculopapular rash* **Other:** *fever,* lupus erythematosus–like syndrome (especially after prolonged administration), myalgia

(continued)

Common adverse reactions in *italics;* life-threatening, in ***bold italics.***

Quick reference to cardiovascular drugs (continued)

Drug	Indications & dosage	Adverse reactions
Procainamide hydrochloride *(continued)*	tachycardia, atrial fibrillation, and paroxysmal atrial tachycardia. Dose is 500 mg to 1 g q 6 hours.	
Propafenone hydrochloride Rythmol Pharmacologic classification: sodium channel blocker Therapeutic classification: antiarrhythmic	*Suppression of life-threatening ventricular arrhythmias, such as sustained ventricular tachycardia* **Adults:** initially, 150 mg P.O. q 8 hours. Dosage may be increased to 225 mg q 8 hours after 3 to 4 days; if necessary, increase dosage to 300 mg q 8 hours. Maximum daily dosage is 900 mg.	**CNS:** anorexia, anxiety, ataxia, dizziness, drowsiness, fatigue, headache, insomnia, syncope, tremor, weakness **CV:** angina, atrial fibrillation, bradycardia, bundle-branch heart block, ***CHF,*** chest pain, edema, first-degree AV block, hypotension, increased QRS duration, intraventricular conduction delay, palpitations, ***proarrhythmic events (ventricular tachycardia, premature ventricular contractions)*** **EENT:** blurred vision **GI:** abdominal pain or cramps, constipation, diarrhea, dyspepsia, flatulence, nausea, vomiting, dry mouth, unusual taste **Respiratory:** dyspnea **Skin:** rash **Other:** diaphoresis, joint pain
Propranolol hydrochloride Apo-Propranolol, Detensol, Inderal, Inderal LA, Ipran, Novopranol, PMS-Propranolol Pharmacologic classification: nonselective beta-adrenergic blocker Therapeutic classification: antihypertensive, antianginal, antiarrhythmic, adjunctive therapy of MI	*Management of angina pectoris* **Adults:** 10 to 20 mg P.O. t.i.d. or q.i.d. Or, one 80-mg sustained-release capsule daily. Dosage may be increased at 7- to 10-day intervals. The average optimum dosage is 160 mg daily. *To reduce mortality after MI* **Adults:** 180 to 240 mg P.O. daily in divided doses. Usually administered t.i.d. to q.i.d. *Supraventricular, ventricular, and atrial arrhythmias; tachyarrhythmias caused by excessive catecholamine action during anesthesia; hyperthyroidism; pheochromocytoma* **Adults:** 1 to 3 mg by slow I.V. push, not to exceed 1 mg/ minute. After 3 mg have been given, another dose may be given in 2 minutes; subsequent doses, no sooner than q 4 hours. Drug may be given by direct injection or diluted in 50 ml D_5W or 0.9% sodium chloride	**CNS:** *fatigue, lethargy,* vivid dreams, hallucinations **CV:** *bradycardia, hypotension,* ***CHF,*** peripheral vascular disease **GI:** nausea, vomiting, diarrhea **Metabolic:** hypoglycemia without tachycardia (in diabetic patients) **Respiratory:** ***bronchospasm*** **Skin:** rash **Other:** *increased airway resistance, fever, arthralgia*

Common adverse reactions in *italics;* life-threatening, in ***bold italics.***

Quick reference to cardiovascular drugs *(continued)*

Drug	Indications & dosage	Adverse reactions
Propranolol hydrochloride *(continued)*	solution and infused slowly. Usual maintenance dose is 10 to 80 mg P.O. t.i.d. to q.i.d. *Hypertension* **Adults:** initially, 80 mg P.O. daily in two to four divided doses or the sustained-release form once daily. Increase at 3- to 7-day intervals to maximum daily dosage of 640 mg. Usual maintenance dosage for hypertension is 160 to 480 mg daily.	
Quinapril hydrochloride Accupril Pharmacologic classification: ACE inhibitor Therapeutic classification: antihypertensive	*Hypertension* **Adults:** initially, 10 mg P.O. daily. Adjust dosage based on patient response at intervals of about 2 weeks. Most patients are controlled at 20, 40, or 80 mg daily, as a single dose or in two divided doses.	**CNS:** somnolence, vertigo, lightheadedness, syncope, nervousness, depression **CV:** palpitations, vasodilation, tachycardia, heart failure, *MI, hypertensive crisis, CVA,* angina, orthostatic hypotension, cardiac rhythm disturbance **EENT:** cough, dry throat **GI:** dry mouth, abdominal pain, constipation, GI hemorrhage, pancreatitis **Skin:** sweating, pruritus, *exfoliative dermatitis, photosensitivity* Other: hyperkalemia, back pain, malaise, elevated liver enzymes
Quinidine bisulfate (66.4% quinidine base) Biquin Durules **Quinidine gluconate** (62% quinidine base) Duraquin, Quinaglute Dura-Tabs, Quinalan, Quinate **Quinidine polygalacturonate** (60.5% quinidine base) Cardioquin **Quinidine sulfate** (83% quinidine base) Apo-Quinidine, Quine, Quinidex Extentabs, Quinora	*Atrial flutter or fibrillation* **Adults:** 200 mg quinidine sulfate or equivalent base P.O. q 2 to 3 hours for five to eight doses with subsequent daily increases until sinus rhythm is restored or toxic effects develop. Administer quinidine only after digitalization to avoid increasing AV conduction. Maximum dosage is 3 to 4 g daily. *PSVT* **Adults:** 400 to 600 mg I.M. gluconate q 2 to 3 hours until toxic adverse reactions develop or arrhythmia subsides. *Premature atrial and ventricular contractions, paroxysmal AV junctional rhythm, paroxysmal atrial tachycardia, paroxysmal ventricular tachycardia, mainte-*	**Blood:** *hemolytic anemia, thrombocytopenia, agranulocytosis* **CNS:** *vertigo, headache, lightheadedness,* confusion, restlessness, cold sweat, pallor, fainting, dementia **CV:** *premature ventricular contractions, severe hypotension,* SA and AV block, *ventricular fibrillation,* tachycardia, *aggravated CHF,* ECG changes *(particularly widening of QRS complex, notched P waves, widened QT interval, ST-segment depression)* **EENT:** *tinnitus, excessive salivation, blurred vision* **GI:** *diarrhea, nausea, vomiting,* anorexia, abdominal pain

(continued)

Common adverse reactions in *italics;* life-threatening, in ***bold italics.***

Quick reference to cardiovascular drugs *(continued)*

Drug	Indications & dosage	Adverse reactions
Quinidine bisulfate **Quinidine gluconate** **Quinidine polygalacturonate** **Quinidine sulfate** *(continued)* Pharmacologic classification: cinchona alkaloid Therapeutic classification: ventricular antiarrhythmic, supraventricular antiarrhythmic, atrial antitachyarrhythmic	*nance after cardioversion of atrial fibrillation or flutter* **Adults:** test dose is 50 to 200 mg P.O., then monitor vital signs before beginning therapy. Quinidine sulfate or equivalent base 200 to 400 mg P.O. q 4 to 6 hours; or initially, quinidine gluconate 600 mg I.M., then up to 400 mg q 2 hours, p.r.n.; or quinidine gluconate 800 mg (10 ml of the commercially available solution) added to 40 ml D_5W, infused I.V. at 16 mg (1 ml)/minute.	**Hepatic:** hepatotoxicity, including granulomatous hepatitis **Skin:** rash, petechial hemorrhage of buccal mucosa, pruritus **Other:** angioedema, acute asthmatic attack, ***respiratory arrest,*** fever, cinchonism
Ramipril Altace Pharmacologic classification: ACE inhibitor Therapeutic classification: antihypertensive	*Essential hypertension (used alone or in combination with diuretics)* **Adults:** initially, 2.5 mg P.O. once daily. Increase dose as necessary based on patient response. Maintenance dose is 2.5 to 20 mg daily as a single dose or in divided doses.	**CNS:** headache, dizziness, fatigue, light-headedness, asthenia, malaise, anxiety, amnesia, *seizures,* depression, insomnia, nervousness, neuralgia, neuropathy, paresthesia, somnolence, tremor, vertigo **CV:** orthostatic hypotension, syncope, chest pain, angina, *MI, arrhythmia,* palpitations **EENT:** epistaxis **GI:** nausea, vomiting, anorexia, abdominal pain, constipation, diarrhea, dry mouth, dyspepsia, dysphagia, gastroenteritis, increased salivation, taste disturbance **GU:** impotence **Respiratory:** dry, persistent, tickling, nonproductive cough; dyspnea **Skin:** urticaria, rash, photosensitivity, pruritus, hypersensitivity reactions, dermatitis, purpura **Other:** *angioedema,* arthralgia, arthritis, edema, increased sweating, myalgia, weight gain
Reserpine Novoreserpine, Serpalan, Serpasil Pharmacologic classification: rauwolfia alkaloid, peripherally	*Mild to moderate essential hypertension* **Adults:** 0.1 to 0.25 mg P.O. daily.	**CNS:** mental confusion, *depression, drowsiness, nervousness, paradoxical anxiety, nightmares,* extrapyramidal symptoms, sedation **CV:** *orthostatic hypotension,*

Common adverse reactions in *italics;* life-threatening, in ***bold italics.***

Quick reference to cardiovascular drugs *(continued)*

Drug	Indications & dosage	Adverse reactions
Reserpine *(continued)* acting antiadrenergics Therapeutic classification: antihypertensive		*bradycardia, syncope* **EENT:** *nasal stuffiness,* glaucoma **GI:** *hyperacidity, nausea, vomiting, dry mouth,* GI bleeding **Skin:** pruritus, rash **Other:** *impotence, weight gain*
Simvastatin Zocor Pharmacologic classification: lactone Therapeutic classification: HMG-CoA reductase inhibitor	*Reduction of LDL and total cholesterol levels in patients with primary hypercholesterolemia (types IIa and IIb)* **Adults:** initially, 5 to 10 mg daily in the evening. Adjust dosage q 4 weeks based on patient tolerance and response; maximum daily dosage is 40 mg.	**CNS:** headache, asthenia **GI:** abdominal pain, constipation, diarrhea, dyspepsia, flatulence, nausea **Other:** upper respiratory infection
Sotalol Betapace, Sotacor Pharmacologic classification: nonselective beta-adrenergic blocker Therapeutic classification: antiarrhythmic	*Documented, life-threatening ventricular arrhythmias* **Adults:** initially, 80 mg P.O. b.i.d. Increase dosage as needed and tolerated; most patients respond to daily dosages of 160 to 320 mg. A few patients with refractory arrhythmias have received as much as 980 mg daily. **Dosage adjustment for patients with renal failure:** if creatinine clearance is above 60 ml/minute, no dosage interval adjustment is necessary; if creatinine clearance is 30 to 60 ml/minute, dosage interval is q 24 hours; if creatinine clearance is 10 to 30 ml/minute, dosage interval is q 36 to 48 hours; if creatinine clearance is below 10 ml/minute, dosage interval is individualized.	**CNS:** *asthenia, headache, dizziness, weakness, fatigue* **CV:** *bradycardia,* **arrhythmias, CHF, bradycardia, AV block** **GI:** *nausea* **Respiratory:** *dyspnea,* **bronchospasm**
Spironolactone Aldactone, Novospiroton, Sincomen Pharmacologic classification: potassium-sparing diuretic Therapeutic classification: management of edema, antihypertensive	*Edema* **Adults:** 25 to 200 mg P.O. daily in divided doses. *Hypertension* **Adults:** 50 to 100 mg P.O. daily in divided doses.	**CNS:** headache **GI:** anorexia, nausea, diarrhea **Metabolic:** **hyperkalemia,** dehydration, hyponatremia, transient elevation in BUN level, acidosis **Skin:** urticaria **Other:** gynecomastia in men, breast soreness and menstrual disturbances in women

(continued)

Common adverse reactions in *italics;* life-threatening, in ***bold italics.***

Quick reference to cardiovascular drugs (continued)

Drug	Indications & dosage	Adverse reactions
Streptokinase Kabikinase, Streptase Pharmacologic classification: plasminogen activator Therapeutic classification: thrombolytic enzyme	*Venous thrombosis, pulmonary embolism, arterial thrombosis and embolism* **Adults:** loading dose is 250,000 IU I.V. infusion over 30 minutes. Sustaining dose is 100,000 IU/hour I.V. infusion for 72 hours for deep vein thrombosis and 100,000 IU/hour over 24 to 72 hours by I.V. infusion pump for pulmonary embolism. *Lysis of coronary artery thrombi after MI* **Adults:** 140,000 IU administered as a loading dose followed by maintenance infusion. Loading dose is 20,000 IU via coronary catheter, followed by a maintenance dose of 2,000 IU/minute for 60 minutes as an infusion. Alternatively, may be administered as an I.V. infusion. Usual adult dose is 1.5 million IU infused over 60 minutes.	**Blood:** *bleeding,* low hematocrit **CV:** transient lowering or elevation of blood pressure **EENT:** periorbital edema **Respiratory:** *bronchospasm* **Skin:** urticaria **Local:** phlebitis at injection site **Other:** *hypersensitivity,* fever, *anaphylaxis,* musculoskeletal pain, minor breathing difficulty, angioneurotic edema
Sulfinpyrazone Anturan, Anturane Pharmacologic classification: uricosuric agent Therapeutic classification: platelet aggregation inhibitor	*Inhibition of platelet aggregation; increase of platelet survival time in treatment of thromboembolic disorders, angina, MI, transient cerebral ischemic attacks, peripheral arterial atherosclerosis* **Adults:** 200 mg P.O. q.i.d.	**Blood:** *agranulocytosis, blood dyscrasias* (rare) **CNS:** dizziness, vertigo, tinnitus **GI:** *nausea, dyspepsia,* epigastric pain, blood loss, reactivation of peptic ulcers **Skin:** rash
Terazosin hydrochloride Hytrin Pharmacologic classification: selective alpha₁ blocker Therapeutic classification: antihypertensive	*Hypertension* **Adults:** initially, 1 mg P.O. h.s., gradually increased according to patient response. Usual dosage range is 1 to 5 mg daily. Maximum recommended dosage is 20 mg/day.	**CNS:** asthenia, *dizziness, headache, nervousness, paresthesia, somnolence* **CV:** *palpitations,* postural hypotension, tachycardia, *peripheral edema* **EENT:** *nasal congestion, sinusitis, blurred vision* **GI:** *nausea* **Respiratory:** dyspnea **Other:** back pain, muscle pain, weight gain, impotence, decreased libido
Timolol maleate Apo-Timol, Blocadren Pharmacologic classification: nonselec-	*Hypertension* **Adults:** initially, 10 mg P.O. b.i.d. Usual daily maintenance dosage is 20 to 40 mg. Maximum daily dosage is 60 mg.	**CNS:** fatigue, lethargy, vivid dreams **CV:** *bradycardia, hypotension, CHF,* peripheral vascular disease

Common adverse reactions in *italics;* life-threatening, in ***bold italics.***

Quick reference to cardiovascular drugs *(continued)*

Drug	Indications & dosage	Adverse reactions
Timolol maleate *(continued)* tive beta-adrenergic blocker Therapeutic classification: antihypertensive agent, adjunct in MI	Drug is used either alone or in combination with diuretics. *Long-term prophylaxis in patients who have survived acute phase of MI* **Adults:** recommended dosage is 10 mg P.O. b.i.d.	**GI:** nausea, vomiting, diarrhea **Metabolic:** hypoglycemia without tachycardia **Respiratory:** dyspnea, ***bronchospasm*** **Skin:** rash **Other:** *increased airway resistance,* fever
Tocainide hydrochloride Tonocard Pharmacologic classification: local anesthetic (amide type) Therapeutic classification: ventricular antiarrhythmic	*Suppression of symptomatic ventricular arrhythmias, including frequent premature ventricular contractions and ventricular tachycardia* **Adults:** initially, 400 mg P.O. q 8 hours. Usual dosage is between 1,200 and 1,800 mg daily in three divided doses.	**Blood:** *blood dyscrasias, including aplastic anemia* **CNS:** *light-headedness, tremor,* restlessness, paresthesia, confusion, dizziness **CV:** hypotension, **new or worsened arrhythmias, CHF** **EENT:** blurred vision **GI:** nausea, vomiting, epigastric pain, constipation, diarrhea, anorexia **Hepatic:** hepatitis. **Respiratory:** ***respiratory arrest,*** pulmonary fibrosis, pneumonitis, ***pulmonary edema*** **Skin:** rash
Urokinase Abbokinase, Win-Kinase Pharmacologic classification: thrombolytic enzyme Therapeutic classification: thrombolytic enzyme	*Lysis of acute massive pulmonary emboli; lysis of pulmonary emboli accompanied by unstable hemodynamics* **Adults:** for I.V. infusion only by constant infusion pump that will deliver a total volume of 195 ml. Priming dose: 4,400 IU/kg of urokinase–0.9% sodium chloride solution admixture given over 10 minutes. Follow with 4,400 IU/kg hourly for 12 to 24 hours. Total volume should not exceed 200 ml. Follow therapy with continuous I.V. infusion of heparin, then oral anticoagulants. *Coronary artery thrombosis* **Adults:** following a bolus dose of heparin ranging from 2,500 to 10,000 units, infuse 6,000 IU/minute of urokinase into the occluded artery for up to 2 hours. Average total dosage is 500,000 IU.	**Blood:** *bleeding,* low hematocrit **Local:** phlebitis at injection site **Respiratory:** *bronchospasm* **Other:** hypersensitivity (not as frequent as with streptokinase), musculoskeletal pain, ***anaphylaxis***

(continued)

Common adverse reactions in *italics;* life-threatening, in ***bold italics.***

Quick reference to cardiovascular drugs *(continued)*

Drug	Indications & dosage	Adverse reactions
Verapamil hydro-chloride Calan, Calan SR, Cordilox Oral, Isoptin, Isoptin SR, Veradil, Verelan Pharmacologic classification: calcium channel blocker Therapeutic classification: antianginal, antihypertensive, antiarrhythmic	*Management of vasospastic angina (Prinzmetal's or variant angina) and classic chronic, stable angina pectoris; control of ventricular response in chronic atrial fibrillation* **Adults:** starting dose is 80 mg P.O. t.i.d. or q.i.d. Dosage may be increased at weekly intervals. Some patients may require up to 480 mg daily. *Supraventricular arrhythmias* **Adults:** 0.075 to 0.15 mg/kg (5 to 10 mg) I.V. push over 2 minutes with ECG and blood pressure monitoring. Repeat dose in 30 minutes if no response.	**CNS:** dizziness, headache, fatigue **CV:** *transient hypotension,* ***CHF,*** bradycardia, AV block, ***ventricular asystole,*** peripheral edema **GI:** *constipation,* nausea (primarily from oral form) **Hepatic:** elevated liver enzymes
Warfarin sodium Coumadin, Panwarfin, Warfilone Sodium Pharmacologic classification: coumarin derivative Therapeutic classification: anticoagulant	*Prophylaxis and treatment of pulmonary emboli; prevention and treatment of emboli associated with deep vein thrombosis, MI, rheumatic heart disease with heart valve damage, prosthetic heart valves, atrial arrhythmias* **Adults:** 10 to 15 mg P.O. daily for 2 to 5 days, or until desired PT is reached. Usual maintenance dosage, based on PT, is 2 to 10 mg P.O. daily.	**Blood:** ***hemorrhage with excessive dosage,*** eosinophilia, leukopenia **GI:** paralytic ileus, intestinal obstruction (both resulting from hemorrhage), diarrhea, vomiting, cramps, nausea **GU:** excessive uterine bleeding **Skin:** dermatitis, urticaria, *rash,* necrosis, gangrene, alopecia **Other:** *fever,* hepatitis, jaundice

Common adverse reactions in *italics;* life-threatening, in ***bold italics.***

Index

E

ECG. *See* Electrocardiography.
ECG strip, analyzing, 54-55, 57. *See also* Electrocardiography.
Echocardiography
  aortic insufficiency and, 184
  aortic stenosis and, 189
  cardiac tamponade and, 320
  cardiogenic shock and, 310
  dilated cardiomyopathy and, 115
  heart failure and, 106
  hypertrophic cardiomyopathy and, 122
  MI and, 90
  mitral insufficiency and, 170
  mitral stenosis and, 177
  mitral valve prolapse syndrome and, 164
  pericarditis and, 141
  pulmonic insufficiency and, 202
  pulmonic stenosis and, 206
  restrictive cardiomyopathy and, 128
  rheumatic fever and, 158
  tricuspid insufficiency and, 193
  tricuspid stenosis and, 198
  ventricular aneurysm and, 316
Edema
  assessing, 12, 38-40
  causes of, 39
Electrocardiogram interpretation, arrhythmias and, 214-232i
Electrocardiography, 46-57
  aortic insufficiency and, 184
  aortic stenosis and, 189
  CAD and, 82
  cardiac tamponade and, 320
  cardiogenic shock and, 310
  continuous, 49, 50-51i, 51-52
  dilated cardiomyopathy and, 115
  heart failure and, 106
  interpreting results of, 52, 54-55, 57
  lead placement in, 48-49i, 50-51i
  mitral insufficiency and, 170
  mitral stenosis and, 177
  myocarditis and, 136
  pericarditis and, 141

Electrocardiography *(continued)*
  pulmonic insufficiency and, 202
  pulmonic stenosis and, 207
  restrictive cardiomyopathy and, 128
  rheumatic fever and, 158
  tricuspid insufficiency and, 193
  tricuspid stenosis and, 198
  12-lead, 46, 48-49i, 49
  variations of, 47
  ventricular aneurysm and, 316
  waveform components in, 53i
Embolectomy, arterial occlusive disease and, 275
Embolism, infective endocarditis and, 150i
Emergency care, implementing, 21
Emotional support, implementing, 21
Enalaprilat, 341-342t
Enalapril maleate, 341-342t
Endocarditis, infective. *See* Infective endocarditis.
Endomyocardial biopsy, myocarditis and, 136
Erythema marginatum rheumaticum, 157
Erythrocyte sedimentation rate, myocarditis and, 136
Esmolol hydrochloride, 342t
Essential hypertension, cause of, 74. *See also* Hypertension.
Ethacrynate sodium, 342t
Ethacrynic acid, 342t
Evaluation, 22-24
Evaluation statements, writing, 23-24
Exercise, patient teaching about, 100
Exercise ECG, 47
  CAD and, 82

F

Family history, health history and, 3
Fatigue
  aortic insufficiency and, 184, 185
  aortic stenosis and, 189, 190
  as nursing diagnosis, 17
  assessing, 40-42
  causes of, 41
  mitral insufficiency and, 171, 174

Fatigue *(continued)*
  mitral stenosis and, 177, 178, 181
  pulmonic insufficiency and, 202, 203
  pulmonic stenosis and, 207
  tricuspid insufficiency and, 194
  tricuspid stenosis and, 198
Felodipine, 342t
Femoral aneurysm, 266-270
  assessing, 266-268
  causes of, 266
  discharge planning for, 270
  evaluating patient's response to therapy for, 269-270
  implementing interventions for, 268-269
  nursing diagnoses for, 268
  patient outcomes for, 268
  patient teaching for, 269
Femoral pulses, assessing, 13
First-degree AV block, ECG characteristics of, 230i
Flecainide acetate, 343t
Fluid, accumulation of. *See* Edema.
Fluid challenge algorithm, 306i
Fluid replacement, hypovolemic shock syndrome and, 305, 306i
Fluid volume deficit
  abdominal aortic aneurysm and, 261
  thoracic aortic aneurysm and, 255
Fluid volume deficit, high risk for, hypovolemic shock syndrome and, 303, 304
Fluid volume excess
  as nursing diagnosis, 17
  dilated cardiomyopathy and, 115, 116
  heart failure and, 107
  hypertrophic cardiomyopathy and, 123
  mitral insufficiency and, 171-172
  pulmonic insufficiency and, 202, 203
  pulmonic stenosis and, 207-208
  restrictive cardiomyopathy and, 128
  tricuspid insufficiency and, 194
  tricuspid stenosis and, 198, 199
  ventricular aneurysm and, 316

Hypertrophic cardiomyopathy *(continued)*
implementing interventions for, 124-126
nursing diagnoses for, 123
patient outcomes for, 123-124
patient teaching for, 124-126
treatment of, 125
Hypovolemic shock syndrome, 302-308
assessing, 302-303
causes of, 302
discharge planning for, 307
evaluating patient's response to therapy for, 307-308
implementing interventions for, 304-307
nursing diagnoses for, 303
patient outcomes for, 303-304
patient teaching for, 307
treatment of, 305

I

Ice water immersion test, 281
Idiopathic hypertension, cause of, 74. *See also* Hypertension.
Idiopathic hypertrophic subaortic stenosis. *See* Hypertrophic cardiomyopathy.
Implementation, 20-22
reviewing, 23
Inactivity as risk factor, 83
Individual coping, ineffective, as nursing diagnosis, 17
Infection, high risk for
aortic insufficiency and, 184
aortic stenosis and, 189-190
mitral insufficiency and, 171, 172, 174
mitral stenosis and, 177, 178, 181
pulmonic insufficiency and, 202
pulmonic stenosis and, 207
tricuspid insufficiency and, 194
tricuspid stenosis and, 198
Infective endocarditis, 147-155
assessing, 148-149, 151
causes of, 147-148
classifying, 148
complications of, 149, 155
discharge planning for, 154

Infective endocarditis *(continued)*
evaluating patient's response to therapy for, 154-155
implementing interventions for, 152-154
nursing diagnoses for, 151
patient outcomes for, 151-152
patient teaching for, 153-154
treatment of, 152
Inflammatory disorders, 134-162
Injury, high risk for
cardiac arrest and, 242, 243
hypertension and, 76-77
infective endocarditis and, 151
thrombophlebitis and, 290, 291
Interventions
developing, 18, 20
therapeutic, 20-21
Intra-aortic balloon counterpulsation, 328t
Intra-aortic balloon pump, 312, 313
insertion of, 98-99
patient teaching for
Intra-arterial pressure monitoring, 58, 61
complications of, 61
Isoproterenol, 346t
Isosorbide dinitrate, 346-347t
Isosorbide mononitrate, 346-347t
Isradipine, 347t

J

J point, 53i
Jugular veins, inspection of, 6
Junctional rhythm, ECG characteristics of, 221i
Junctional tachycardia, ECG characteristics of, 222i

K

Knowledge deficit,
abdominal aortic aneurysm and, 261-262
arrhythmias and, 213
as nursing diagnosis, 16
CAD and, 83, 84
chronic venous insufficiency and, 295, 297
dilated cardiomyopathy and, 115, 116
femoral aneurysm and, 268
heart failure and, 106
hypertension and, 76, 77
MI and, 90, 93

Knowledge deficit *(continued)*
mitral valve prolapse syndrome and, 166
popliteal aneurysm and, 268
Raynaud's disease and, 281
restrictive cardiomyopathy and, 128, 129
rheumatic heart disease and, 158
thoracic aortic aneurysm and, 255, 256
thrombophlebitis and, 290, 291
varicose veins and, 284, 285

L

Labetalol hydrochloride, 347t
Laser angioplasty, 85, 328t
Laser surgery, arterial occlusive disease and, 275
Lead placement
in cardiac monitoring, 50-51i
in 12-lead ECG, 48-49i
Left ventricular failure, 105. *See also* Heart failure.
Legs, assessing, 12
Levarterenol bitartrate, 353t
Lidocaine hydrochloride, 348t
Life-style factors, health history and, 3
Life-style modifications, hypertension and, 77-79
Lignocaine hydrochloride, 348t
Limb lead placement, 48i
Lisinopril, 348t
Liver, percussing, 11
Lovastatin, 348-349t
Lumbar sympathectomy, arterial occlusive disease and, 275

M

Manual compression test for valve incompetence, 286
Medication history
heart failure and, 105
hypertension and, 74-75
Metaraminol bitartrate, 349t
Methyldopa, 349t
Methyldopate hydrochloride, 349t
Metolazone, 350t
Metoprolol succinate, 350t
Metoprolol tartrate, 350t
Mexiletine hydrochloride, 350-351t
MI. *See* Myocardial infarction.
Minoxidil, 351t

i refers to an illustration; t, to a table